Basics of Planning and Management of Patients during Radiation Therapy

Ashutosh Mukherji

Basics of Planning and Management of Patients during Radiation Therapy

A Guide for Students and Practitioners

Springer

Ashutosh Mukherji
Department of Radiotherapy
Regional Cancer Centre, JIPMER
Puducherry
India

ISBN 978-981-13-3888-5 ISBN 978-981-10-6659-7 (eBook)
https://doi.org/10.1007/978-981-10-6659-7

Softcover re-print of the Hardcover 1st edition 2018

Printed on acid-free paper

This Springer imprint is published by Springer Nature
The registered company is Springer Nature Singapore Pte Ltd.
The registered company address is: 152 Beach Road, #21-01/04 Gateway East, Singapore 189721, Singapore

I would like to dedicate this work to my parents for their guidance and love through all my life; my wife and my daughter for their patience; and my patients for having placed their belief in me.

Dr. Ashutosh Mukherji

Preface

What This Book Is About

Radiation medicine has now progressed from a volume and anatomical landmark-guided approach to an image- and function-guided therapy which takes into account possible routes of tumour spread, biologically active tumour volumes and critical normal structures lying in or near target volumes with a focus on delivering maximal tumouricidal doses and sparing of surrounding normal structures. In the last three decades, the quantum of advancement in the field of radiation oncology has been immense with the availability of better diagnostic tools, immobilization methods and treatment machines. No longer are large regional volumes treated, but the field is fashioned and the dose sculpted depending on the tumour volume, location and tumour activity. The addition of imaging modalities to therapy machines has enabled near and real-time tracking of tumour even during the delivery of therapy, thus enabling the radiation oncologist to "see what volume he is treating and where he is delivering radiation".

With fast-changing parameters, the modern radiation oncologist has to keep in touch with all modalities falling in his domain. *This book tries to fill the gap between standard textbooks of radiation therapy and pocket handbooks on practice guidelines*. It describes how to approach a cancer patient, what investigations to order and how to decide upon a treatment schedule. It deals with the various modalities of delivering radiotherapy and then takes the reader through the steps of a radiation treatment planning algorithm – on how to image, immobilize, contour, plan, evaluate and deliver radiation therapy.

This book is divided into various sections mainly in the order in which a radiation oncologist sees a cancer patient. It takes the reader from diagnosis to investigation, treatment decision and planning, evaluating and delivering radiotherapy. It talks about the latest modalities in radiation therapy as well as other types of radiation as well as combining radiation with biomolecules and chemotherapy in today's world of combined modality treatment. This book describes also the use of adjunctive radiosensitizers as practical points. Finally, this book covers aspects of handling a patient while on radiation, what problems a practitioner can face and how to solve various accompaniments of radiotherapy. In addition, the last few chapters also cover post radiation sequelae and follow-up evaluations.

Objective of This Book

- How to approach a cancer patient
- Deciding a treatment modality
- How to use newer modalities of radiotherapy
- Ways of correctly evaluating a radiation schedule and delivering treatment correctly
- Care of patient during treatment
- Managing complications and sequelae of treatment
- Counselling of patients

The author of this book has tried to explain by the use of charts and diagrams especially the role of immobilization, target volume contouring, plan evaluation and sequelae to provide the readers with an appreciation of what issues they are likely to face during planning and delivering radiotherapy. This book discusses the general background, radiobiology, radiophysics and clinical applications of radiation therapy in the management of cancer. This handbook is an up-to-date and comprehensive survey on how to use the latest radiotherapy techniques such as stereotactic and adaptive radiotherapy, particle beam therapy, concurrent and sequential chemotherapy, etc. The chapters also cover the impact of different treatment techniques and toxicities on quality of life and the relationship of toxicity prevention, rehabilitation and supportive care to quality of life after treatment.

Who Should Read This Book

Over the past three decades, cancer has become a major cause of morbidity and mortality cutting across both developed and developing nations. Cancer is therefore a major component of the cases a medical postgraduate student encounters in surgery, gynaecology, orthopaedics, neurosurgery, ENT, haematology as well as many other disciplines of medicine and of primary concern to nurses and allied health workers. This work is designed as a quick reference volume of the dos and don'ts of managing a patient receiving radiotherapy for practitioners of the field of radiation oncology as well as on how to manage common day-to-day situations that one comes across in radiation oncology practice. This book is *not* designed as a textbook of oncology, but merely as a guide for practising radiation oncology. This book has been planned as a useful reference for young radiotherapists in their daily dealings with cancer patients and also as a useful guide for practical exams. This book is primarily meant as a ready guide to clinical use for practising radiation oncologists as well as those in allied fields such as medical physicists, radiation technologists, medical oncologists and even surgeons primarily dealing with cancer patients. It is intended to serve as a basic *how and why* of the irradiation treatment planning process especially for young oncologists and also hoped to help them ask more questions on the processes involved.

Puducherry, India Ashutosh Mukherji
January 2018

Acknowledgements

Working in oncology can be a very satisfying career, though one must be prepared to take on and internalize a lot of challenges both intellectually and emotionally. It is particularly satisfying to be able to help people with this most distressing and worrying disease, and the sense of satisfaction one feels when one declares a patient to be in remission is beyond expression. But there is also the frequent acknowledgement of defeat and the emotionally draining experience of delivering bad news to hopeful ears. At such times we have to remember that in oncology while many patients are cured, all can be helped.

This book has been my first attempt and I am grateful to all my teachers, who have fashioned my beliefs and knowledge and have always been there to help and guide me: Dr. Bhowmik of Safdarjung Hospital, Delhi, and Drs. Rathi and Kishore Singh of MAMC, Delhi, as well as Dr. Manoj Sharma of MAMC, Delhi; Dr. Veena Gupta of Safdarjung Hospital, Delhi; Dr. Vinod Nimbran, Mohali; and Dr. KS Reddy and Dr. S Vivekanandam of JIPMER Puducherry, to name a few. I would like to acknowledge their presence in my life and thank them deeply for their blessings. I thank the present director of our institute, Dr. SC Parija, and the previous director Dr. TS Ravikumar for having constantly given direction and motivation to all faculties. I would also like to thank my colleagues and friends across the country for providing valuable inputs during our many discussions. Like all teachers, we are inspired by our students as we not only pass on knowledge to them but also learn from them. To have interested and enthusiastic students is a real stimulus and privilege, and their doubts and questions were one of the guiding factors when I decided to first pen down my ideas and frame them for this book. I would also like to thank the untiring efforts of Dr. Naren and Dr. Eti from Springer Nature for giving shape to my ideas and guiding my vision towards the final manuscript. They have been constantly with me, checking my work and offering their inputs which I feel have added to this work. Also my acknowledgements would not be complete without thanking my patients who have through their experiences provided me valuable insight and humility in my short years in clinical practice.

Finally, both clinical practice and academic activities are demanding of time and energy in our lives. This is the time and energy for which our wives, families and friends have so often had to make allowances for our absence. Without the love, support and acceptance of the conditions of my work from my family, this work would have been severely affected and may not have seen the light of the day.

My family has stood up both for and with me during the preparation of this manuscript. I especially owe my family a debt of thanks and gratitude for this work and would like to dedicate this work to my parents, my wife Meetu and my daughter Arnavi for their patient tolerance of my frequent absence from their lives.

Dr. Ashutosh Mukherji
Puducherry, India
January 2018

Contents

Part I

Approaching a Cancer Patient

1 Taking a Decision and Ordering Investigations

The primary aim of radiotherapy in treating cancers is *Achieving Maximum Possible Tumour Remission with Minimum Possible Side Effects*. This question is partly answered by tumour staging and patient performance status, as well as other factors like physician's exposure to various modalities, availability of options, financial implications and socio-religious factors. However, achieving maximal dose to tumour tissue with complete sparing of surrounding normal tissue may not always be achievable, and compromises may need to be done. The oncologist has to examine and stage the tumour in the patient and decide the aims and objectives of his treatment clearly at the start so as to identify and treat patients correctly.

(a) **History and physical examination**: The first step when a patient presents with symptoms suggestive of underlying malignancy is a complete and thorough history and physical examination which can then suggest a possible diagnosis or point to a possible site of primary.
(b) **Confirmation of malignancy**: This is the first and foremost step when a patient first presents with a suspicion of malignancy.
(c) **Histopathological typing and characterization.**
(d) **Identifying the organ of primary location.**
(e) **Intent of treatment**: What treatment to offer, whether to give radical or palliative treatment, how to sequence different modalities of cancer treatment to tailor that particular patients' needs and how to avoid treatment related sequelae as best as possible.
(f) **Follow-up of the patient, managing treatment-induced sequelae and psychological support.**

When a patient first presents, the clinician must recognize initial signs or symptoms which might suggest towards a diagnosis of an underlying malignancy. These could be a lump or ulcer which has suddenly increased in size or shown change in consistency with or without associated pain, unnatural bleeding or discharge from body orifices, difficulty in undertaking daily acts of life not explained by any

A. Mukherji, *Basics of Planning and Management of Patients during Radiation Therapy*, https://doi.org/10.1007/978-981-10-6659-7_1

existing long-term illness, sudden onset of loss of function of a vital organ, change in bowel or bladder habits, swelling of any body part, persisting pain not explained by any injury or somatic cause, difficulty in breathing/swallowing/change in voice/micturition and unexplained and significant loss of weight. Any of the above symptoms could also be due to many other debilitating or infective disorders, but always a malignancy should be ruled out. Sometimes the malignancy itself may not manifest any primary symptoms but could give rise to a host of metabolic, endocrinological or haematological manifestations. These are known as paraneoplastic syndromes and usually patients present with conditions like long-standing anaemia, hyper- or hypocalcemia, hyperkalemia or hypokalemia, SIADH, thrombocytopenia or hyperthrombosis, hyperuricemia, hypoglycemia or hyperglycemia, skin eruptions, myoclonic disorders, abnormal involuntary movements or even unexplained pathological fractures.

Modern medicine gives the clinician valuable tools in the form of a plethora of diagnostic and confirmatory investigations including biochemical, physiological and imaging investigation of the patient. However, what is most essential initially is a good clinical examination starting with a complete history taking. This gives the clinician a good indication of the possible diagnosis and enables him to selectively focus examination more thoroughly. An assessment of the patient's disease status should also include ascertaining for any existing risk factors or family history and determining the disease stage and burden as well as any co-morbid factors. An assessment should also be made of the patient's psychosocial status and expectations from treatment. This is particularly useful in the present era of educated patients and legal liabilities of clinicians. The clinician should also interact with patients and their families to educate them about the disease, treatment options, likely sequelae of therapy and follow-up requirements and find out the patient's treatment preferences. Based on the history and examination, the oncologist then has an idea of the possibility of presence of malignancy and the likely primary site of origin. The next step is confirming the presence and type of malignancy and assessing the stage.

1.1 Staging

Staging of a tumour is the sequence of investigations or assessments done to describe the extent or spread of the disease at the time of diagnosis and has a vital bearing on determining the choice of therapy as well as predicting prognosis and in various statistical or descriptive analyses. A stage basically signifies the tumour burden in the body and the extent of its spread. It is assessed by measuring or *mapping* the primary tumour's size, its location with respect to organ of origin, regional draining lymph nodes or spread to adjoining organs/tissues or distant sites. The invasiveness of a cancer depends on its penetration of the basement membrane of the tissue of origin; if penetrated then it is an invasive cancer (even if there is a single point of invasion), but if not invaded and localized within the membrane, then it is a cancer in situ. Invasive cancers can be further categorized into localized if the cells are confined to the organ of origin, locally advanced or regional if the cells have spread beyond their original site to nearby lymph nodes or surrounding organs or tissues and metastatic if they have spread to organs or non-draining lymph nodes which are away from the primary site. There are different staging systems described in literature to classify tumours. The TNM staging system was first described by Pierre Denoix in 1944 [1] and is still the most widely used. In this system, tumours are divided on basis of size and extent of the primary tumour (T), absence or presence of regional lymph nodes (N) and absence or presence of distant metastases (M). Grading is defined by degree of differentiation in the tumour tissue such as G1, well differentiated and looks like tissue of origin; G2, moderately well differentiated; G3, poorly differentiated; and G4, undifferentiated tumours; Gx is used when it is not possible to determine grading, such as in a damaged specimen. GB signifies a borderline malignant tumour.

Principles of stage grouping: Once the T, N and M individual stages are determined, a composite stage of I, II, III, or IV is assigned, in which stage I is early stage and stage IV is usually metastatic disease. This division of tumours is based on certain clinical principles. Early-stage tumours generally denote masses limited to organ of origin with no lymphatic involvement clinically and which can be surgically removed. Stage II tumours are those locally advanced cancers which may have spread to first-station nodes or cancer encroaching on the immediate tissues surrounding point of origin. Even these can be surgically removed, but there may be microinvasion into tumour capsule or lymphatics. Stage III cancers denote extensive primary lesions involving surrounding tissues, bone or vasculature or extensive regional nodal involvement. These cancers may still be operable, but complete resection may not be possible in this stage. Finally stage IV cancers indicate primary lesion which may be unresectable or metastatic involvement of no regional nodes or distant organs.

Another system of classification is the WHO's "*International Classification of Diseases for Oncology* or ICD-O system" [2]. This is a numerical coding system based on anatomical location and morphology with the main deciding parameters being type of tumour and the dominant grade therein. Over the last few decades, many other staging and classification systems have come into effect. The two main organisations involved with such activities, namely, the American Joint Committee for Cancer (AJCC) [3] and the International Union against Cancer (UICC) [4] mainly use the above two described systems, the TNM for anatomical staging and the ICD-O for histopathological classification. However, TNM staging systems are mostly in use for adult non-gynaecological solid tumours. Gynaecological cancers use FIGO (Federation Internationale Gynecologique Oncology) system, while haematological malignancies have their own varied systems. Even many sarcomas and paediatric malignancies have their systems for staging.

The validity of a staging or classification system is usually denoted by its *Certainty or C-factor* [5]. This classification reflects the trueness of the staging system used based on levels of investigative techniques. The levels are from C1-C5 and increase with increasing certainty based on investigative parameters. In C1, evidence is based on standard diagnostic tools like clinical examination, basic radiography or endoscopy; C2 is based special investigations like CT/MR/biopsy/

endoscopy/ultrasound or lymphangiography; C3 is based on surgical exploration and tissue report; C4 is based on histopathological review of received tissue after definitive surgery; and C5 is based on autopsy findings.

One of the most common changes seen in any staging is the rate of conversion due to migration between stages as the certainty factor improves. This phenomenon is called the *Will-Rogers Phenomenon* and is based on interpolations between the clinic-diagnostic staging and the final surgico-pathological staging and affects cancer response reporting. Basically this means that after pathological staging following surgery, many advanced cancer patients are upstaged. These cases then are removed from their previous diagnosed earlier-stage groups, and as a result there may be thus artificially creating improved results for the remaining cases. This is seen as a discrepancy as the overall survival remains the same. Therefore, this difference between the clinically derived stage and the pathologically determined stage is usually expressed as a *Conversion Rate*. It is important at the time of staging to know this conversion rate as it may have a bearing on the prognosis and therefore in determining the aggressiveness of therapy. Cancers with low conversion rate like skin cancers can be treated by local therapy or single-modality therapy alone, while others like lung, GI, breast or ovarian cancers need multimodality therapy.

1.2 Histopathological Diagnosis

After a patient is examined and a suspected lesion identified either as a lump, nodule, induration, ulcer or suspected haematological malignancy, the first step is confirm by either biopsy or cytology or blood or bone marrow smear examination. The histological diagnosis and classification determine the aggressiveness, natural history and likely pathways of spread of the tumour. A pathology report should contain both a macroscopic description of the gross tumour specimen along with its size, margins and anatomical relationships, as well as a microscopic description after appropriate staining of the tumour, including features such as areas of necrosis, nodes, lympho-vascular invasion, capsule breach, neural bundle invasion, mitotic rate of tumour cells and any other special feature seen. Such a description based on pathological findings also requires description of adequacy of excision of the relevant lymph node compartment which can be assessed by a defined minimum number of nodes for each site, a ratio of negative to positive as well as size of the nodes and also if possible identifying sentinel node.

This entire information is relevant for prognostic stratification and helps choose appropriate treatment strategies. It provides a clue to the clinician about what to expect in that particular tumour, what are the treatment options to be utilized and what are the chances of response and remission in that particular tumour. Histological diagnosis can also be made by biopsy, cytology, immunohistochemistry and bone marrow examination.

Tissue biopsy: It can include core biopsies, frozen sections, endoscopic and laparoscopic biopsies, excision biopsies and incision biopsy as well as image-guided biopsies. There is however some points a surgeon should remember before planning any biopsy procedure. These include planning the biopsy in such a way that will not hamper any future composite resection and reconstructive surgery. There should be minimal disruption of normal tissue, and unless definitive surgery is being planned, the suspected lesion should not be entirely removed as it can affect cosmesis. Sometimes an open biopsy should be preferably be done along with definitive surgery rather than delaying it. Also the specimen should be properly oriented, marked and accurately described so that he pathologist can properly take sections. Various biopsy procedures done include:

1. **Core needle biopsy**: This procedure removes cylinders of tissue 3–4 mm wide and 1–2 cm long. Can be done from both accessible tissues or from deeper organs using image-guided means. Advantage of doing this method is that it can be done on outpatient or minor OT basis with adequate tissue sample available for both histology and immunocytochemistry. The disadvantage is that it can cause needle track seeding of tumour cells leading to later recurrences. Also there is the risk of increased bleeding if the patient has a coagulation defect which has not been detected before in history and pre-biopsy work-up.
2. **Excision biopsy**: Is useful both in diagnosis and therapy. Small tumours in accessible areas like skin, oral cavity, breast or subcutaneous tissue can be excised with minimal margins. The extent of excision and amount of margin taken would depend on the site of lesion and its likely diagnosis and hence natural history. This type of biopsy usually gives the best information regarding the tumour. The main disadvantage is that in spite of being a planned procedure, adequate margins are many times missed, and the surgeon has then to go in again and do a wide local excision if that would have been the initial treatment planned for that site.
3. **Incision biopsy**: This is the procedure of choice when radiotherapy or chemotherapy is the definitive treatment or when excision biopsy is not possible. The amount of tissue sample is larger than needle biopsy but less than excision biopsy. Also tissue sample from the edges should be taken with care after ascertaining that it is the malignant tissue that is being sampled and not the surrounding normal tissue. Also care should be taken to avoid damage to surrounding or underlying normal structures.
4. **Laparoscopic biopsy**: This is especially important in case of intraperitoneal tumours where traditionally an open laparotomy and staging used to be done. But before a biopsy is done, the patient should undergo proper imaging with both a CECT scan and an abdominal ultrasound (USG). The CT scan gives an idea of the tumour extent and which site to put in the laparoscope. USG then helps in estimating tumour thickness as well as location of solid and necrotic areas. After the representative area is identified, multiple pieces are taken with a biopsy forceps. Video assisted procedures are used in thoracoscopy and mediastinoscopy.
5. **Frozen section**: These provide fast diagnoses in the operation theatre whether a given piece of tissue removed is actually malignant and if yes whether margins taken are adequate or not. In this technique a sample of tissue removed during surgery is frozen and then examined by the pathologist who can give his opinion

within minutes. The advantage is that the patient is spared a second surgery with its attendant risks. The main problem is in quickly and correctly sampling tissue and the expertise of the pathologist.

6. **Endoscopic biopsy**: This technique helps in visualizing intraluminal tumours like in nasal, bronchial, oesophageal, stomach, biliary tract, colon or anal canal. Usually fibre-optic and sometimes even rigid endoscopes are used to visualize, examine and then sample tumours. Procedures that are commonly done include nasal and nasopharyngeal endoscopy, direct laryngoscopy, esophagoscopy, bronchoscopy, cystoscopy, upper GI endoscopy, colonoscopy, sigmoidoscopy, proctoscopy, ERCP, etc. The tissue which is obtained is then fixed immediately in formalin and sent for pathological review.

Cytologic review: Exfoliative cytological examinations for detection of cancer as well as aspiration cytology for diagnosis are useful tools for quick diagnosis and confirmation of malignancies as well as for record of response (to differentiate between post-therapy fibrosis and residual/recurrent disease) and for staging procedures (like FNAC neck nodes, axillary nodes, bronchial wash or ascitic cytology):

1. **Pap smear**: It was first devised by Papanicolaou and is used extensively both as a screening tool for early detection of cervical cancer and for post-treatment follow-up for reviewing response. The principle of this technique is that cancer cells lose adherence from the surrounding cells and are exfoliated from the tissue; which can then be stained and identified. This technique is also used in bronchial washing for lung cancers, oral cavity scrapings, peritoneal exudates, gastric washes, sputum and urine sampling.
2. **Fine-needle aspiration cytology**: In this technique, cells are aspirated from a mass by needle aspiration and then examined for presence of malignant cells. It can be done for both superficial tumours under direct palpation or for deep-seated tumours under image guidance. This method however cannot confirm a malignancy; it only indicates the likelihood of a mass lesion being malignant. Further confirmation with a biopsy has to be done. This is because an FNAC if negative cannot rule out cancer as the area sampled may not have had representative cells. Other disadvantages of FNAC are risk of implantation of cancers cells in needle track and risk of bleeding.
3. **Fluid cytology**: Cancer cells on histopathological examination exhibit characteristic loss of differentiation (anaplasia) and orientation. These cells also show pleomorphism, increased mitotic activity, large nucleus to cytoplasmic ratio and hyperchromatism. These cells are exfoliated due to loss of adherence into the pleural, peritoneal or pericardial spaces or part of exudates.

Bone marrow aspiration and biopsy: This technique is widely used in many haematological malignancies as well as many paediatric malignancies like neuroblastoma, Ewing's sarcoma. It is used both as a prognostic and staging tool. The marrow is aspirated from the iliac crest with a specialized needle under local anaesthesia. If aspiration is dry, then a bone marrow biopsy is attempted.

Immunocytochemistry: This is the technique of biologically identifying specific tissue constituents which are markers of specific tissue types and hence specific cancers by antigen-antibody reactions. This technique identifies expression of specific tissue antigens especially in tumours which are poorly differentiated and thus helps in diagnosis of cancer.

1.3 Imaging

Imaging plays an important role both in the mapping and staging of cancer patients. ***Mapping*** refers to the estimation of the extent of local spread of the tumour mass which would be useful for planning both surgical extirpation and deciding on the radiotherapy portals, target volume contours and dose prescription. ***Staging*** is the process of estimation of the tumour load in the body, to identify areas involved, areas at risk of subsequent involvement and whether disease has spread to distant organs. Staging helps in deciding modality of therapy and intent of therapy, has prognostic significance and gives an idea about expected biological course of the tumour. Various imaging modalities used are:

1. **X-rays**: These are still the most common initial imaging investigation ordered along with ultrasonography. A tumour present in the chest on X-rays will be relatively brighter and more opaque (radio-dense) compared to normal dark shadow from the air-filled lungs. On the other hand, an osteolytic tumour present in a bone and causing bone destruction will be seen as relatively dark areas surrounded by white coloured bone shadow caused by radio-opacity of normal bone to X-rays, while an osteoblastic lesion seen in certain cancers like breast or prostate will be seen as increased whiteness compared to surrounding bone.
2. **Barium contrast films**: Barium compounds, usually a barium sulphate mixture, are radio-opaque and are used to outline hollow organs such as in the GI tract as soft tissues cannot be otherwise seen in a plain X-ray film. Various barium studies commonly performed include barium meal, barium follow through and barium enema, which are used to visualize the stomach, small intestines and colon/rectum, respectively. These compounds fill the lumen of the organ being studied, and the lining of these organs can then be made out. In case there is a mass lesion, then it is seen as a filling defect, while an ulcerative lesion is seen as an out-pouching of the barium into the defect in the wall lining.
3. **Air contrast barium studies**: Even using barium studies in many cases may not adequately distinguish a small tumour or ulcer from surrounding mucosal rugae. In many such cases, air is then pushed into the GI tract along with barium sulphate so that the barium mixture forms a thin lining over the wall of the GI tract, while air fills the lumen. This allows even more precise visualization of the bowel lumen and any small lump or ulcer. Air encephalograms used to be done before CT/MRI became common. In this technique, air replaces partly the

fluid in the ventricles, and this is used to detect some brain lesions by comparing the difference in penetration of X-rays in air and in tumour.

4. **Iodine contrast films**: Iodine compounds are excreted by the kidneys and therefore are used as contrast in studies requiring outlining of the kidneys or bladder as well as assessing their functional status. Iodine compounds can also be injected into the bladder or the kidneys through the urethra or the ureters and X-rays taken (retrograde pyelograms or retrograde urograms) or into other body cavities such as myelograms in the thecal sac to detect filling abnormality if tumour is present or to outline the shape and inner dimensions of the gall bladder (cholecystogram) or even bile ducts (cholangiogram). Injection of contrast into the pancreatic duct from the ampulla of Vater after endoscopically passing a tube into the duodenum is known as endoscopic retrograde cholangiopancreatogram (ERCP). All these tests help in locating a lesion by filling defects.
5. **Mammography**: While X-rays are used characteristically to visualize bony structures or soft tissue in relation to bone or air-filled organs, mammograms are X-rays of the breast which assess the soft tissue of the breast based on architectural patterns, lobularity and calcification patterns. Malignant lesions of the breast are identified specifically by their calcification patterns and by disruption of breast tissue architecture. This study is a useful, safe and inexpensive tool for screening women having or at risk of breast cancer. These X-rays deliver small radiation doses but even these have increased risk of mutation in foetal cells in pregnant women or in actively functioning ovarian tissue. Therefore, mammography is not routinely recommended in women younger than 40 years age. Also caution should be used in interpreting results as a negative scan may not mean absence of disease.
6. **Isotope scan**: In these technique radioactive isotopes tagged to proteins or other ligands are distributed in the bloodstream after they are injected into the patient. Examples are use of radioactive iodine in the thyroid gland or technetium in bone scans, especially in areas with increased cellular activity or growth. Similar scans are used in the liver and spleen. Gallium isotopes are used to help differentiate between normal and pathologically involved lymph nodes. The pattern of distribution of these ligands is picked up by imaging, and they provide useful information during initial staging for extent of disease dissemination as well as in assessing response to therapy.
7. **CT scans**: CT scanning is used in modern-day oncology practice as a diagnostic, staging, therapeutic and prognostic tool. Cross-sectional pictures of the body part examined allow for the reconstruction of a three-dimensional image in which the position, size and shape of various tissues and organs, major blood vessels, bones and muscles in the imaged region can be visualized and their relations studied. Also the position, size and density of any abnormal tumour or tissue can be identified and assessed. In modern-day medical practice, use of CT scanning helps in visualizing many otherwise inaccessible areas of the head, abdomen, chest and limbs for which surgical exploration may have been

difficult. CT scanning also helps in obtaining guided tissue samples for diagnosis, in radiotherapy planning process, as a guidance tool in planning surgery and in response assessment.

8. **Ultrasound**: This imaging technique is based on the use of ultrasound waves which penetrate the body and are reflected back by the various tissues depending on their densities so as to present a cross-sectional picture of body tissues and organs in the study window. Ultrasound scans can be more accurate in showing the position and type of lesion in organs like the breast as well as intra-abdominal organs. It is also safe for use during pregnancy or ovulation.
9. **MRI scan**: An MRI scan is also an anatomical scan based on the computer analysis of patterns of absorption or penetration of high-frequency radio waves by water molecules when a strong magnetic field is applied. The advantages of an MRI over CT scan include avoidance of exposure to X-rays, availability of images in various cross sections from any angle (axial/coronal/sagittal/oblique, etc.) allowing for detailed assessment, better visualization of soft tissues as well as fascial planes from tumour mass especially in the brain, muscles or wherever fat component is higher and less likelihood of allergic reactions to contrast compared to CT scan. The scan is usually performed as an outpatient procedure, and no anaesthetic is required, except in small children to immobilize them. Disadvantages include higher cost, feeling of claustrophobia which may unsettle many patients and more time required for scanning and may not be suitable for patients with pacemakers or metallic implants because of use of a powerful magnetic field while scanning.
10. **PET scan**: PET scan is a method of physiological imaging based on different chemical activity in different types of tissues and cells. The basic principle in this imaging modality is that cancer cells consume more glucose than normal cells because of uncontrolled growth and division, and therefore the glucose uptake in these cells would be higher than normal tissues. Thus, PET scans demonstrate physiological activity of the cancer and any changes occurring in the cancerous tissue by treatment given such as necrosis or fibrosis which may not be apparent anatomically or give a false anatomical impression of non-responding residual tumour. In cancers like lymphomas, GI cancers or lung cancers, a PET scan is better able to demonstrate distant metastases compared to anatomical imaging which might suggest small nodes or deposits as being non-significant but which might be otherwise intensively PET-avid [6–8]. Thus, with respect to staging, a PET scan helps in establishing regional, nodal or distant metastases but provides little anatomic staging information for primary site. A PET scan can also indicate whether a cancer has completely or partially responded to therapy or whether it might be starting to recur after treatment. More recently combined imaging of PET and CT or PET and MRI have been used to more precisely demonstrate both anatomical and functional activity of cancer deposits. This helps in identifying areas of biologically active tumour as well as areas of necrosis and quiescent cells and is useful both for staging and planning radiotherapy or surgery.

1.4 Tumour Markers

These are biological compounds which are produced by specific tumour and used as markers for tumour diagnosis, response and recurrence. Examples of regularly used markers include PSA in prostate cancer; carcinoembryonic antigen (CEA) for cancers of the GI tract, especially large bowel cancers; alpha-foeto-protein (AFP) for primary liver cancer and germ-cell tumours of yolk sac, human chorionic gonadotropin (HCG) and lactate dehydrogenase (LDH) in choriocarcinomas; and CA125 in epithelial ovarian cancers.

Tumour markers as mentioned before both as diagnostic and as prognostic tools. They help estimate the success or failure of a particular treatment regime and also in recognizing late recurrences after apparent earlier remission. In some cancers like prostate, choriocarcinoma and ovarian carcinoma, monitoring levels of these agents are linked to treatment decisions. These agents are broadly classified as:

1. **Oncofoetal antigens**: These markers are based on the principle that in malignant cells, the foetal genetic structure is expressed, and therefore placental-foetal antigens are studied. Commonly used ones are **carcinoembryonic antigen** (CEA) which is expressed in embryonic GI tract, pancreas and liver. It is a complex glycoprotein and is found to be elevated in 60–90% colorectal cancers, 50–80% pancreatic cancers and about 25% gastric and breast cancers. It is also elevated in inflammatory conditions and cirrhosis. **Alpha foeto-protein** (AFP) was the first tumour marker identified in this group and is commonly raised in hepatocellular carcinomas and in yolk sac tumours. Some elevation is also seen in gastric, pancreatic, colorectal and lung cancers and also elevated slightly in cirrhosis, foetal death in pregnancy and hepatitis. Another commonly studied antigen is the **prostate-specific antigen** (PSA), which is used in the screening and diagnosis of prostate cancers. The normal level is below 4 ng/mL in a normal patient, but it rises both in cancer and benign hypertrophy. To differentiate, PSA velocity is calculated, and it is found to be around 3.5 ng/cm^3/gm in cancers and 0.5 ng/cm^3/gm in benign hypertrophy.
2. **Cell surface antigens**: These include CA125 (ovarian cancers), CA 19.9 (pancreas and GI cancers), CA 15.3 (breast, ovary, GI and lung cancers) and CA 27.29 (breast cancers). These are usually carbohydrate antigens expressed by epithelial derived tumour tissue.
3. **Hormones**: Include various hormones like β HCG (in gestational trophoblastic tumours), calcitonin (medullary thyroid cancer), catecholamines (pheochromocytoma) and oestrogen and progesterone receptors (breast cancer, uterine cancers). They help both in diagnosis as well as therapy.

1.5 Blood Investigations

1. **Haemoglobin and red cell count (RCC)**: Anaemia, detected either as decreased haemoglobin or red blood cell counts, is a common accompaniment of cancer. Persistent anaemia can also be considered as a marker in the diagnosis of many cancers like gastric or caecal cancers, myeloma and renal cell carcinoma.

2. **White blood counts**: They are used in diagnoses of leukaemias, staging of lymphomas, as a marker of tolerance to therapy with chemotherapy or radiotherapy and as a marker for radio- or chemosensitivity. The total white cell count and type of white cells might be the first direct indication of leukaemia and also might be present as a reaction to some types of cancer.
3. **ESR**: The ESR is an index of red blood cell sedimentation and increases with elevation of certain proteins in the blood in conditions of ill health. It is basically an indicator of an ongoing inflammatory process in the body. Many organic disease processes, including cancer, are associated with a raised ESR. This test can also be useful for indicating response to treatment given.
4. **Biochemistry**: Many cancers can be associated with biochemical parameter derangements such as an increase in the enzyme serum acid phosphatase in prostate cancers; advanced breast cancer may cause elevation of serum calcium, and papillary adenocarcinoma of the large bowel may cause loss of potassium from the bowel resulting in fall in serum potassium. Hypercalcemia is seen in squamous cell cancers of the lung. Tests like serum electrolytes, urea and/or creatinine also help in assessing fitness of patients to receive cytotoxic drug therapy as well as their tolerance to therapy. It also gives us an idea about the underlying state of the body, as well as an indication of any serious events due to happen. Continuous monitoring also helps in avoiding life-threatening situations caused by sudden cancer debulking or effect of renal/hepatic functions or fluid/electrolyte balance.

1.6 Genotyping

These are the methods of molecular diagnosis and prognostic classification. In future they are also expected to have a role in the deciding of treatment protocols. The basic principle lies in identification of specific mutations or genes expressed by various cancer types and correlating them with the responses seen to standard therapy; based on which individualized treatments can be tailored. Various techniques used are:

1. **Polymerase chain reaction (PCR)**: It is used for the detection of genetic abnormalities in haematological malignancies, in prognostic analysis of tumours for chromosomal abnormalities, in the differential diagnosis of haematological malignancies from other dysplastic conditions, in the detection of minimal residual disease not possible by routine imaging and in the diagnosis of many soft tissue malignancies.
2. **Fluorescent in situ hybridisation (FISH)**: This is a method of cytogenetic analysis in which full or part of chromosome is labelled with fluorochrome-bound molecules and then analysed by fluorescent microscopy. It is used in detection of chromosomal abnormalities which helps in diagnosis of tumours uncertain by routine histopathology, prognostic marking, response to therapy and confirmation of diagnosis.
3. **Telomerase activity**: Telomeres are short repeated segments of DNA forming the linear ends of chromosomes. Telomerase are RNA enzymes which generate

telomere sequences; and their activity is highest in germ cells and actively dividing cells. Cancer cells have reactivation of telomerase with telomere elongation leading to continuous active division. Thus, there is expected heightened telomerase activity in cancer cells which can be used for detection.

1.7 Deciding on the Treatment

Once a diagnosis has been made and patient has been staged, a decision on what treatment to offer to the patient is made. Many factors decide what treatment is offered to the patient. These are:

- Stage of the disease
- Patient age
- Performance status of the patient
- Prognostic features

Broadly treatments for cancer are either curative or palliative, though the word "cure" should be used with caution in most cancers. Studies have shown that most cancers relapse most frequently within 2 years, with some relapses possible even up to 5 years post-therapy and in rare cases even after 10–15 years. Therefore in general the word "remission" is used to denote disappearance of disease clinically, biochemically and on imaging at least till up to 10 years post-therapy after which the word "cure" may be used in most cases. Basically in rapidly growing cancers after treatment, remission for more than 5 years may be considered as having achieved cured, while tumour types which are indolent or slow growing (thyroid, salivary glands) require disease-free periods of up to 15–20 years before they can be considered as having being cured.

Biological cure of cancer refers to the state of absence of disease in a former cancer patient who would then have the same life expectancy as someone who has never had a cancer. Generally curable cancers are those which are rapidly dividing, more radio- or chemosensitive or, in early stage (1 or 2), non-infiltrative locally advanced. Cancers which are relatively radio- or chemo-resistant or infiltrative type locally advanced or metastatic are generally incurable.

Indicators of the patient's health such as performance status or quality of life have of late become surrogate markers for response to treatment. They are used to help to decide whether a patient is likely to tolerate a particular treatment, whether doses of treatment need to be adjusted or whether the provided treatment has been effective. These parameters are assessed by using determined scoring systems which themselves are based on patient responses to framed questionnaires. The pretreatment status of all patients should be recorded using these scoring systems both at presentation and after completion of treatment. There are various scoring systems, of which the most commonly used are the Karnovsky and WHO scales for adults and the Lansky score for children. The EORTC Quality of Life Questionnaires have become a valid and commonly used tool and are available in many different languages. They consist of a series of questions with answers for which grading and scoring is done to assess changes in a cancer patient's global, emotional, physical, social and psychological health during and after treatment. EORTC has specific questionnaires for specific tumour sites and symptomatology. Another commonly used scale in quality of life assessment is the HADS (Hospital Anxiety and Depression Scale) which is used to measure changes in mental and emotional well-being during treatment or with progression of disease.

Various studies have noted that cancers which have been detected during population-based screening like breast, rectum or cervix have a better prognosis than tumours presenting symptomatically because diagnosis is made in an earlier stage. But in many other cancers, screening has not demonstrated clear prognostic benefit (like screening chest X-ray for detecting early lung cancer). Histological tumour type, grading and staging have an important bearing in determining outcome for individual patients, and use of new techniques of tumour detection and assessment can yield more information such as on gene expression which may affect prognosis. Other factors which must also be considered include age; sex; lifestyle factors such as smoking, alcohol and other drug use; obesity; and family history of disease. Biological factors such as performance status also have to be considered. Biochemical tumour markers can have either specific prognostic value (β-hCG levels in testicular cancer) or may have relative poor correlation only (CEA in colon cancer), but these markers are useful for indicating treatment response or disease progression.

There has been a recent propagation of the concept of risk assessment and "personalized medicine." This implies use of predictive tools which can be based on population datasets or on specific risk factors within a framed population from which a risk percentage is calculated using predetermined risk-based scoring frames. These variables are determined before treatment and give information on the probability of a response to a specific treatment (such as p53 expression denotes increased recurrence risk). Other examples are of such predictive tools which include the estimation of MYCN amplification in neuroblastoma, oestrogen/HER2 receptor status for assessing response to hormone therapy or trastuzumab and risk estimation of patients with Li-Fraumeni syndrome to develop second tumours. These predictive indices are important in determining strategies for treating different tumour subsets in guidelines and protocols. Sometimes specific genetic profiles are also designed which correlate with natural history of disease or outcome of treatment like the use of Rotterdam Signature in breast cancer risk determination.

Curative treatment: When a patient presents in early-stage cancer, with a tumour type considered well responsive to therapy, a variety of options can be considered. Surgery, radiotherapy and chemotherapy, all options are available in cases where curative or radical intent is used for treatment. Surgery can be considered upfront or after downstaging the tumour post-neoadjuvant chemotherapy or radiotherapy so as to get better margins. Likewise, radiotherapy can be delivered radically, concurrently with chemotherapy, as neoadjuvant preoperatively or adjuvant post-operatively. Preoperatively radiotherapy is given to decrease tumour size and hence prevent mutilative surgery. It also helps in preventing of tumour cell seeding which would have otherwise occurred during surgery of a large bulky tumour. Post-operative radiotherapy is contemplated to account for micro-metastases or sterilize positive or close surgical margins or even sometimes ablate any residual disease left behind. Likewise chemotherapy is also administered pre- and post-operatively, as only therapy, sequentially or concurrently with radiotherapy or even as post-intensive phase maintenance therapy in many cancers. The prime aim with all these interventions remains the optimal killing of cancer cells and prevention of recurrences while ensuring acceptable levels of toxicity and post-treatment sequelae.

Palliative treatment: Many patients present in stage where the cancer has disseminated such that cure is no longer a possibility. Some patients may also present in conditions which can be life threatening (tumour lysis, dyselectrolytemia, severe cancer cachexia, respiratory distress due to tracheal compression/lung collapse, sudden severe haemorrhage, cardiac tamponade) or threatening vital functions (acute cord compression, brachial plexopathy, severe pain from tumour bulk). In such cases the priority shifts to controlling the acute event or symptom, ensure stabilization of the patient's general condition and provide for symptom relief. In many cases also, the patients present in a terminal stage with no active measures possible. The care giver's role in such cases remains to provide best possible symptomatic relief and comfort the patient. The aim thus is improve the patient's quality of life. In cases where the acute event is in a curable stage, the patient has to be subsequently re-evaluated and restaged and treated accordingly. At all times the physician should keep in mind the overall picture of the patient's disease stage and decide accordingly on whether to proceed with curative or palliative intent. A sudden event should not divert the clinician from what has to be done.

References

1. Denoix P. TNM classification. Bull Inst Nat Hyg (Paris). 1944;1:1.
2. World Health Organisation. International classification of diseases for oncology. 2nd ed. Geneva: World Health Organisation; 1999.
3. AJCC cancer staging manual. 7th ed. Philadelphia: Lippincott-Raven Publishers; 2007.
4. International Union against cancer: TNM classification of malignant tumours. 5th ed. Berlin: Springer; 1997.
5. Rubin P. Clinical oncology: a multidisciplinary approach for physicians and students. 8th ed. Philadelphia: WB Saunders Publishers; 2001. p. 20.
6. Tucker R, Coel M, Ko J, et al. Impact of fluorine-18 fluorodeoxyglucose positron emission tomography on patient management: first years' experience in a clinical centre. J Clin Oncol. 2001;19:2504–8.
7. Schoder H, Meta J, Yap C, et al. Effect of whole body ^{18}F FDG PET imaging on clinical staging and management of patients with malignant lymphoma. J Nucl Med. 2001;42:1139–43.
8. Fong Y, Saldinger PF, Akhurst T, et al. Utility of ^{18}F FDG positron emission tomography scanning on selection of patients for resection of hepatic colorectal metastases. Am J Surg. 1999;178:282–7.

2 Role of Surgery in Cancer Management

The use of surgery in the treatment of *growing sores or ulcers* which may have been malignant has been reported from ancient times. There are records from ancient Egypt around 1600 BC and also from ancient Sumeria, India and China. Cancer surgery is an important tool and one of the principal methods of management of this scourge of cancer. Some famous people associated with development of surgical principals of cancer management of various sites include Albert Theodore Billroth for surgery of larynx, oesophagus and stomach, William Stewart Halsted for breast and Emil Theodore Kocher for thyroid. Other famous procedures designed include radical neck dissection by Crile, head and neck radical surgery by Martin and prostate by Charles Huggins [1]. In the present day of multidisciplinary management of cancer patients, surgery plays an important role in all stages of cancer management be it screening or even end-stage palliative care. The aims of a surgeon differ when he is operating for a benign lesion than when he is operating on a cancer. In a benign lesion, the surgeon tries to remove the least amount of tissue required to achieve surgical aims which would leave the patient with function as near a normal as possible. On the other hand, in cancers, the surgeon aims to remove the maximal amount of involved tissue possible to achieve either clear margins or preserve tissue function as near as normal possible.

Role in cancer screening and prevention: Various conditions such as precancerous ulcers, chronic scars, keloids or even certain normal body tissues can undergo cancerous transformation when exposed to repeated stimuli such as inflammation, food habits, living styles, genetic make-up or endocrinal disorders. Examples include development of skin cancers over chronic burn scars or mucosal cancers in areas exposed to chronic irritation and inflammation such as Barrett's oesophagus causing adenocarcinoma of the oesophagus or irritable bowel disease predisposing to colon cancer or even chronic cervicitis leading to cervical cancers. These organs undergo the entire spectrum of dysplastic to premalignant to malignant changes over a long period of usually 10–15 years and are amenable to surgical treatment during this period.

A. Mukherji, *Basics of Planning and Management of Patients during Radiation Therapy*, https://doi.org/10.1007/978-981-10-6659-7_2

Thus there are established protocols wherein surgery is indicated in the treatment of precancerous lesions such as in:

(a) MEN syndromes in which prophylactic total thyroidectomy is done usually before 5 years of age in MENS 2A and first year of life in MENS 2B to prevent the development of medullary thyroid carcinoma (MTC) later in life [2].
(b) Prophylactic mastectomy and surgical oophorectomy have been recommended as treatment options to reduce risk of development of breast cancer (80% lifetime risk) and ovarian cancer (23–54% lifetime risk) in patients with BRCA1 and BRCA2 mutations [3].
(c) Patients with high risk of development of colon cancer due to expression of several high-penetrance genetic mutations can be advised prophylactic resection of the colon and rectum [4, 5].
(d) Even in patients who have developed cancer in situ or intra-epithelial cancers such as in breast, cervix or oral cavity can lead normal lives with substantial risk reduction after surgery [6].
(e) With improvement in treatment outcomes, there are increasing numbers of cancer survivors with long-term survivals who are at increased risk of developing second malignancies or recurrences as a result of genetic predispositions or due to effects of chemotherapy or radiotherapy [7].
(f) Increasing prevalence of obesity worldwide [8] has brought into focus bariatric surgery for weight management [9] which may also aid in cancer prevention.

Role in cancer diagnosis and staging: In suspected cancerous lesions, surgical excision is often used to procure tissue for histopathological diagnosis. This exercise provides valuable biological evidence of disease as well as information on the disease subtype and tissue make-up. This information is extremely useful in designing treatment protocols. Surgery also helps in assessing the disease stage in which surgical procedures are often used along with imaging modalities to map the disease. Laparotomy and surgical staging are established methods of cancer staging for GI cancers like stomach, pancreatic cancers, ovarian cancers and even endometrial cancers. In fact the AJCC staging manual describes staging as *clinical classification* which is based on examination, investigation findings and even minor surgical procedures that have taken place before definitive surgery, *pathological classification* depending on the pathological assessment of the resected specimen as well as preoperative staging, *retreatment classification* based on the restaging of a recurrent tumour and *autopsy classification* which is based on the autopsy findings.

Cancer treatment: In the present era, cancer requires treatment approach by a combined team of surgeons, radiation and medical oncologists, dieticians, critical care specialists, nursing care psychologists and even physicians. The involvement of the various disciplines depends on the stage of the disease and the condition of the patient. Present trend is towards organ and function preservation. Cancer patients may also require minor surgical procedures such as a chemoport insertion for vascular access for chemotherapy [10], feeding procedures in patients unable to feed orally or planned for radiotherapy of the oesophagus or hypopharynx, patients planned for debulking surgery before other definitive cancer therapy [11] or even for surgical management of cancer treatment complications such as strictures or acute bowel or airway obstruction.

The Halstedian era of the late nineteenth century and the early part of the twentieth century was the first major advancement in surgical treatment of cancerous lesions. Radical enbloc resection of the tumour mass along with draining lymph nodes as well as full compartmental resections of the affected organs resulted in significant improvements in tumour control rates. However, these could not stand the test of time in all stages and especially advanced stages. The discovery of irradiation as a treatment modality and advances in irradiation procedures as well as availability of modern chemotherapeutic drugs has enabled function preservation with limited resections followed by adjuvant therapy to prevent or reduce recurrences. But even these multimodality therapeutic modalities are effective only if adequate surgery has been done. They cannot compensate for poor surgery. The watchword in organ preservation surgery is adequate surgery removing maximum required involved tissue without significantly affecting organ function.

In spite of organ preservation being a major aim in cancer surgery, there may be significant associated cosmetic defect which may then require reconstruction. This is another aspect of radical cancer surgery in the present day and one which requires team-based approach between not only the cancer surgeon and the plastic surgeon but also other specialized surgical disciplines where required. For example, extensive craniofacial resection requires coordination between the cancer/ENT surgeon, plastic surgeon and even neurosurgeon. Extensive pelvic tumours may require exenterations which may require reconstruction of the bladder or rectum and may need a joint team of cancer surgeons with a surgical gastroenterologist or even a urological surgeon.

Palliative care and rehabilitation: Surgery is also an important modality of treatment in cases of advanced or disseminated cancer which may not be amenable for curative treatment. In these cases, the aim of surgery is improve the patient's quality of life and try to improve the expected survival period. Cancer surgery is not just indicated in the radical setting to take out tumours and save the patient. It plays also an important role in patients whose tumour cannot be taken out or irradiated. Bypass surgeries in patients with inoperable cancers which would allow for physiological functions or even a simple creation of stoma or insertion of feeding tubes can significantly improve the quality of life of these terminally ill patients. Surgical interventions in patients who have had treatment-related complications such as release of strictures or treatment of lymphedema or even complex procedures such as face/limb or breast reconstruction help reduce morbidity of cancer treatment and improve patient compliance and satisfaction.

Surgical palliation can help relieve symptoms of patients beyond cure. It involves treatment options designed to enhance quality of life rather than eliminating disease [12]. Surgically removal of a large primary tumour mass even in a metastatic setting or even a large metastatic deposit causing distressing symptoms can result not only in improved quality of life due to symptom relief but may even result in an increment in the survival. Other examples may include the surgical excision of fungating lymph nodes which otherwise would have led to social ostracism of the patient, increased susceptibility to infections as well as psychological distress. Surgical interventions as explained in the previous paragraph can help improve patient quality of life, self-esteem and self-care [12]. As described earlier these procedures include nerve or plexus blocks to relieve pain, release of strictures, wound care, creation of stoma or bypass surgery or insertion of feeding tubes to help improve patient nutrition or care of blocked hollow organs, tracheostomy for airway obstruction as well as surgery to provide for passage for urine or stools in case of compromised urinary or rectal function or incontinence. Orthopaedic interventions in similar situations include use of prosthesis or rods/plates to stabilize spine/weight-bearing bones to avoid collapse and/or compression of the spinal cord or vital nerves or vessels.

Cancer emergencies: Specific conditions in cancers like severe haemorrhage, spinal cord compression, rupture of tumour or perforation of viscera, sudden lung collapse following massive pleural effusion, cardiac tamponade or secretory carcinoids require emergency intervention to save the life of the patient, relieve pain or prevent organ deterioration and failure [13].

2.1 Future of Surgery in Cancer Management

As seen in the preceding sections, surgery plays an important role in the treatment of various cancers and is often the definitive treatment in various solid tumours. Through the last century, surgical interventions have become more limited in the extent of tissue damaged and with the advent of various imaging (both anatomical and physiological) as well as changes in surgical protocols themselves and the incorporation of latest techniques such as robotic or even real-time image guidance in surgery; the extent of surgery is becoming progressively less mutilating with function preservation remaining an important goal. In developing countries, surgical interventions are still one of the most common definitive interventions for solid tumours [14].

References

1. Kufe DW, Pollock RE, Weichselbaum RR, et al., editors. Cancer medicine 6. Hamilton: BC Decker; 2003.
2. Ogilvie JB, Kebebew E. Indication and timing of thyroid surgery for patients with hereditary medullary thyroid cancer syndromes. J Natl Compr Canc Netw. 2006;4:139–47.
3. Narod SA, Offit K. Prevention and management of hereditary breast cancer. J Clin Oncol. 2005;23:1656–63.
4. Adebamowo CA, Adeyi O, Pyatt R, et al. Case report on hereditary non-polyposis colon cancer (HNPCC) in Nigeria. Afr J Med Med Sci. 2000;29:71–3.
5. de la Chapelle A. Genetic predisposition to colorectal cancer. Nat Rev Cancer. 2004;4:769–80.
6. Bertagnolli MM. Surgical prevention of cancer. J Clin Oncol. 2005;23:324–32.
7. Aziz NM. Cancer survivorship research: challenge and opportunity. J Nutr. 2002;132:3494S–503S.

8. Hedley AA, Ogden CL, Johnson CL, et al. Prevalence of overweight and obesity among US children, adolescents, and adults, 1999-2002. JAMA. 2004;291:2847–50.
9. Gasteyger C. Bariatric surgery for morbid obesity. N Engl J Med. 2007;357:1158–9.
10. Tilney NL, Kirkman RL, Whittemore AD, et al. Vascular access for dialysis and cancer chemotherapy. Adv Surg. 1986;19:221–70.
11. Al-Shammaa HA, Li Y, Yonemura Y. Current status and future strategies of cytoreductive surgery plus intraperitoneal hyperthermic chemotherapy for peritoneal carcinomatosis. World J Gastroenterol. 2008;14:1159–66.
12. Desai MJ, Kim A, Fall PC, et al. Optimizing quality of life through palliative care. J Am Osteopath Assoc. 2007;107:ES9–14.
13. Adebamowo CA. Topical formalin for management of bleeding malignant ulcers. World J Surg. 2000;24:518–20.
14. Ozgediz D, Riviello R. The "other" neglected diseases in global public health: surgical conditions in sub-Saharan Africa. PLoS Med. 2008;5:e121. https://doi.org/10.1371/journal.pmed.0050121.

3 Radiotherapy in Cancer Care

Role of Radiotherapy: Radiotherapy is along with surgery one of the principal modalities of treatment of patients with solid tumours and plays an important part also in the treatment of hematolymphoid malignancies. It has been studied that the principal advantage with radiotherapy is that this modality is relatively inexpensive if the infrastructure investment amount is calculated according to the amount spent per patient [1] and therefore with respect to the prevalent response and survival rates in different cancers with radiotherapy can be considered the most cost effective. This aspect has been studied and documented by the NHS in the UK in which radiotherapy costs account for only 10% of the cancer budget, while chemotherapy accounted for about 15% and surgery more than 30% [2]. It is also universally accepted and studied that about two-thirds of cancer patients will require some form of radiotherapy during the course of their cancer treatment [3], including nearly four-fifths of breast cancer patients and nearly all head and neck cancer as well as cervical cancer patients [4]. The intent and extent of radiotherapy required for a patient is influenced by the extent of disease at presentation. Indications for use of radiotherapy differ in early cases compared to locally advanced disease or even metastatic cases.

Palliative radiotherapy: The word *Palliate* means to relieve a symptom. There are at least in one-third to one-half of cases requiring radiotherapy where in the disease cannot be cured. In such cases, the intent of radiotherapy is to deliver a smaller dose that will relieve the symptoms a patient has presented with or will address an impending catastrophic cancer presentation. In these cases, as described, a shorter treatment protocol is used often for as less as a single short or at the most for 2–3 weeks. The dose per fraction is larger than curative radiation, and while this has the risk of higher late effects, these are usually not encountered because of the decreased expected survival. The duration of the palliative radiotherapy course is dictated by patient's performance status and expected survival with those expected to survive more than 10 weeks receiving longer duration protocols. Examples of the use of palliative radiotherapy include single or few doses for the treatment of painful bone metastases or malignant spinal cord compression, dyspnoea caused by lung

A. Mukherji, *Basics of Planning and Management of Patients during Radiation Therapy*, https://doi.org/10.1007/978-981-10-6659-7_3

or thoracic tumours compressing the bronchus or causing superior vena caval obstruction, dysphagia caused by a hypopharyngeal or oesophageal cancer, bleeding from advanced pelvic malignancies or even headache and symptoms of raised intracranial pressure from brain tumours or metastases. Relief of these symptoms would result in improved patient quality of life which is one of the primary goals of palliative radiotherapy.

Radiotherapy alone: Radiotherapy has also been used in the curative intent either as a single-modality definitive treatment or along with surgery (usually post-operative) for early-stage or locally advanced malignancies or with chemotherapy. Curative radiotherapy protocols are longer-duration treatments lasting 5–8 weeks and can range from a simple parallel opposed beam disposition to complex multi-field techniques. Adjuvant radiotherapy is routinely used in breast cancer after breast-conserving surgery or in selected patients after mastectomy and has been shown to reduce local relapse and improve overall survival [5–7]. Adjuvant radiotherapy is also indicated in stomach, rectal cancers, gliomas, sarcomas, gynaecological malignancies and some situations in head and neck cancers as well as many other cases [8–10]. Radical radiotherapy alone may be delivered for early laryngeal, oropharyngeal, hypopharyngeal and paranasal sinus tumours with the intent to cure while preserving function and avoid surgery [11] as well as in prostatic cancers. Neoadjuvant radiation has been advocated in many cancers of rectum, stomach, oesophagus, sinuses and sarcomas as a means of decreasing tumour size and treating potential sites of micrometastases before surgery especially in locally advanced cases to improve surgical clearance and ensure less morbid surgery [12].

Chemo-radiation: Radiotherapy is either given sequentially before or after chemotherapy in many radiosensitive tumours like lymphomas or testicular germ cell tumours in place of surgery and has shown to achieve even high rates of remission. In many head and neck cancers, lung cancers, bladder, cervix as well as GI cancers, concurrent chemo-radiation has been shown to achieve remission rates rivalling that of extensive radical surgery and adjuvant radiotherapy with preservation of organ and function with more recent trend towards decreasing normal tissue toxicity by better RT techniques [13–15].

Safety of radiotherapy: In the first few decades of its use, radiotherapy was frequently associated with morbid sequelae limiting its use and effectiveness. However, the development since the 1960s of high-energy (megavoltage) ionizing radiation beams has been useful in sparing the surface tissue. Treatment techniques have evolved from single direct or parallel opposed dual beams which would irradiate large amounts of normal tissues in the field to the use of multiple planar or even non-planar beams which can be shaped to match even an irregular target volume by the use of custom-made lead blocks or multileaf collimators. Thus, more normal tissue can be spared which in recent times can be increased even further by the use of beam modulation, differential beam penetration, image guidance in planning and beam delivery and even better immobilization and image reproduction. CT-based simulation, contouring and planning methods as well as imaging the treatment areas before treatment are delivered. These improvements in radiotherapy technology and equipment have resulted in the ability to deliver higher doses with better normal tissue sparing. This is turn has allowed for higher response rates even for tumours considered previously less radio-responsive and better compliance and survival. But for everything there is a cost. These improvements have come at the cost of higher maintenance and service protocols, more strict quality assurance protocols and a higher risk of catastrophic errors.

Recent developments: The advent of computer-based calculation models and modern imaging has brought in a sea of change in radiation therapy. These new changes include changes in dose fractionation, availability of newer generations of machines, newer techniques, rapid integration of modern imaging and radiation therapy as well as newer calculation models. Various studies showed that existing conventional fractionation techniques were not giving desired results, and with the availability of radiobiological models, the reasons were understood. These led to formulation of techniques of dose fractionation such as altered fractionation of radiotherapy in head and neck cancer and Continuous Hyperfractionated Accelerated Radiotherapy (CHART) in non-small cell lung cancers (with no weekend break). These have been shown to be superior to single daily treatments [16]. In other cases hypofractionation in breast, prostate and rectum has been studied and validated, and with the advent of IMRT, Simultaneous Integrated Boost (SIB) has been studied in head and neck, prostate and pelvic tumours. Similarly with better imaging and immobilization and even real-time positional corrections being available, a new branch of radiotherapy, namely, stereotactic radiotherapy, has come into prominence which very precisely delivers multiple beams into a small very precise target volume, and daily doses ranging from 4–5 Gy to up to 20 Gy are achieved. These help in treating small malignant and non-malignant lesions especially relatively less radio-responsive lesions such as arteriovenous malformations, schwannomas, isolated metastases, prostate cancer and early lung cancers.

Such precise therapy has also been possible not only due to new and very precise immobilization techniques but also with the advent and integration of new imaging techniques such as 4 D-CT, MR or PET with the linear accelerator. Respiratory gating and real-time imaging is now available as an add-on to modern linear accelerators. These new megavoltage treatment units have built in cone beam CT scan capability (Tomotherapy™) or high-precision stereotactic treatment capability (Cyberknife™). In the last two decades, researchers have studied the properties of other radioactive particles and compared them with the photon beams used traditionally. New particle beam therapies such as proton beams and heavy ion beams such carbon ion treatment have been found to be more precise than photon beams and affect much as normal tissue. Also these are usually not affected by the radioresponsiveness of a tissue and therefore would provide better response. These therapies have been proven in the management of some orbital tumours and base of skull sarcomas. Presently the cost of installation of such units is very high, but as with any technology, the next generation of cyclotrons and particle beam machines are both less costly and less bulky and are finding greater user acceptance in many centres around the world.

In conclusion: Radiotherapy is a branch of medicine which is to a very large extent technologically driven and has benefitted in the last three decades with the advent of computers and new technology. New modalities of therapy and new technology have allowed for increase in dose delivery with tighter margins while at the same time limiting the sequelae of therapy; and what were once deadly but common sequelae such as acute pneumonitis, radio-necrotic fractures of rib and jaw and even radiation-induced brachial plexopathy from breast radiotherapy technique are now rarities. But all this comes at a cost. High-quality precision radiotherapy requires significant upfront infrastructure investment in the form of a functioning megavoltage unit with facilities for adequate beam shaping, facilities for real-time or near real-time imaging for treatment planning, beam placement and treatment delivery, a basic planning computer system as well as trained and dedicated medical, physics and technology staff with routine and strict protocols for quality assurance both for planning fidelity and treatment delivery fidelity. Radiotherapy is an integral part of the multimodality and multidisciplinary management of cancer patients and is essential for good cancer care.

References

1. Ploquin NP, Dunscombe PB. The cost of radiation therapy. Radiother Oncol. 2008;86:217–23.
2. Richardson M. Lead clinician for cancer, NHS England; 2008. Oral Presentation.
3. Delaney GP, Jacob S, Featherstone C, et al. Radiotherapy in cancer care: estimating optimal utilization from a review of evidence based clinical guidelines. Sydney: Collaboration for Cancer Outcomes Research and Evaluation (CCORE); 2003.
4. Scottish Executive Health Department. Cancer in Scotland. Radiotherapy activity planning for Scotland 2011–2015. http://www.scotland.gov.uk/Publications/2006/01/24131719/0. 18 Nov 2008.
5. Group EBCTC. Effects of radiotherapy and of differences in the extent of surgery for early breast cancer on local recurrence and 15-year survival: an overview of the randomised trials. Lancet. 2005;366:2087–106.
6. Nielsen HM, Overgaard M, Grau C, et al. Study of failure pattern among high-risk breast cancer patients with or without postmastectomy radiotherapy in addition to adjuvant systemic therapy: long-term results from the Danish Breast Cancer Cooperative Group DBCG 82 b and c randomized studies. J Clin Oncol. 2006;24:2268–75.
7. Overgaard M, Jensen MB, Overgaard J, et al. Randomized trail evaluating postoperative radiotherapy in high risk postmenopausal breast cancer patients given adjuvant tamoxifen: results from the DBCG 82c trial. Lancet. 1999;353:1641–8.
8. Smalley SS, Gunderson L, Tepper J, et al. Gastric surgical adjuvant radiotherapy consensus report: rationale and treatment implementation. Int J Radiat Oncol Biol Phys. 2002;52:283–93.
9. Vigliotti A, Rich TA, Romsdahl MM, et al. Postoperative adjuvant radiotherapy for adenocarcinoma of the rectum and rectosigmoid. Int J Radiat Oncol Biol Phys. 1987;13:999–1006.
10. Stupp R, Mason WP, van den Bent MJ, et al. Radiotherapy plus concomitant and adjuvant temozolomide for glioblastoma. N Engl J Med. 2005;352(10):987–96.
11. Mendenhall WM, Werning JW, Hinerman RW, et al. Management of T1-T2 glottic carcinomas. Cancer. 2004;100:1786–92.
12. Higgins CA, Humphrey EW, Dwight RW, et al. Preoperative radiation and surgery for cancer of the rectum: Veterans Administration Surgical Oncology Group trial II. Cancer. 1986;58:352.
13. Keys H, Bundy B, Stehman F, et al. Cisplatin, radiation, and adjuvant hysterectomy compared with radiation and adjuvant hysterectomy for bulky stage IB cervical carcinoma. N Engl J Med. 1999;340:1154–61.

14. Kaufman DS, Winter KA, Shipley WU, et al. The initial results in muscle invading bladder cancer of RTOG 95-06: phase I/II trial of transurethral surgery plus radiation therapy with concurrent cisplatin and 5-FU followed by selective bladder preservation or cystectomy depending on the initial response. Oncologist. 2000;5:471–6.
15. Soresi E, Clerici M, Grilli R, et al. A randomized clinical trial comparing radiation therapy versus radiation therapy plus cis-dichlorodiammine platinum (II) in the treatment of locally advanced non-small cell lung cancer. Semin Oncol. 1988;15(Suppl 7):20–5.
16. Saunders MI, Dische S. Continuous hyperfractionated accelerated radiotherapy (CHART) in NSCLC. Int J Radiat Oncol Biol Phys. 1990;il2:1211–5.

4 Role of Chemotherapy in Management of Cancers

4.1 General Principles

Chemotherapy is the modality of treatment of cancers with administration of cytotoxic chemical agents or biological extracts or biomolecules. These agents act on the rapidly dividing tumour cells in the body and cause cell death by various mechanisms. Unfortunately they also act on the actively dividing bone marrow stem cells, mucosal lining cells and cells of the hair follicles thereby giving rise to the various sequelae seen with chemotherapy. The requirement for systemic therapy in cancer patients arises both in the locally advanced and in the metastatic settings. Systemic spread of cancer cells through the vascular or lymphatic channels puts these patients beyond the purview of local or even regional therapy, while in locally advanced disease, any micro-metastases that could have occurred are dealt with by the use of systemic chemotherapy or biotherapy. Here the chemotherapy acts to decrease the size of micro-metastases in locally advanced cancers like in breast, rectum, stomach and paediatric cancers; after which local treatment with surgery or radiotherapy can be started with lesser normal tissue toxicity. The early classification of the various systemic chemotherapeutic drugs was based on the mechanism of action of these drugs on cultured or in vivo mouse tumour model systems. These had a high proliferation rate, short doubling times and a large proportion of cycling cells and thus predisposed the screens to selecting inhibitors of DNA synthesis [1]. Various existing classes of chemotherapeutic agents are:

1. **Antimetabolites**: This class of drugs is composed of chemicals which structurally bear similarity with existing normal physiological metabolites which are required for certain essential pathways such as cellular energy production/DNA synthesis or reproduction. These chemicals replace the normal body metabolite, and being physiologically inactive, they act by blocking critical cellular pathway and cause cell death. An example is methotrexate which inhibits the enzyme dihydrofolate reductase (DHFR) and prevents the formation of tetrahydrofolate required for synthesis of the DNA building block thymidine. Similarly

A. Mukherji, *Basics of Planning and Management of Patients during Radiation Therapy*, https://doi.org/10.1007/978-981-10-6659-7_4

5-fluorouracil is metabolized by cancer cells to 5-flurodeoxyuridine monophosphate and inhibits the enzyme thymidylate synthase [2] which is required for DNA synthesis. Cytosine arabinoside and gemcitabine act by depleting intracellular deoxycytidine, while thioguanine and mercaptopurine inhibit enzymes involved in synthesis of guanine.

2. **DNA adductors**: These drugs are called adductors as they form reactive species in the body after their first-pass metabolism. These species then bind to the DNA helix or "adduct" to it, and after this they can distort the DNA structure by forming either bands or crosslinks which prevent the uncoiling of the DNA and thus its replication. This class includes alkylating agents (cyclophosphamide nitrosoureas), platinum analogues (cisplatin, carboplatin and oxaliplatin) and mitomycin C.
3. **Mitotic inhibitors**: The anaphase phase of the mitotic cycle results in the formation of the mitotic spindle which is a key step for subsequent cell division and duplication. This class of drugs prevents this step either preventing the formation of the tubulin network or preventing its dissolving thus preventing cell division. Common drugs causing this effect include the taxanes (taxol and taxotere), the vinca alkaloids (vincristine and vinblastine) and the emerging class of epothilones.
4. **Prevention of DNA unwinding**: This class of drugs includes inhibitors of the enzyme topoisomerase which is responsible for uncoiling of the DNA prior to its replication. Drugs such as doxorubicin [3], etoposide (both topoisomerase II inhibitors), irinotecan and topotecan (topoisomerase I inhibitors) prevent uncoiling of the DNA leading to apoptosis of the cancer cells.
5. **Hormone receptor antagonists**: Cancers such as breast, uterine and prostate are dependent on hormone manipulation, and drugs which can modulate production of steroid hormones can be used to prevent the growth and spread of these tumours. Drugs such as tamoxifen, letrozole, anastrozole and flutamide have shown action by directly influencing the expression of the hormone receptors in the target tissues. Also other drugs such as LHRH agonists can act on the pituitary and cause the release of LHRH thereby reducing production of testosterone or oestrogen by feedback inhibition and depriving cancer cells of hormonal stimulation for cancer cell proliferation.

Chemotherapy toxicity: Thus, as is seen from the above section, most anti-cancer drugs act by preventing cell replication or interfering with the energy cycle. Thus, these drugs by default would be selectively concentrated by actively dividing tissues (both the actively dividing cancer and normal tissues), and thus the common toxicities that we see from cancer chemotherapy are usually those affecting these actively dividing tissues such as skin, mucosa and bone marrow, leading to bone marrow suppression causing effects like neutropenia, anaemia and thrombocytopenia, hair follicle cell damage leading to alopecia, death of gastrointestinal crypt cells leading to diarrhoea and oral mucositis. Some of these anti-cancer drugs also cause very specific toxicities because of their mode of action (e.g. heart myocytes affected by anthracyclines or nerve damage from vinca alkaloids)/active metabolite formed in the body (cyclophosphamide causing haemorrhagic cystitis or lung toxicity from bleomycin) or manner of excretion (cisplatin causing renal damage). Also these drugs may interact with other medication the patient might be taking, or there may be complications of drug administration (fluid overload with cisplatin or capillary leak with docetaxel) especially in patients who are elderly with compromised hepatic and renal functions. In such cases the magnitude of drug induced reaction would be more severe than in an otherwise normal patient.

Combination therapy: Most chemotherapy protocols used are a combination of two or more drugs so as to achieve maximal tumour kill and at the same time minimize the side effects. This can be achieved in a combination by choosing drugs which may supplement or complement each other in their actions thus reducing the dose of drug otherwise required singly to achieve tumour cell kill. Also it is important to choose drugs so that their sequelae are not overlapping and thus do not reach the threshold dose required to cause toxicity. Also two different combinations can be added in a protocol to alternate between the two regimes so that tumour kill can be achieved with prevention of the rise of drug resistance such as the alternate use of VAC/IE regime in sarcomas or FEC/taxanes in breast cancer. Studies have also explored the duration of treatment like in patients with colorectal cancer in whom "chemotherapy holidays" of 2–3 months provide improved quality of life without having a negative impact on patients' survival compared to continuous chemotherapy [4].

Markers of effectiveness: The aim of chemotherapy or any other cancer treatment is generally to cure the patient. However, different regimes have different effects, and therefore it becomes necessary to develop common markers to assess the usefulness or efficacy of a chemotherapeutic regimen. The best such marker of drug efficacy would be the overall survival, but since this can take a long time to assess (up to even 10 years in breast cancers), surrogate markers have been identified to quickly determine the efficacy of a treatment regime. These include response rates after therapy, disease- or progression-free survival rates, toxicity profile, quality of life scoring and patient compliance rates. These may have to be correlated with complication rates and cost of therapy. The majority of common solid cancers can be palliated with chemotherapy, associated with significant prolongation of survival, but not cure [5]. However, the use of multimodality therapy in cancers such as breast, colon and stomach in which chemotherapy with or without irradiation given in the adjuvant setting has led to significant improvement in survival [6].

4.2 Novel Agents

In recent years there has been renewed interest in the study of intracellular and intercellular signalling and growth pathways as well as the role cancer genomics [7]. This has been the direct offshoot of the Human Genome Project which has made available the entire genetic database of the human body. New molecules developed now target the growth and signalling pathways between cells as well as cell membrane complexes, and these molecules act by binding to receptors present of the cell membrane and activating cellular processes either by the kinase/phosphorylase signalling pathways or through the activation of steroid receptor pathways. These pathways in turn activate or deactivate genes such as ras (cell proliferation). Thus, newer agents can act at any of these points and trigger either increased cell apoptosis or decrease the rate of proliferation or even interfere with the process of cell proliferation and cause cell death. A common target for many of such drugs is the EGFR (epidermal growth factor receptor) commonly expressed by cancers of the head and neck, lung, bladder and colorectal cancer. These drugs either block the receptor itself or its tyrosine kinase signalling pathway such as cetuximab/gefitinib (external surface of the EGF receptor) or lapatinib/erlotinib (tyrosine kinase inhibitor).

Tumour-induced blood vessel growth differs from normal anatomical microvasculature in its organization. Normal microvasculature proceeds orderly from arteries to arterioles to capillaries and then again back to venules and veins. In this way, oxygen is supplied to all body tissues. In tumours however there are clumps of half-formed or ill-formed vessels which may not reach the entire tissue. Oxygen from these vessels can diffuse to maximum of 50–100 μm beyond which the tissue becomes hypoxic and may even necrose. Therefore, some tumours secrete cytokines such as the vascular endothelial growth factor (VEGF) which stimulates the growth and invasion of new blood vessels into the tumour nodule, improving its proliferative capacity. Drugs have been designed to block the action of this factor (bevacizumab) by binding to its receptor and thus prevent tumour growth. This drug has been used in patients with advanced colorectal, breast and lung cancer [8].

Other improvements in the field of cancer genetics and molecular medicine are in the field of personalized therapy especially with the introduction of nanoparticles which can be used as carrier agents or even as molecular drugs. Specific markers for drug or radiation sensitivity have been developed using RNA signatures, micro-RNA sequences, specific DNA mutations or even patterns of phosphorylation of specific proteins which are used to target specific genetic or physiological pathways and thereby specifically act on the cancer cells rather than on the entire gamut of proliferating cells which results in higher chemotherapy-induced toxicities. Thus, people with specific DNA or RNA sequences can theoretically be treated by specific biomolecules affecting those sequences thus choosing patients who would benefit the most from such therapy [9].

References

1. Graham MA, Riley RJ, Kerr DJ. Drug metabolism in carcinogenesis and cancer chemotherapy. Pharmacol Ther. 1991;51:275–89.
2. Goldberg JA, Kerr DJ, Willmott N, et al. Pharmacokinetics and pharmacodynamics of locoregional 5-fluorouracil (5FU) in advanced colorectal liver metastases. Br J Cancer. 1988;57:186–9.
3. Kerr DJ, Wheldon TE, Kerr AM, et al. The effect of adriamycin and 4′-deoxydoxorubicin on cell survival of human lung tumour cells grown in monolayer and as spheroids. Br J Cancer. 1986;54:423–9.

4. Maughan TS, James RD, Kerr DJ, et al. Comparison of intermittent and continuous palliative chemotherapy for advanced colorectal cancer: a multicentre randomised trial. Lancet. 2003;361:457–64.
5. Midgley R, Kerr D. Colorectal cancer. Lancet. 1999;353:391–9.
6. Quasar Collaborative Group, Gray R, Barnwell J, et al. Adjuvant chemotherapy versus observation in patients with colorectal cancer: a randomised study. Lancet. 2007;370:2020–9.
7. Nair P. Epidermal growth factor receptor family and its role in cancer progression. Curr Sci. 2005;88:890–9.
8. Kerr DJ. Targeting angiogenesis in cancer: clinical development of bevacizumab. Nat Clin Pract Oncol. 2004;1:39–43.
9. Chan R, Kerr DJ. Can we individualize chemotherapy for colorectal cancer? Ann Oncol. 2004;15:996–9.

5 Principles of Management of Cancers in Paediatric Patients

Cancers in the paediatric age group may be due to genetic alterations and environmental influences, with no known preventive measures available. Metastatic disease is seen in 80% cases. Combined modality management with intent for organ and function preservation with reduction in treatment-related toxicity is of prime importance. The sequencing of treatment modality is important. Most treatment protocols for paediatric cancer start with induction chemotherapy followed by definitive therapy in the form of radiation therapy/surgery followed by maintenance chemotherapy. Most of these tumours are extremely responsive to therapy with remission rates in the region of 60% on an average.

These tumours can be divided broadly into:

- **Embryonal**: Tumour arises from embryonic tissue.
- **Lymphomas**: Lymphatic tissue.
- **Leukemias**: Blood.
- **Sarcoma**: Seen in the bone, cartilage, nerve and fat.

Cardinal signs of a malignancy in a paediatric patient are:

- Unusual mass or swelling
- Unexplained paleness and loss of energy
- Spontaneous bruising
- Prolonged, unexplained fever
- Headaches in morning
- Sudden eye or vision changes
- Excessive, rapid weight loss

Pretreatment evaluation:

1. Haematological:
    - Hb, TC, platelets
    - Liver function tests (LFT)

A. Mukherji, *Basics of Planning and Management of Patients during Radiation Therapy*, https://doi.org/10.1007/978-981-10-6659-7_5

- Renal function tests (RFT)
- Erythrocyte sedimentation rate (ESR)
- Bone marrow biopsy
- Urine analysis

2. Radiological evaluation:
   - CXR
   - X-ray of involved site
   - CT/MRI scan of primary site
   - Bone scan
3. Biopsy:
   - H&E
   - Immunohistochemistry
   - FISH
   - RT PCR

Patients are staged and treatment policy (sequence of multimodal therapy) is decided for each individual case. Post-induction imaging, surgery dates and radiotherapy are scheduled. After each planned modality of treatment is completed, patients are re-evaluated in the joint clinic for continuation or any change in the treatment policy. At completion of planned therapy, response rates and treatment-related side effects are documented. Follow-up schedule is explained to the patient and strictly adhered to. Any child with relapse is evaluated for salvage therapy.

5.1 General Principles of Treatment

1. Aim at long-term cure.
2. Multidisciplinary approach.
3. Minimize functional and cosmetic deficit.
4. Surgery – Should be reasonable, i.e. removal of tumour bulk with maximum preservation of organ and function.
5. Chemotherapy – Judicious use of multi-agent chemotherapy to minimize toxicity and maximize tumour control.
6. Radiotherapy – Optimize external radiotherapy use (3DCRT). Brachytherapy should be used wherever applicable [1].
7. Minimizing risk of secondary cancers in cases where complete cure possible by use of small RT fields if possible and avoiding chemotherapy drugs which have such risk.
8. Lifetime follow-up to detect secondary malignancies especially after use of extended field RT for Hodgkin's lymphoma and use of certain chemotherapy drugs like procarbazine.
9. Bone marrow transplant: Haematopoietic stem cell transplant (HSCT) depends on the patients' disease, disease status and general physical condition. It involves umbilical cord blood and parent's stem cells.

5.2 Principles of Radiotherapy in Paediatric Patients

1. Many paediatric tumours are radio-responsive and require relatively low doses, especially as chemotherapy is also used.
2. Growing tissues in children are likely to suffer more damage from radiotherapy than their adult counterparts, and radiotherapy may sometimes have to be delayed. In general radiotherapy is not used for children below 3 years of age [2].
3. Immobilization of young children is a major issue. Target volumes are generally well defined, with narrow margins, and hence immobilization is necessary. Children below 5 years of age may require anaesthesia [3].
4. Ideally the child should undergo pretreatment immobilization cast preparation and simulation in a child-friendly environment with tools available for distraction like toys.
5. Centres in many countries have video films as cartoons or in child-friendly format explaining the procedure to be followed and various steps that would be taken; this is done so that the element of apprehension is taken care of and the child readily cooperates with the treating personnel.
6. As far as possible, the child should be treated daily on the same machine so that he/she is familiar with the treating personnel.
7. There should be a two-way communication device during simulation and treatment delivery so that the child does not feel isolated in the treatment/simulation room.
8. Daily set-up verification of portals prior to delivery is a must especially in conformal radiotherapy and hypofractionated treatments where margins are minimal.
9. In case of extended field portals or those involving more than one bone, twice weekly blood counts should be done to detect marrow depression early.
10. In case of chemotherapy given concurrently or sequentially with radiotherapy, extra care has to be taken as the reactions to both are expected to be more severe. There should be prophylaxis for infections, treatment-induced diarrhea and vomiting as well as monitoring and correction of fluid and electrolyte imbalance.
11. Growth and development of the child has to be continuously monitored long after completion of treatment.
12. Late effects expected after treatment like intellectual deficits, visual loss, hearing loss, endocrine dysfunction, sexual issues and risk of second malignancies should be discussed and explained before commencement of therapy [4].

5.3 Principles of Chemotherapy in Paediatric Patients

1. Goals of chemotherapy include reducing the primary tumour size, destroying cancer cells and preventing metastases and microscopic spread of the disease.
2. Multiple classes of drugs like alkylating agents, antibiotics, vinca alkaloids, etc. are used.

3. Minimal possible cycles of chemotherapy are used to prevent long-term side effects especially in the more curable malignancies.
4. Chemotherapy is used where possible in combination with surgery or radiotherapy to maximise gains and minimise sequelae.
5. Chemotherapy can decrease immunoglobulin concentrations, and children with cancer become immune impaired. This can be also due to alteration of lymphocyte production and splenic dysfunction which prevents maturation of blood cells and alteration in inflammatory response.
6. Significant neutropenia can develop during chemotherapy creating an increased risk of infection in the child with cancer [5].
7. In immunosuppressed child with no history of varicella infection or varicella immunization having direct contact with an individual with chickenpox or shingles, varicella zoster immune globulin should be administered. Immunization against varicella may be considered 3 months after chemotherapy especially after patient is off prednisone.
8. Central venous access devices (CVAD) are an integral part of paediatric oncology and used to deliver chemotherapy, blood components, antibiotics, fluids, TPN, medications and blood sampling. Aseptic technique is used for dressing changes and heparin flushing. One should avoid trauma to devise and observe for catheter occlusion.
9. Cells most affected by chemotherapy are rapidly growing cells such as hair follicles, reproductive system, bone marrow and gastrointestinal tract mucosa.
10. Mucositis is more frequently seen in this age group. Thrombocytopenia or physical trauma may lead to bleeding and further mucosal damage. Neutropenia and poor dental hygiene predispose the oral mucosa to secondary infection.
11. Malnutrition occurs in 8–32% of the paediatric oncology population. Nutritional goals focus on maintaining normal growth and development as well as preventing nutritional deficiencies.
12. Growth and development of the child has to be continuously monitored long after completion of treatment and achievement of remission.

References

1. Kortmann RD, Timmermann B, Taylor RE, et al. Current and future strategies in radiotherapy of childhood low-grade glioma of the brain. Part II: treatment-related late toxicity. Strahlenther Onkol. 2003;179:585–97.
2. Duffner PK, Horowitz ME, Krischer JP, et al. Postoperative chemotherapy and delayed radiation in children less than three years of age with malignant brain tumors. N Engl J Med. 1993;328:1725–31.
3. Evans P, Chisholm D. Anaesthesia and paediatric oncology. Curr Anaesth Crit Care. 2008;19:50–8.
4. Ris MD, Packer R, Goldwein J, et al. Intellectual outcome after reduced-dose radiation therapy plus adjuvant chemotherapy for medulloblastoma: a Children's Cancer Group study. J Clin Oncol. 2001;19:3470–6.
5. Mason WP, Grovas A, Halpern S, et al. Intensive chemotherapy and bone marrow rescue for young children with newly diagnosed malignant brain tumors. J Clin Oncol. 1998;16:210–21.

6 Palliative and Supportive Care of Cancers

Supportive care includes symptom control, psychosocial support and rehabilitation and is an important component of cancer care as it has the ability to modify the course of disease irrespective of the possible outcomes. If the patient is intended for curative therapy, then good supportive care will ensure good compliance and hence good response. A subset of supportive care for cancer patients is palliative care in cases where anticipated life is shortened as a result of cancer as well as terminal care of dying patients aiming to improve their physical distress and symptoms [1–3]. Discussing the entire gamut of interventions required in palliation and supportive care of cancer patients would a separate volume by itself; this chapter only attempts at introducing various concepts important and relevant in palliative services and supportive care in cancer patients.

Health professionals engaged in oncology practice in recent times are now expected to be able to provide cancer-related therapy whether curative or palliative, should be able to achieve symptom control as well as limit treatment-related complications and should have an understanding of the patient's needs whether physical, psychological, social and financial. The aim of good cancer care should be to eradicate the disease if possible with minimum sequelae and hence to optimize a person's functional abilities. Therefore any definition of comprehensive cancer care includes the contribution of supportive and palliative services.

It is important also to include supportive and palliative care programmes into cancer research and education. The aim should be to develop new protocols for patient care and palliation of symptoms, develop new drug delivery systems as well as to educate and make aware clinicians of the importance of both palliative and supportive care services in the management of cancers. These will over a period of time lead to changes in the approach of clinicians from a regimen or guideline-based option to patient requirement-based care and will reflect in some measure the patient's informed choice. These decisions are important to help modify the course of the illness (either as a direct result of the cancer, the treatment of cancer or intercurrent co-morbid disease).

A. Mukherji, *Basics of Planning and Management of Patients during Radiation Therapy*, https://doi.org/10.1007/978-981-10-6659-7_6

6.1 Need for Supportive and Palliative Care Services

A diagnosis of cancer in a person has profound physical, psychological, social and economic effects on the patient and his/her family. The disease itself may have its attendant symptoms and loss of physiological function, cosmetic derangement and even loss of life expectancy. Psychologically the patient looks at the diagnosis as a death sentence. The family has to come to terms with a member being subjected to prolonged therapy with various adverse effects and if an earning member then to loss of earnings and expenditure on therapy as well. Frequently in uninformed societies, these people face social ostracism as well, and these can lead to depression and loss of self-esteem. Hence it is important for all healthcare providers to combat this gamut of issues a cancer patient faces and try to provide relief to them [4].

Principles of symptom relief in palliative care services include recognizing the right of every patient and the duty of every caregiver to offer such services when required of them, taking patient-centric decisions and establishing a relationship with both patients and their relatives, as cancer treatment requires the clinician to be associated with patients and their relatives for extended periods of time during which the clinician for his/her own mental well-being and for better patient compliance cannot afford to remain "clinically detached". Indeed the patients and their attendants should be encouraged to come up with their problems, opinions as well as fears, and there should be a free environment for mutual discussion. Also effective palliative care requires that the clinician promptly and accurately identifies the root cause of symptoms and starts treatment which should not be standard doses or regimes but tailored to the patient's needs and goal of such treatment should be realistic with regular assessment and monitoring.

6.2 Measuring Supportive and Palliative Care

The requirement for need for supportive and palliative care in cancer patients in a given population has to be estimated by using various statistical tools. These include the incidence of various cancers and their stage-wise distribution which would help define the magnitude of care required, prevalence rates of various cancers and their association if any with various causal factors and lifestyles which indicates the risk of morbidities and frequency of interventions required, mortality rates, survival rates, cause-specific death rates and disease-free survivals. These metrics will give an idea of the magnitude of the problem encountered and their likely response to various interventions.

The goals of palliative care are to provide for a continuum of support for the cancer patient's physical, social, emotional, sexual and financial needs and not just for uncontrolled physical symptoms [5]. Therefore since this care is a continuum throughout the spectrum of the natural history of the disease, measurement of outcomes also needs to be done throughout this period and not just in the terminal phase and includes those of the cancer patient and their caregivers before, during and after the terminal event in the disease [6].

6.3 Benefits of Palliative and Supportive Care

There are four levels at which effect of palliative care can be assessed:

- The person with cancer
- Family caregivers
- Health service providers
- Populations studied

The impact of good supportive and palliative services can be evident on entire populations and is the sum total of each aspect of cancer care and forms an integral part of quality healthcare provision at the community level, especially with end-of-life issues [7]. Setting up of a good supportive care programme has to take into account issues such as cancer control, symptomatic care, future planning and resource allocation and setting up the required infrastructure. For all of this, dedicated staff, material, finances, administration, planning and good management are required [8]. Also at the community level, patient point of view issues such as legacy, relationships, decision on home or hospice care and finalizing personal affairs have to be looked into [8–10].

Thus while setting up a good palliative care facility is indeed very demanding, there are a lot of benefits for the patients from these specialized services especially for patients with advanced cancer. These include:

- Comfort and care towards end of life whether in home care or hospice care [11, 12]
- Effective pain palliation [13]
- Protocolled management of dying cancer patients who have been institutionalized [14]
- Proper symptomatic treatment for cancer patients requiring hospital admission [15]
- Patient satisfaction with care [16–19]

It has also been seen that providing effective palliative care services not only helps cancer patients but has a positive effect on the clinicians, paramedical staff and patient caregivers. It helps through the following:

- It provides a sense of satisfaction at having helped someone and gives value to one's actions [16, 18].
- With caregivers having constantly to deal with morbid patients, satisfaction with good palliative care helps adjusting to relinquishing the role after death of patient [20, 21].
- It helps reduce stress, feeling of hopelessness and anxiety [19].
- It is associated with improved caregiver survival having relinquished the role [22].

Better palliative care also helps cancer care administrators through the following:

- It decreases admission loads for any and every symptom [17, 23, 24].
- It reduces the overall cost of cancer care [17, 25].

- With better hospice care, patient may choose his own place of death reducing burden on primary treating units [26].

One also has to overcome wrong perceptions about palliative care both in caregivers and patient attendants. It is usually perceived that referring a patient for palliative or hospice care means giving up on the patient and that after this the patient's condition would only worsen. This is one of the reasons why many physicians do not refer patients for palliative care. This perception has however not been supported by evidence such as in one large population-based study, it was found that survival was longer in 16 separate diagnoses studied of which 12 were advanced cancers [27]. Similarly systematic reviews on the benefits of good palliative care have reported that there is benefit for domains studied such as pain [28–31]; satisfaction with services, reduced hospital bed days and overall costs [32]; and potential benefits for caregivers [33]. Also follow-up has been easy and more informative for patients who have been referred for palliative care services than for patients left on their own [34–36].

6.4 Globally Available Supportive and Palliative Care Services

Even with all such proven benefits, there is however a wide variation in the availability and structure of services around the world, and this may be because of various reasons such as difference in treating philosophies worldwide, cultural differences, different healthcare philosophy, differential availability of funding and/or differential healthcare priority (developing countries may be more focused on population control, provision of safe water/food or infection control), availability of trained staff as well as social outlook towards dying people especially in resource-poor countries [37, 38]. In many of these countries, even the access to opioids for pain relief is a struggle and reflects poorly on the health regulatory systems in many countries [39]. However it is evident that many countries have started investing in palliative care and countries which already have an advanced program are funding and providing manpower and training to develop programmes in other countries by training of manpower, providing core manpower to train others in the field, provision of medicines especially opioids, infrastructure development and planning for future needs.

6.5 Dealing with Difficult Situations and Breaking Bad News

One of the most unpleasant or difficult situations for an oncologist is when they have to convey decisions regarding either inability of patient to tolerate or respond to definitive care or news of failure of therapy and disease progression. The clinician may have to deal with not only abject dejection on part of the patient but also denial, anger or even outright hostility. They may also face a patient who might completely break down and require emotional support.

While this aspect of oncology care has been spoken of often, there is little to prepare the doctor in the actual situation. A few guiding points include first acknowledging the importance of the statement or question to the patient and asking the patient where he/she would like to be talked to. The setting is important to allow adequate privacy and allows the patient to choose their comfort zone. The clinician must approach the patient directly maintaining eye contact, speak firmly but softly and lay before the patient all facts and options clearly. There should not be any attempt at patronization or glossing over of facts. Before presenting facts, however the clinician must try to understand the patient's level of cognizance, knowledge and cultural orientation as then he/she could explain to the patient in terms more easily understandable and culturally less shocking.

Also important for the oncologist is to keep the patient and their attendant (depending on the patient's mental faculties and wishes regarding privacy) informed at all steps during a management decision or regime and to proceed after adequate consent has been taken. End-of-life issues can be discussed if the patient is intellectually and culturally comfortable. The clinician has to understand that denial for consent or to news delivered is not due to lack of understanding but generally because of difficulty in coping with understanding of disease state. Therefore these people have to be treated with empathy, but at the same time their right to take their own decision has to be respected.

References

1. Sepulveda C, Marlin A, Yoshida T, et al. Palliative care: the World Health Organization's global perspective. J Pain Symptom Manage. 2002;24:91–6.
2. WHO. Cancer control: knowledge into action: WHO guide for effective programmes. Module 5: palliative care. Geneva: World Health Organization; 2007.
3. Lynn J, Adamson DM. Living well at the end of life: adapting health care to serious chronic illness in old age. Santa Monica: Rand; 2003.
4. Maguire P. Barriers to psychological care of the dying. Br Med J (Clin Res Ed). 1985;291:1711–3.
5. Johnson CE, Girgis A, Paul CL, et al. Cancer specialists' palliative care referral practices and perceptions: results of a national survey. Palliat Med. 2008;22:51–7.
6. Hearn J, Higginson IJ. Outcome measures in palliative care for advanced cancer patients: a review. J Public Health Med. 1997;19:193–9.
7. Bodenheimer T. The Oregon Health Plan—lessons for the nation. First of two parts. N Engl J Med. 1997;337:651–5.
8. Cancer care during the last phase of life. J Clin Oncol. 1998;16:1986–96.
9. Steinhauser KE, Christakis NA, Clipp EC, et al. Factors considered important at the end of life by patients, family, physicians, and other care providers. JAMA. 2000;284:2476–82.
10. Smith TJ, Schnipper LJ. The American Society of Clinical Oncology program to improve end-of-life care. J Palliat Med. 1998;1:221–30.
11. Currow DC, Ward AM, Plummer JL, et al. Comfort in the last 2 weeks of life: relationship to accessing palliative care services. Support Care Cancer. 2008;16:1255–63.
12. Wallston KA, Burger C, Smith RA, et al. Comparing the quality of death for hospice and non-hospice cancer patients. Med Care. 1988;26:177–82.

13. Miller SC, Mor V, Teno J. Hospice enrollment and pain assessment and management in nursing homes. J Pain Symptom Manage. 2003;26:791–9.
14. Miller SC, Mor V, Wu N, et al. Does receipt of hospice care in nursing homes improve the management of pain at the end of life? J Am Geriatr Soc. 2002;50:507–15.
15. Jack B, Hillier V, Williams A, et al. Hospital based palliative care teams improve the symptoms of cancer patients. Palliat Med. 2003;17:498–502.
16. Teno JM, Clarridge BR, Casey V, et al. Family perspectives on end-of-life care at the last place of care. JAMA. 2004;291:88–93.
17. Brumley RD, Enguidanos S, Cherin DA. Effectiveness of a home-based palliative care program for end-of-life. J Palliat Med. 2003;6:715–24.
18. Hughes SL, Cummings J, Weaver F, et al. A randomized trial of the cost effectiveness of VA hospital based home care for the terminally ill. Health Serv Res. 1992;26:801–17.
19. Kane RL, Wales J, Bernstein L, et al. A randomized controlled trial of hospice care. Lancet. 1984;1:890–4.
20. Abernethy AP, Currow DC, Fazekas BS, et al. Specialized palliative care services are associated with improved short- and long-term caregiver outcomes. Support Care Cancer. 2008;16:585–97.
21. Aoun SM, Kristjanson LJ, Hudson PL, et al. The experience of supporting a dying relative: reflections of caregivers. Prog Palliat Care. 2005;13:319–25.
22. Christakis NA, Iwashyna TJ. The health impact of health care on families: a matched cohort study of hospice use by decedents and mortality outcomes in surviving, widowed spouses. Soc Sci Med. 2003;57:465–75.
23. Costantini M, Higginson IJ, Boni L, et al. Effect of a palliative home care team on hospital admissions among patients with advanced cancer. Palliat Med. 2003;17:315–21.
24. Shelby-James TM, Currow DC, Phillips PA, et al. Promoting patient centred palliative care through case conferencing. Aust Fam Physician. 2007;36:961–4.
25. Taylor DH Jr, Ostermann J, Van Houtven CH, et al. What length of hospice use maximizes reduction in medical expenditures near death in the US Medicare program? Soc Sci Med. 2007;65:1466–78.
26. Ahlner-Elmqvist M, Jordhoy MS, Jannert M, et al. Place of death: hospital-based advanced home care versus conventional care. A prospective study in palliative cancer care. Palliat Med. 2004;18:585–93.
27. Connor SR, Pyenson B, Fitch K, et al. Comparing hospice and non-hospice patient survival among patients who die within a three-year window. J Pain Symptom Manage. 2007;33:238–46.
28. Finlay IG, Higginson IJ, Goodwin DM, et al. Palliative care in hospital, hospice, at home: results from a systematic review. Ann Oncol. 2002;13(Suppl 4):257–64.
29. Goodwin DM, Higginson IJ, Edwards AG, et al. An evaluation of systematic reviews of palliative care services. J Palliat Care. 2002;18:77–83.
30. Higginson IJ, Finlay I, Goodwin DM, et al. Do hospital-based palliative teams improve care for patients or families at the end of life? J Pain Symptom Manage. 2002;23:96–106.
31. Higginson IJ, Finlay IG, Goodwin DM, et al. Is there evidence that palliative care teams alter end-of-life experiences of patients and their caregivers? J Pain Symptom Manage. 2003;25:150–68.
32. Hearn J, Higginson IJ. Do specialist palliative care teams improve outcomes for cancer patients? A systematic literature review. Palliat Med. 1998;12:317–32.
33. Harding R, Higginson IJ. What is the best way to help caregivers in cancer and palliative care? A systematic literature review of interventions and their effectiveness. Palliat Med. 2003;17:63–74.
34. Christakis NA, Iwashyna TJ, Zhang JX. Care after the onset of serious illness: a novel claims-based dataset exploiting substantial cross-set linkages to study end-of-life care. J Palliat Med. 2002;5:515–29.
35. Currow DC, Abernethy AP, Fazekas BS. Specialist palliative care needs of whole populations: a feasibility study using a novel approach. Palliat Med. 2004;18:239–47.

36. McNamara B, Rosenwax LK, Holman CD. A method for defining and estimating the palliative care population. J Pain Symptom Manage. 2006;32:5–12.
37. Joranson DE, Rajagopal MR, Gilson AM. Improving access to opioid analgesics for palliative care in India. J Pain Symptom Manage. 2002;24:152–9.
38. Rajagopal MR, Joranson DE. India: opioid availability. An update. J Pain Symptom Manage. 2007;33:615–22.
39. Brennan F, Carr DB, Cousins M. Pain management: a fundamental human right. Anesth Analg. 2007;105:205–21.

Part II

Principles of Application of Radiotherapy

7 Radiobiological Principles

Various early works in the field of therapeutic uses of ionizing radiation to treat malignant diseases led to the gradual formulation of some basic principles of radiotherapy planning, dose prescription and treatment durations, giving rise to concepts of time-dose-fractionation. While most of these early works were trial-and-error formulations, some were based on radiobiologically tested experiments.

The spectrum of electromagnetic radiation is commonly used for the treatment of cancer patients with radiotherapy and usually is referred to as ***ionizing radiation*** (IR). Typical energies of such radiation that are used medically range from 4 to 25 MV. This irradiation conducts its effects by its ability to ionize, or excite electrons, from the outer shells of molecules within cells and also by direct damage to irradiated molecules. A major part of the effects of ionizing irradiation that is important in cancer medicine is because of the effects of this "electron ionization/excitation" which with repeated collisions in molecules and further ionizations in these molecules gradually lose energy and get deposited in increasing bunches or clusters towards the end of their tracks or lead to formation of ionized free radicals which are inherently unstable and cause a chain of ionizations [1, 2]. These resultant ionized molecules or free radicals are highly reactive and can cause damage to the structure of macromolecules like DNA or RNA. Ionizing radiation, depending on the frequency of inter-electron collisions, deposits its energy randomly causing damage to all molecules in the cell which lie in the path of these ionized active electron or free radical clusters. But while most molecules like RNA or proteins may have multiple copies and can undergo continuous rapid turnover thus limiting the damage caused, DNA having limited turnover with a large molecular size provides an easy target, and the consequences of significant damage to cellular DNA can be often lethal for the cell.

The action of ionizing radiation on cellular structures is usually by two pathways, direct damage and indirect damage [1, 2]. The pathway of indirect damage occurs in four stages: initially a physical stage where the radiation passes through the tissue and reacts with cellular water leading to formation of a variety of free radicals. This is followed by a physiochemical stage where these charged molecules

A. Mukherji, *Basics of Planning and Management of Patients during Radiation Therapy*, https://doi.org/10.1007/978-981-10-6659-7_7

react further to form either other stable reactive molecules or commonly more reactive radicals like the hydroxyl radical. Next is the chemical stage where these radical species react with intracellular molecules like proteins, RNA or DNA leading to structural or reproductive cellular damage. Finally comes the biological phase where the result of these changes can lead to either cell death, loss of reproductive ability, apoptosis or mutation. Direct damage to cell constituents is caused by direct action of ionizing radiation leading to direct DNA damage with resultant expression of the effect. This damage can lead to loss of base pairs, uncoupling of DNA strand, breaking of hydrogen bonds of DNA helix or formation of cross linkages. Thus the end result of these changes may be faulty transcription of genetic information leading to mutation, metabolic disturbance and defective repair of cell damage or even direct cell death caused by disruption of cellular environment or activation of certain genes. These changes are caused most easily in the G2M phase of the cell cycle when the cell is undergoing division and is extremely susceptible to damage. This process of "direct action" or direct damage is commonly seen when high LET particles interact with tissues as being highly ionized with heavy particles there is dense clustering of ionizing in the tissues, leading to direct damage.

The process of damage to cellular DNA is brought about by various ways which could involve:

1. Damage to single bases or single-strand breaks (SSBs): In this type of damage, single or few base pairs are affected and can be quickly repaired by base excision. This type of damage does not contribute significantly to the radiosensitivity of a tissue.
2. Double-strand breaks (DSBs): Repaired by a process of homologous recombination repair (in late S/G2, when a DNA template is available) which is accurate or non-homologous end joining which is error-prone. DSBs are believed to be the significant event in the expression of radiosensitivity; and it is estimated that accumulation of about 40 DSBs can kill a cell.
3. Chromosomal aberrations: Result from unrepaired or wrongly repaired DSBs. Symmetric chromosome damage, i.e. those occurring on both the chromatids (such as translocations), is usually nonlethal, while an asymmetric damage (such as a ring chromosome) can be lethal because of the loss of significant amount of DNA.

7.1 Cell Survival and Effect of Linear Quadratic Function

A cell survival curve could be defined as a plotted graph which describes the relationship between that fraction of cells in an irradiated tissue which are able to maintain their reproductive integrity or *clonogenic/surviving cells* and the absorbed dose [3, 4]. This ratio of surviving cells or cell survival which can be reported diagrammatically as a function of the delivered radiation dose by plotting this surviving cell fraction on a logarithmic scale on the ordinate against the irradiation dose on the abscissa. A study of various types of cell survival curves shows that the shape of this curve and hence the pattern of survival can be influenced by the type of radiation delivered, with survival curves seen after exposure to densely ionizing radiations exhibiting an almost exponential function of dose, shown by an almost straight line on the log-linear plot; while after exposure to sparsely ionizing radiation, tissues exhibit an initial slope followed by a shoulder region which then later nearly straightens out at higher doses [3, 4].

The linear quadratic model is presently the widest used mathematical model for explanation of radiobiological effects and had been introduced in the 1980s [5]. But even this model can predict dose effects to up to 6 Gy per fraction reasonably accurately and up to 8 Gy per fraction with little less accuracy [5]. Beyond this fractionation, there are as yet no mathematical models, and most calculations are based on extrapolations. This model is used to calculate equivalent doses between various fractionation schedules for comparison of effects or even for conversion of brachytherapy dose to its equivalent conventional radiotherapy dose. The simplest adequate mathematical description of these data is provided by a linear-quadratic function:

$$\mathrm{SF} = \mathrm{e}^{-\alpha \times d - \beta \times d^2}$$
$$\left(\mathrm{SF}: \text{surviving fraction of cells}; d: \text{dose}\right)$$

This principle as its name implies is based on the interaction between the two components of cell kill by radiation—a linear component and a quadratic component. The **linear component** of this complex phenomenon is made up of single-hit cell damages or cell kills in which the damage produced is directly proportional to the dose the cell is exposed to, but its repair probability is independent of dose; both these effects are within the limits of clinically relevant doses. This equation is depicted as equal to $\alpha \times d$. The **quadratic component** of the cell kill does not cause lethal damage by itself and affects *sublethal damage (SLD)*. However with increasing dose exposure, the probability of a combination of two or more SLDs causing a lethal event to the cell increases proportional to square of the dose. This effect is also assumed to be within the range of clinically relevant doses and is expressed as equal to $\beta \times d^2$.

As mentioned previously, a typical cell survival curve for tissues irradiated with medically used ionizing radiation have an initial slope which then bends linearly with higher doses with the steepness of this linear (straight) part proportional to the dose. The curvature of the initial slope also depends on the type of irradiation used and has been mentioned in preceding paragraphs. This curved part or the initial slope is the quadratic part of the curve while the steep part is the linear part. The slope of this linear-quadratic curve is a depiction of the relative components of cell kill and is denoted by the ratio of α/β. **When α/β is large, the linear term predominates, so the slope of the log (SF) against d curve is relatively straight**. This means that there is higher number of lethal cell events even with single hits, and this is seen with either high LET radiations, tissues with less repair potential or with higher dose per fraction (doses above 6–8 Gy per fraction may straightway cause ablation with minimal quadratic component). **On the other hand, if the α/β is**

small, it means that there is more likelihood of double hits required for lethal events, and hence the curved part of the plot may predominate. The main benefit in this linear-quadratic formula is in demonstrating a difference in the repair potentials of various tissues with high ratio tissues showing less repair potential and low ratio tissues able to repair damage better, indicating a benefit with dose fractionation. Also tissues which have a lower α/β ratio are more sensitive to the effects of fractionation and fraction size as doubling the dose will lead to square of effects (more than double) on the log (SF) curve. An earlier multi-target single-hit model described the slope of the survival curve by D0 (*the dose to reduce survival to 37% of its value at any point on the final near exponential portion of the curve*) and the extrapolation number *n* (*the point of intersection of the slope on the log survival axis*) [1, 6]. *D*q was the quasi-threshold dose. However, this model does not have any current biological basis.

The linear quadratic model describes the two components to cell kill by radiation by the following equation:

$$S(D) = \mathrm{e}^{-\alpha D - \beta D^2}$$

where S(D) is the fraction of cells surviving a dose D, alpha is a constant describing the initial slope of the cell survival curve and beta is a smaller constant describing the quadratic component of cell killing [6].

The ratio of α/β gives the dose at which the linear and quadratic components of cell killing are equal and is an important component in estimating fractionation schedules [6]. A high α/β (straighter curve) ratio is seen in cells with little repair capability such as cancer cells while a low α/β (more curved) ratio is seen in cells with a high repair potential such as well-differentiated (late responding) normal tissue. This difference in the cell survival curves provides window for achieving higher cancer cell kill compared to differentiated tissue cells and thus provides the explanation for the radiobiological advantage of fractionated radiation therapy treatment. The biological equivalent dose (BED) refers to the effective total absorbed dose (in Gy) for any given fractionation scheme in terms of early or acute effects and late sequelae (BED3 or BED10), while the term EQD2 is another value often used to compare fractionation regimes, and it basically refers to the effective absorbed dose or BED if it were given by standard fractionation (1.8–2.0 Gy/day).

Withers (1975) suggested four basic mechanisms that contribute to the diverse reactions of different tissues to irradiation (Table 7.1) [7, 8]:

- Redistribution of cells in the cell cycle
- Reoxygenation of hypoxic cells in the tumour
- Repair of cellular radiation damage
- Repopulation of surviving cells during radiotherapy treatment

Redistribution: Cells may not be radiosensitive all the time, but during certain periods when they are in specific phase of the cell cycle, cells are more vulnerable to lethal damage by radiation. An exposure of radiation has the effect of killing off

Table 7.1 Effect of fractionated radiotherapy on tissues

	Effect of fractionated radiotherapy	
Effect	Tumour cells	Normal tissue
Repair of damage (sublethal)	There is some amount of tumour cell repair as well, but additional sublethal damage from each fraction increases lethal damage	Improves repair and prevents increased damage
Reoxygenation	Decreased bulk of tumour after fractions allows oxygen to penetrate deeper and increase tumour kill	Increased oxygenation improves cell defences of normal tissues also
Redistribution	After each fraction, surviving cells move from non-proliferative to proliferative phase as dividing cells are lost	Some dividing normal tissues also suffer same effect; however scale is less
Repopulation	With increased killing of labile cells, few resistant cell lines may emerge	Increase in dividing cells leads to more damage
Inherent radiosensivity	Rapidly dividing tumour cells are more radiosensitive	Tissues with more turnover suffer more compared to differentiated tissues

the cells in the sensitive phases (G2M) of the cycle leaving behind the quiescent cells. This has the effect of moving a large part of the cells to determined phases of the cell cycle which in effect leads to redistribution of these cells [9]. Thus this phenomenon results in a determined fraction of cells being killed with every dose of radiation and if calculated properly will have minimal effect on normal tissues. Thus assuming that a proliferating tumour is surrounded by non-proliferating normal tissue, small doses per fraction and time intervals sufficient for redistribution should result in an improved therapeutic differential between the tumour and normal tissue with better control and lesser toxicities.

Reoxygenation: Hypoxic cells have been found to be more resistant to photon beams (X- or gamma rays) than normally oxygenated cells. This is because oxygen is presence ingredient required for the formation of free radicals which play an important role in radiation-induced cell kill. Irradiation preferentially sterilizes cells that are adequately oxygenated. Hypoxic cells are seen especially in the central portions of tumours or wherever the vascularization is not adequate and is due to the imbalance between the rate of production of new cells, the predominant glycolytic pathway of cellular respiration and the vascularization of the tumour (Thomlinson and Gray, 1955) [10, 11]. Various studies have demonstrated that oxygen diffuses from the blood in the capillary network into the cells, and this diffusion capability is dependent on the capillary density in a tissue. If the cells are within 100 μm from a capillary, there is good oxygenation; but this level falls at distances more than 150 μm and beyond 200 μm mostly anoxic cells are seen. When a tissue is thus irradiated, the dose kills off the oxygenated cells. In the period between the two fractions, there is some tumour shrinkage, and vessels grow into the previous anoxic area. With subsequent fractions, this process is repeated, and each dose kills off the part which has been freshly oxygenated.

Repair of Cellular Radiation Damage: This was proposed by Elkind and Sutton in 1960 [12]. The response of various cellular repair mechanisms in response to a dose of irradiation is usually depicted in the linear-quadratic equation and iso-effect curves. The effect of linear-quadratic equation on cell kill has been explained in the section on sublethal damage in this chapter. As explained previously, this phenomenon has an application in fractionation in radiotherapy. The dose is fractionated or divided into a number of smaller daily exposures with a time interval in between; there is the likelihood of repair of sublethal damage in the normal tissues in the inter-fractional period.

The benefit of fractionated radiotherapy can be explained on the basis of the radiobiological principles of the dose-survival curves. When a dose is given as a total single fraction dose, there is an initial shoulder in the curve, and for higher effect, higher dose may have to be given which could cause severe tissue effects. On the other hand, when a total dose is divided into a number of equal daily fractions and the interval between these fractions is enough theoretically to allow for SLD repair to minimize tissue toxicities but not allow tumour cell repopulation, the shoulder of the survival curve is repeated many times; and the effective survival curve becomes an exponential function of fractional dose and is seen as a straight line through that point on the single-dose survival curve which corresponds to the daily dose. This dose D0 (the reciprocal of the slope) has been calculated as close to 3 Gy for human cells.

Repopulation: This was proposed by Hermens and Barendsen in 1969 [13]. Tissue can be divided based on their ability to regenerate and grow. Thus there can be either highly proliferative tissue with a large number of cell actively dividing or slowly proliferative tissues with most cells being quiescent unless they receive a stimulus to proliferate. Since these proliferative tissues have many actively dividing cells, they are sensitive to radiation-induced damage and express these damages early. These tissues are the early-reacting tissues such as the skin, mucosa and gonads. In addition, proliferation of surviving tumour cells during treatment is one of the main factors that determine the outcome of fractionated radiotherapy and is thought that in general cancer cells are intermediate to fast in their proliferative potential though some such as prostate cancers or melanoma are slowly proliferative cancers. While increase in the treatment duration may lead to a decrease in the acute reactions, there may also be a corresponding increase in the number of viable tumour cells between fractions or during treatment interruptions which is assumed to result in a failure to control the tumour especially after the fourth or fifth week of irradiation [7, 8]. Hence it is important to know the SF2 (surviving fraction at 2 Gy) probability for tumour cells which is *defined as the probability of any cell surviving a single dose of 2 Gy, the most commonly used fraction size* [7]. This is because radiation-induced cell kill is a random event with all cells (tumour or acutely reacting) at equal probability for experiencing a lethal event. It is these surviving cells which lead to repopulation and treatment failure.

Inherent Radiosensitivtiy: This is based on the law of Bergonie and Tribondeau (1906) [14] which states that tissues are more radiosensitive if their cells are less well differentiated, have greater proliferative capacity and divide more rapidly. The clinical importance of this principle is that it accounts for variable response of tumours to radiotherapy. Curative dose is proportional to log of cell number; hence subclinical disease needs smaller dose.

Effect of Oxygen, LET and RBE: As explained previously in this chapter, the presence of oxygen in a tissue has a major effect on the radiation-induced response in that tissue, and this correlation between the effects of presence of oxygen in causing radiation-induced damage is expressed as an oxygen enhancement ratio (OER). Broadly this is defined as the ratio of radiation dose that would cause the same amount of tissue damage in an oxygenated tissue compared to a deoxygenated tissue. The OER for X-rays and electrons is about three at high doses and falls to about two for doses of 1–2 Gy.

Another term used is the linear energy transfer or LET. This term provides an idea about the ionization potential, mass and subsequently the penetrating power in an irradiation beam. This means that beams which ionize more or are heavier can penetrate less or have a defined range of tissue penetration. For example, heavy alpha particles or protons deposit energy densely during their course through a tissue and have a less penetrating power compared to a neutron beam which may not ionize in the tissue and can penetrate very far. Beam types which are very heavy or ionize more depend less on the oxygen concentration in a tissue and therefore have a low OER. Thus the OER decreases as the LET increases and approaches OER = 1 at about LET = 150 keV/mm.

Another term to describe a radiation type is the relative biological effectiveness (RBE), which compares a test radiation to a standard radiation type for equivalent doses to produce the same biological effect. The usually recommended standard type of irradiation beam used for testing now is that of Co-60 gamma rays; while 250 kVp X-rays have been used historically. This RBE is dependent on the type of radiation, the type of cell or tissue, biologic effect under investigation, dose, dose rate and fractionation. In general, it has been seen that the RBE increases with the LET to reach a maximum RBE of 3–8 at LET @ 200 keV/m and then decreases because of energy overkill.

7.2 Types of Cell Damage

In mammalian cells, three types of radiation damage are described:

- **Lethal damage**: This type of cell damage can neither be reversed nor repaired and leads to cell death.
- **Potentially lethal damage**: In this type of cellular damage, the cell suffers grievous injury but which is not sufficient to cause death. However addition or effect of cellular environmental factors could worsen the injury leading to cell death.
- **Sublethal damage**: In this type of DNA damage, under normal circumstances, it can be repaired within 24 h. However in case the cell suffers further injury in less than the time taken for repair, the two sequential injuries can have an additive effect leading to lethal cell damage. Thus this type of radiation-induced cellular damage is the principal method of differential tumour cell kill as the normal tissue cells are expected to repair their sublethal damage before the cancer cells and underlines the benefits of fractionated radiotherapy.

7.3 Importance of Dose Fractionation

During irradiation of a tissue, an important point to be considered is whether the total dose required can be given in a single shot or should it be divided into a number of smaller components called fractions. As has been explained before, the effect of tissue irradiation can be explained in terms of a cell survival curve in which there is an initial shoulder which denotes tissue repair followed by a slope denoting increased cell kill. Thus when a total dose is divided into a number of smaller fractions separated by a time interval, more cells survive than for the same total dose given in a single fraction, because of tissue repair occurring every time the shoulder of the curve is repeated for each fraction. The time interval between each fraction of dose delivered also has a bearing on the surviving fraction (SF). The SF increases rapidly if the interval between dose fractions increases, especially for some late-responding tissues. Also if the time interval between fractions exceeds a cell cycle period the resultant cell number increase will result in an increase in the SF.

Therefore conventional fractionation helps spare normal tissues by the process of repair of sublethal damage between each fraction and cell repopulation. This process of sublethal damage repair helps in protecting slow-growing or late-reacting tissues, while cell repopulation is largely responsible for repair in rapidly dividing or early-reacting tissues. In addition, dividing the total dose into a larger number of smaller dose fractions helps in improving tumour cell kill by better oxygenation (explained in previous section) and also due to a time gap helps in movement of otherwise quiescent tumour cells into the actively dividing phases of cell cycle when they are more prone to fatal injury following exposure (redistribution). Therefore fractionation allows difference in the response to irradiation by tumour as well as early- and late-reacting normal tissues. Smaller doses of irradiation will spare slow-growing or late-reacting tissues, and the time gap between each dose fraction will allow regeneration of early-reacting tissues and tumour reoxygenation.

Thus dose fractionation leads to an increase in therapeutic ratio with maximum probability of tumour control and minimum complications due to decompression of blood vessels caused by tumour shrinkage leading to better oxygenation and decreased hypoxic cells. It exploits difference in recovery rate between normal tissues and tumours and results in improvement in acute toxicity with fractionation [15, 16].

Dose-rate effect is typically seen in brachytherapy practice, and it is the phenomenon of repair of SLD taking place during the process of tissue irradiation when it is occurring over a prolonged period. As explained earlier with each fraction, there is a repetition of the shoulder of the cell survival curve with the slope being dependent on the magnitude of the fractional dose. In case of continuous low-date irradiation, for example, in permanent implants (with gold or iodine-125 seeds), the slope can be considered to represent a very large number of very small fractions and leading to a cell survival curve which has little or no shoulder and has a shallow slope. There is also an inverse dose effect which occurs when decreasing dose rate can lead to an increase in cell killing because the higher dose rates would block the tumour cells in radioresistant phases of the cell cycle by arresting further cell redistribution or division [17].

7.4 Clinical Radioresistance

A tumour can be regarded as radioresistant if it fails to show response after irradiation with the maximum tolerable dose. Since the normal tissue sensitivity limits the success of radiotherapy, it is very important to deliver the maximum possible dose to tumour while sparing normal tissues to the maximum possible extent. Tumours have been classified by Paterson into three categories: **radioresponsive**, these include lymphomas and seminomas; **radioresistant**, which include sarcomas, melanomas and tumours of GI tract; and those with **limited sensitivity**, such as adenocarcinomas and squamous cell carcinoma.

Human tumour cell lines have been classified into five categories in decreasing order of sensitivity: (1) lymphoma, myeloma and neuroblastoma; (2) medulloblastoma and small cell lung cancer; (3) breast, bladder and cervical carcinoma; (4) pancreatic, colorectal and squamous lung cancers; and (5) melanoma, osteosarcoma, glioblastoma and renal carcinoma. The SF2 (surviving fraction for 2 Gy) varied from 0.2 to 0.6.

Many different factors are responsible for the radioresistance of tumours. These are:

1. **Intrinsic radioresistance**: Some tumour cells are more resistant than others according to their Do values as well as the initial shoulder width of survival curves. Survival at low doses of the order used in single fraction in radiotherapy (2 Gy) decides the outcome of treatment. Radioresistant melanomas and sarcomas not only show a higher Do value but also large extrapolation number and shoulder width. On the other hand, radiosensitive tumour cells show near-exponential survival curves with very small shoulder width.
2. **Proliferation kinetics**: Tumours in which a large proportion of the cells are in nonresponsive phases such as Gl, Go or S phase may be radioresistant. Tumours with a large fraction of cells in proliferation compartment and tumours in which the redistribution of cells occurs rapidly are radioresponsive. Tumours in which repopulation occurs rapidly are radioresistant. There is evidence of rapid repopulation in Burkitt's lymphoma, inflammatory breast cancers, laryngeal cancers and malignant melanoma. In such cancers, overall treatment time is reduced to improve response. In general slowly proliferating tumours are radioresistant. This may be due to low growth fraction and large fraction of quiescent cells. Radioresistant tumours are also characterized by low cell proportion of clonogenic cells.
3. **Tumour size**: Large tumours are generally radioresistant as these may contain a large fraction of non-proliferating quiescent cells or even hypoxic areas. Thus they need larger doses and larger field size resulting in higher normal tissue complications.

4. **Ability to recover from potentially lethal damage**: Radioresistant tumours may have a greater ability to recover from PLD. This is seen in cases of melanoma cells and osteosarcoma cells. Particularly, tumour in which a large fraction of non-proliferating cells are present may recover from PLD significantly.
5. **Acquired radioresistance**: Tumours with a large fraction of hypoxic cells may be difficult to cure. Hypoxic cells may persist throughout the treatment in tumours which are slow shrinkers and which reoxygenate poorly.
6. **Metastases**: Tumours which metastasize extensively cannot be cured with radiotherapy alone. Those tumours which are difficult to be locally controlled are the ones which metastasize rapidly. Persistent and recurrent tumours are believed to metastasize more frequently. Hence, improvement of local control by aggressive methods of treatment can help to reduce metastatic dissemination of tumours and can improve cure rate. This has been demonstrated clinically in the case of cervical cancer and oral cavity cancers.
7. **Technical factors**: Under-dosage of tumours due to dosimetric problems, non-uniform irradiation of tumours and errors in the localization of tumours can also lead to failure of response.

References

1. Hall E, Giaccia A. Radiobiology for the radiologist. Philadelphia: Lippincott, Williams & Wilkins; 2006.
2. Ward JF. Complexity of damage produced by ionizing radiation. Cold Spring Harb Symp Quant Biol. 2000;65:377–82.
3. Puck TT, Marcus PI. Action of x-rays on mammalian cells. J Exp Med. 1956;103:653–66.
4. Puck TT. Action of radiation on mammalian cells III. Relationship between reproductive death and induction of chromosome anomalies by x-irradiation of euploid human cells in vitro. Proc Natl Acad Sci U S A. 1958;44:772–80.
5. Bentzen SM, Joiner MC. The linear-quadratic approach in clinical practice. In: Joiner MC, van der Kogel AJ, editors. Basic clinical radiobiology, vol. 4. London: Edward Arnold; 2009. p. 120.
6. Fowler JF. The linear-quadratic formula and progress in fractionated radiotherapy. Br J Radiol. 1989;62:679–94.
7. Withers HR. The 4 R's of radiotherapy. In: Lett JT, Alder H, editors. Advances in radiation biology, vol. 5. New York: Academic; 1975. p. 241.
8. Steel GG, McMillan TJ, Peacock KH. The 5Rs of radiobiology. Int J Radiat Biol. 1989;56:1045–8.
9. Kogelnik HD. Gottwald Schwarz. In: Ellegast HH. Kogelnik HD. Strasser E. eds. Hundert Jahre Medizinsche Radiologie in Osterreich. Wien. Munchen. Bern: Verlag Wilhelm Maudrich (Hundred years of medical radiology in Austria. Vienna. Munich. Bern: Publisher Wilhelm Maudrich). 1995;65–71.
10. Thomlinson RH, Gray LH. The histological structure of some human lung cancers and possible implications for radiotherapy. Br J Cancer. 1955;9:539.
11. Gray LH, Conger AD, Ebert M, et al. The concentration of oxygen dissolved in tissues at the time of irradiation as a factor in radiotherapy. Br J Radiol. 1953;26:638.
12. Elkind MM, Sutton H. Radiation response of mammalian cells grown in culture. I. Repair of x-ray damage in surviving Chinese hamster cells. Radiat Res. 1960;13:556–93.

13. Barendsen GW. Responses of cultured cells, tumors and normal tissues to radiations in different linear energy transfer. Curr Top Radiat Res. 1968;4:295.
14. Bergonie J, Tribondeau L. Intrepretation de quelques resultats de la radiotherapie et essai de fixation d'une technique rationnelle. Compt Rend Acad Sci. 1906;143:983–5.
15. Thames HD, Peters LJ, Withers HR, et al. Accelerated fractionation vs. hyperfractionation: rationale for several treatments per day. Int J Radiat Oncol Biol Phys. 1983;9:127.
16. Withers HR. Biologic basis for altered fractionation schemes. Cancer. 1985;55:2086.
17. Hall EJ. Radiation dose-rate: a factor of importance in radiobiology and radiotherapy. Br J Radiol. 1972;45:81.

8 Patient's Positioning and Simulation: Do's and Don'ts

Modern photon beam radiotherapy uses various beam energies and field sizes. In conventional radiotherapy, treatment is delivered using a constant source-treatment surface distance (SSD) in which the distance between the irradiation source and the patient surface is same for all beams or a constant source-axis distance (SAD or isocentric) set-up in which the isocentre of the treatment beams, i.e. the point where they intersect, is the centre of the target volume. This is done to ensure reproducibility of daily treatments. Field shapes and sizes used in therapy range from very small precise fields used in radiosurgery to standard rectangular or irregular fields to very large fields used for magna-field irradiation.

The main principle behind delivery of irradiation is to achieve the best possible coverage of the target volume by a specific dose of irradiation while minimizing exposure of the surrounding normal tissues. This prescribed dose depends on the primary or involved sites, disease stage and the histopathological type of the tumour. The dose can be delivered in daily fractions over a time period lasting usually 5–8 weeks, or in cases where the intent is not curative, a lesser dose can be delivered over a short time period to produce relief from distressing symptoms [1]. Two important principles of patient's positioning for radiotherapy are immobilization and reproducibility. This means that the patient's position should be fixed during the beam-on time and movement should be the minimum possible or even nil. Reproducibility means that the same field should treat tissue volume in the same position day after day during radiotherapy and which can be daily assessed and checked against the previous day's position. Mismatch between planned treatment volume and treated volume has been an overriding concern with modern conformal techniques like IMRT [2, 3] which allows for tight margins and dose concavities in an attempt to spare critical surrounding uninvolved tissues. Also sites, like the lung, require either increased margins for respiratory motion or compensation to negate the tissue movement. Thus techniques for image-guided delivery of irradiation to the target volume such as deep inspiration breath hold (DIBH) [4], robotic tracking and respiratory gating (RG) [5] are used to track the target volume and spare normal tissues.

A. Mukherji, *Basics of Planning and Management of Patients during Radiation Therapy*, https://doi.org/10.1007/978-981-10-6659-7_8

8.1 Positioning of the Patient

This is the essential first step at the start of the treatment planning process after a decision has been made to treat a patient by radiotherapy. Points to consider are:

- Patient comfort is the most important factor; if the patient is comfortable during the simulation process, chances of error and movement are much reduced.
- Patient's position should ensure that minimum untreated tissue is exposed to the treatment beams. This can be achieved in many ways such as in thoracic tumours positioning the arms over the head rather than by the side will prevent exposure to the beams. Similarly prone position may be considered for posterior fossa brain tumour patients.

Patient's positioning is achieved and maintained by using many types of devices or supports which can be either customized or commercially available such as head and neck supports, breast boards, pillows, as well as various types of straps (Fig. 8.1a, b). The aim of such positioning is to best expose and immobilize the treated area and ensure reproducibility. Routine treatment fields can have standard positioning and immobilization protocols, while in cases of non-routine cases or special positions, the protocol needs to be discussed by the clinician with the physicist and therapist to ensure proper planning and delivery.

8.2 Immobilization

After deciding treatment position, it is necessary to ensure that patient is treated in the same position daily during entire treatment schedule. For this it is necessary to use an immobilizing device to strap the patient comfortably in the treatment position. These devices should also be CT compatible to enable simulation in treatment position. Various immobilizing devices used are:

1. **Plaster casts**: The patient is made to lie in the position in which the irradiation would be best delivered to target volume while minimally involving surrounding tissues and wet plaster of Paris bandages are used to create a cast around the body section to be immobilized. After the pieces are completely dry, the cast is cut into two-halves to allow removal from patient, and then clamps are used to join the pieces. On the day of the treatment, the patient is immobilized by being placed in the treatment position and the two sections clamped together. As these casts may cause beam attenuation, if they are in the treatment beam, an opening is made by cutting away a piece of the cast.
2. **Thermoplastics**: These are rigid at room temperature, but when heated in water to temperatures in the range of up to 70 °C, the material softens and becomes malleable [6]. The softened sheet can be moulded around the body part to be treated and ends of the mask clamped to the supporting board. When the thermoplastic cools, it hardens and forms a rigid mask in the shape moulded (Fig. 8.2).

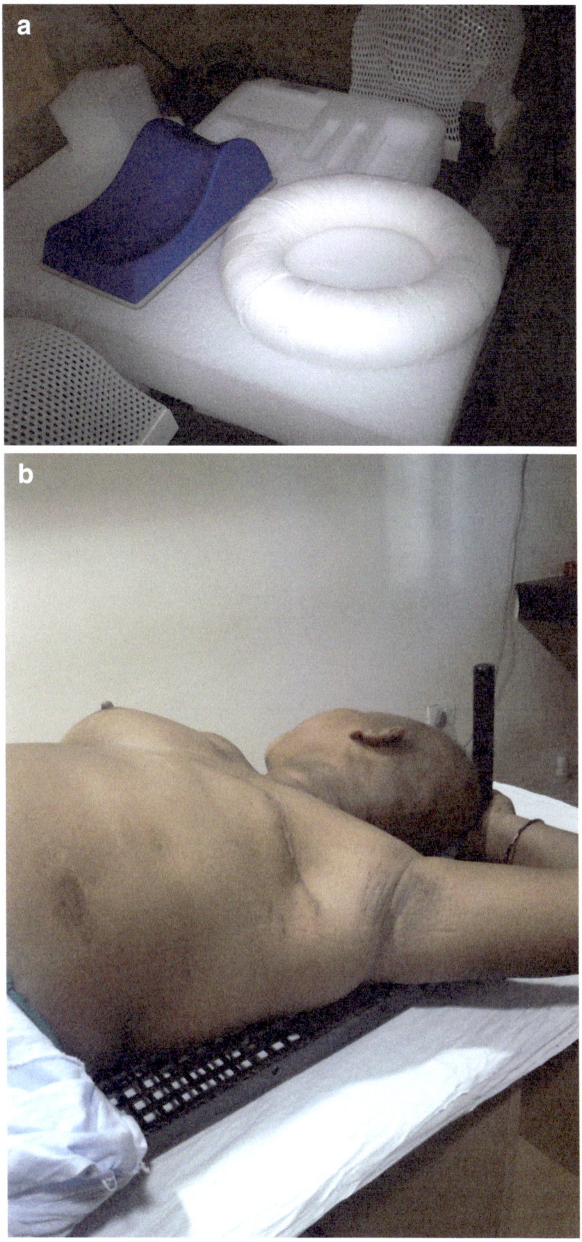

Fig. 8.1 (**a**) Headrest and head-ring. (**b**) Patient's positioned on breast board

Patients in a supine position on a headrest are immobilized with a thermoplastic mask that attaches to a carbon fibre baseplate fixed to the treatment couch. The combination of a baseplate and mask provides a system of accurate patient immobilization.

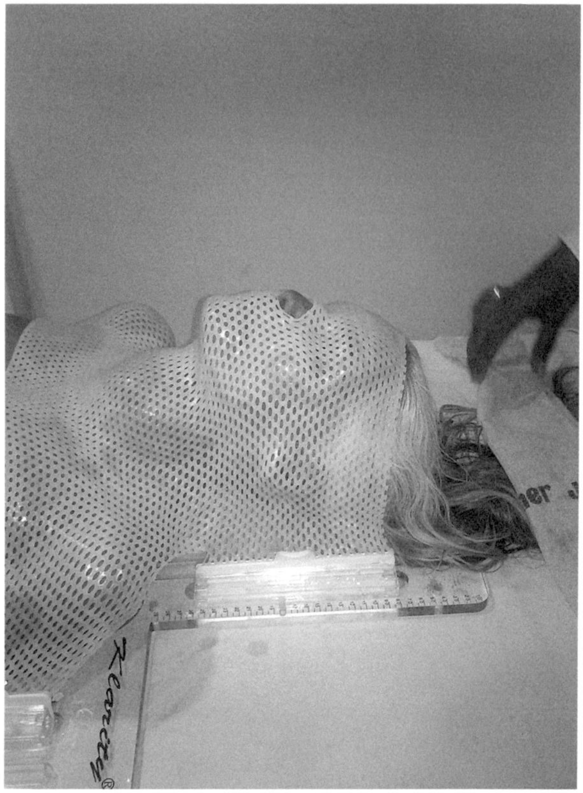

Fig. 8.2 Patient immobilized in thermoplastic mask

3. **Polyurethane foam**: In this case, a cast is made by mixing two foaming agents (trade name Alpha Cradle Mold Maker; Smithers Medical Products, Inc., North Canton, OH), in a plastic bag. The patient is positioned on the top of this bag in the treatment position. As the two chemicals mix, foam is formed that fills up the bag. The bag conforms to the patient's body shape. In about 15 min, the foam hardens, providing a body cast. These casts are lightweight and provide rigid body support.
4. **Vacuum-forming mould**: This device consists of a lightweight plastic mattress that is loosely filled with radiolucent polystyrene beads. This flexible mattress can be moulded around the patient, and then as air is removed from the bag by a vacuum pump, the beads are drawn together and form a rigid mould around the patient. As long as the vacuum is maintained, the mould retains its shape. After completion of the treatment, the bag is cleaned and recycled for the use of other patients (Fig. 8.3).

Sometimes the immobilizing device can lie in the pathway of the treatment beam and, if sufficiently thick, can cause loss of skin sparing. Thermoplastics generally are stretched thin but have been known to increase skin dose by up to 10%. Vacuum cradles are lightweight and do not cause beam attenuation. The baseplates have to be calibrated before treatment for their attenuation values.

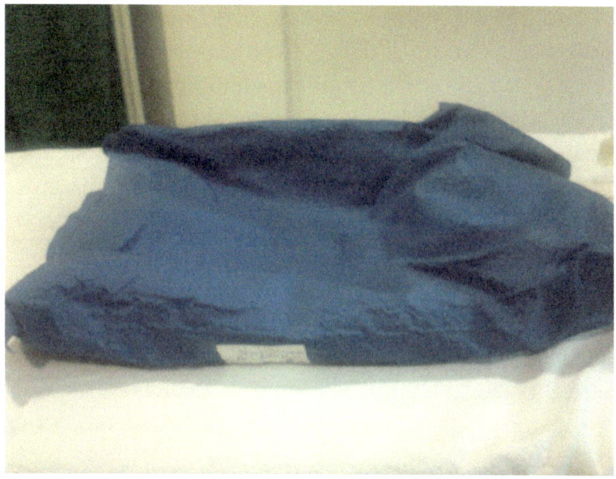

Fig. 8.3 Vacloc immobilization frame

Immobilization of Paediatric Patients: Special boards with straps that immobilize small children are commercially available as are vacuum-forming moulds in small sizes. If the use of these devices is unsuitable and the child is too young to cooperate, it may be necessary to use anaesthesia during the simulation, CT and treatment.

8.3 Simulation

Simulation is the process which mimics the actual treatment delivery and is therefore important in planning for proper delivery of radiation therapy. Thus the simulation process is helpful in tackling the following important issues:

- How is the patient positioned during treatment delivery?
- What immobilization process is required to achieve and maintain the desired treatment position?
- Determination of the direction of treatment beams.

Aims of this patient simulation process include:

- Determine the best possible patient's treatment position with respect to beam placement and target volume coverage.
- Identify the target volumes and delineate areas of normal surrounding structures.
- Determine and verify treatment field geometry.
- Generate simulation films for treatment beams for comparison with treatment port films to enable quality assurance and prevent patient's positioning errors during treatment delivery.
- Acquire patient data in the form of radiological imaging for treatment planning.

Acquiring patient's position and body structure/imaging data is important for proper simulation as this will be required for beam placement, target volume and critical structure delineation, isocentre placement, generating dosimetric data, treatment planning, plan approval and set-up verification. Therefore according to the treatment technique being planned, the requirement for this data varies, and hence there is difference in the simulation process. This process of data collection should consider the following:

- The area to be treated (patient dimensions/contoured volumes) is always required to be presented as a measurable quantity for treatment time or monitor unit (MU) calculation. The amount of data required from a patient will depend on the treatment technique and type of dosimetric calculations required in the planning process.
- Landmarks such as bony or fiducial marks are often used to match positions in the planning images with those on the patient.
- Simulation is done on a conventional simulator or a virtual simulation with CT simulator, with either wall-mounted or movable lasers to help in the patient's alignment.

Various methods used in the simulation process of radiotherapy planning include:

A) **Conventional or 2D simulation**:
   - This machine is a low-energy diagnostic X-ray unit with a couch and a tube mounted on a gantry capable of all the movements of a high-energy X-ray therapeutic unit (Fig. 8.4a).
   - This simulator is where most of the pre-planning patient data such as immobilization techniques, position, body contours, beam placement and isocentre is determined and helps save treatment machine time.
   - The simulator head is basically a diagnostic X-ray unit which has a central axis and is capable of all head and couch movements as a treatment unit diagnostic X-ray tube with the additional ability to record the images and show the field size and location to the planner through a set of movable blades called collimator. The gantry head has crosswires which help to define field shape and size.
   - The crosswires are used to define field size, while the collimator blade positions determine the image size (Fig. 8.4b). A light source in the head projects a central cross marking also called the cross hairs (which denotes the field centre) and the crosswires (denoting field boundaries) onto the patient's skin and helps in marking out the treatment field on the patient's skin/immobilization mask.
   - The field isocentre can be measured by the help of an optical distance indicator.
   - The collimator head of the simulator like the actual treatment machine also has facilities to mount various accessories or beam-modifying devices such as wedges, blocks or electron cones whenever required and in the same position as in actual treatment machine. A graticule tray with marking grids and

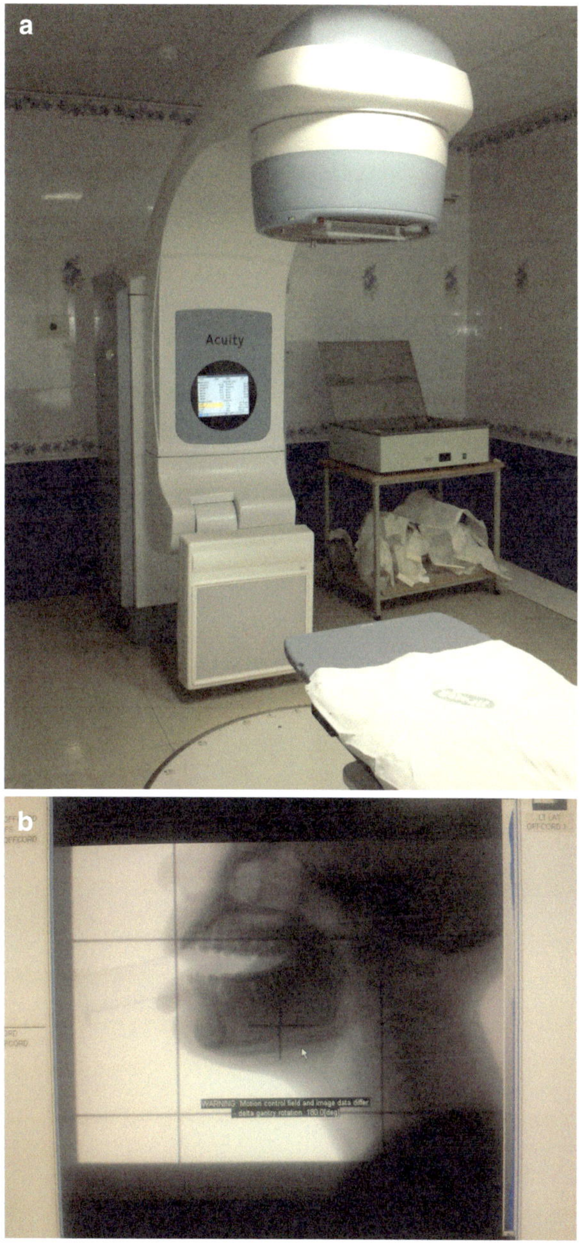

Fig. 8.4 (**a**) Conventional simulator. (**b**) Cross-wires and collimator blades seen showing field borders and imaged area

radiopaque markers is present also on the head for use as a marking scale for the field borders and field centre.

- As defined before, a simulator resembles a treatment couch in its movements but is used to project the field on to the patient surface and images for record.

Therefore this machine has an isocentre, image intensifier, fluoroscopy unit with video for real-time simulation and the means to record and print simulation images. These are in the form electronic storage or radiographic film cassettes for hard copies.

- These simulators are also equipped with collision sensors to prevent accidental collision and damage to the image intensifier during rotational movements around the couch; there is also a hand pendant to allow the operator to make changes to couch or collimator settings during patient's positioning without having to enter the console room every time for positional adjustments. Finally there is control console which allows the operator to see into the simulator room through a lead glass window without being exposed to irradiation.

B) **Alignment lasers**: Lasers are mounted on the simulator room walls in such a way (transverse, sagittal and coronal planes) so that the crossing laser beams intersect at the isocentre on the treatment surface or at depth depending on the matching technique used (Fig. 8.5). The intersections of these light beams on

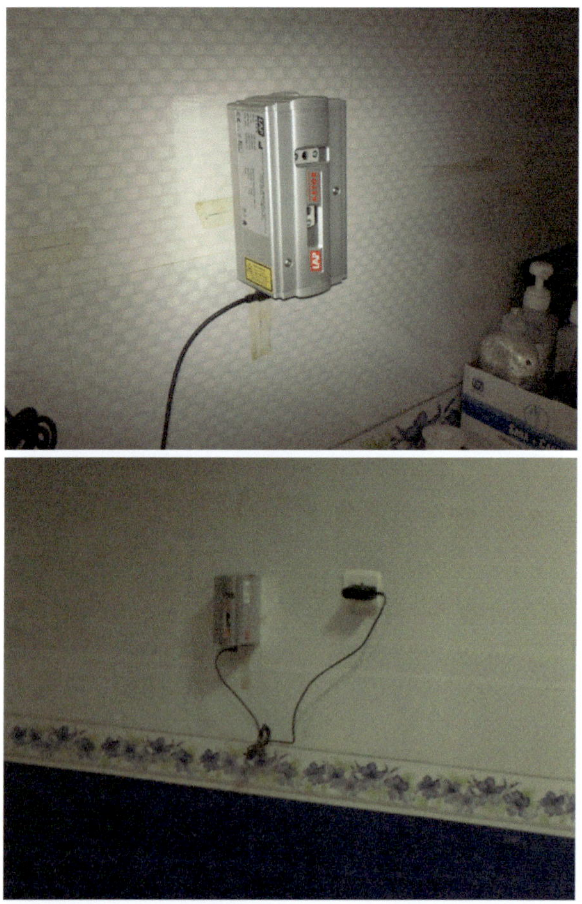

Fig. 8.5 Alignment laser

Fig. 8.6 CT simulator

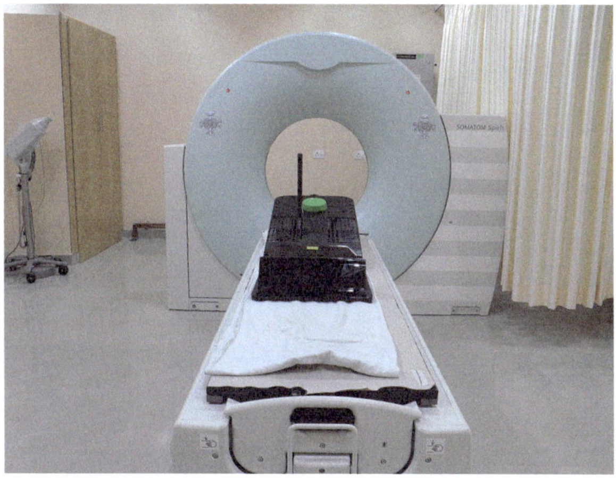

the patient's skin help in marking the triangulation points on the skin. Generally, at the end of the simulation, these triangulation points are tattooed. This laser system both in the X-ray and in the CT simulation rooms mirrors the alignment in the treatment room so that there is correct patient's positioning (with respect to x-, y- and z-axis) during treatment.

C) **CT simulation**: Most modern radiotherapy departments have shifted to CT-based simulation for most cases (Fig. 8.6). This has the advantage of better localization of tumour and delineation of normal structures by direct visualization. A spiral CT scanner when compared with a standard scanner is better able to collect CT data with the patient in the immobilized treatment position within a shorter time frame and to create coronal and sagittal reconstructions with finer details. The importance is given to immobilizing the patient for the shortest possible period in order to get as near as possible actual patient data. The requirements for a therapy CT scan are [7, 8]:
   (a) Patients for radiotherapy undergo their CT simulation on a flat-topped couch which mimics the treatment couch surface. A CT simulator differs from a conventional imaging CT scan in that its aperture is much larger so that the patient along with his/her immobilization device can pass through in the treatment position (especially for cases such as breast cancer) and with a flat couch top as well as laser markers to triangulate the anterior and lateral isocentric points marked on the skin to which radiopaque beads are taped so that these can be seen in the CT image. These marks provide the first reference points for patient's positioning and the basis for couch position error calculations (Fig. 8.7).
   (b) The treatment volume along with a sufficient margin of tissue craniocaudally is then scanned in the treatment position so that not only the full extent of the tumour is delineated but also the surrounding normal structures can be contoured in their full extent. This volume scan also helps in providing value tissue scatter margin for beam placements during treatment planning.

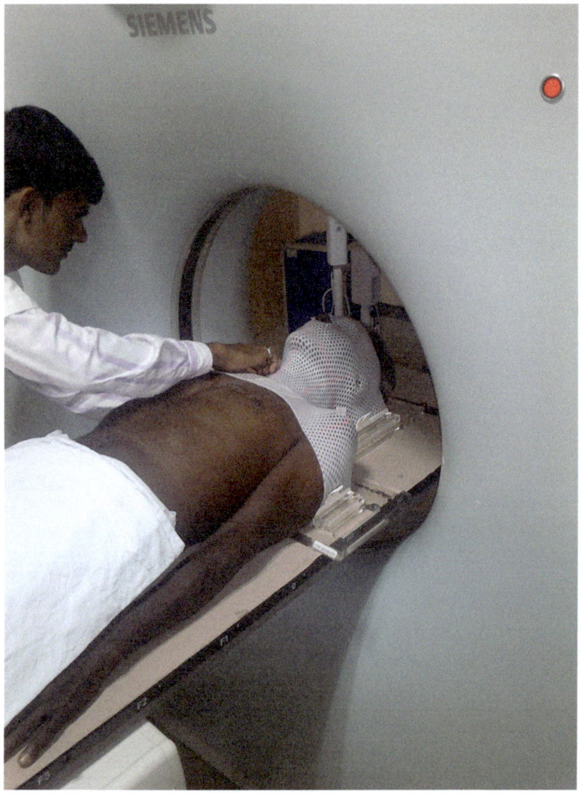

Fig. 8.7 Patient being positioned with lasers and radiopaque markers

Ideally the brain, head and neck can be simulated with 3 mm cuts, while the abdomen and pelvis for 3D-CRT can be imaged with 5 mm cuts. SBRT requires 1 mm cuts. IMRT or VMAT plans should be simulated also with 3 mm slices, while reconstruction for the inner ear and base of skull structures requires 1 mm slices.

(c) Initial anterior-posterior and lateral scout images are obtained to check for treatment position, alignment and the volume being selected. Thereafter the volume is scanned in the required slice thickness and is then reconstructed digitally to obtain a full-volume image. The position of the radiopaque markers is checked before transferring the scanned image to the planning system.

(d) Specific areas require specific imaging protocols. For example, simulation for the prostate requires multiparametric MRI including T2-weighted and diffusion-weighted images; thoracic malignancies and breast planning require shallow breathing to simulate near real patient data, while pelvic malignancies may need specific bladder filling protocols. Respiratory motion can be accounted for by techniques such as active breathing control, deep inspirational breath-hold and respiratory gating.

D) **Virtual simulation**: This process was described by Sherouse and colleagues [9–11] and is a computer-based simulation process that allows users to carry out simulation at a computer workstation instead of a real simulator. This method has the advantage that target volumes and anatomic structures, outlined on the CT scans, are used to decide about the position of the isocentre, field sizes, beam directions and shielding blocks. CT scans provide better visualization of the disease and normal tissues, resulting in better target coverage and normal tissue shielding. The virtual simulator system has the ability to display and execute all the functions of a conventional radiotherapy machine.

Process:

- As in CT simulation, image data is obtained by a CT scan in treatment position which is transferred to the TPS after which the target volume and organs at risk are contoured. From this data, a three-dimensional model is created which shows the relative positions of the various structures and target volume. To this model, the physicist puts in the required parameters such as gantry angle, field size, collimation, MLCs as well as beam modifications required such as wedges, etc.
- The system creates a beam's eye view (BEV) of the field to check for the field projection on to the patient as well as confirm that no body tissue or treatment couch or immobilization device attachment is coming into the field (Fig. 8.8); after checking this BEV, the fields are confirmed and digitally reconstructed radiographs (DRRs) produced for each treatment field [12]. These DRRs are computer-designed radiographic images which use beam attenuation data from the CT scan. The 3D model of the patient scanned image is used then to generate various planning data such as beam angles, various dose parameters and templates for beam modification. The treatment ports are verified finally by matching the DRRs with the localization ports.

E) **Computed tomographic simulator**: The CT simulator is a whole-body CT scanner designed for radiation therapy simulation [13, 14] and consists of three

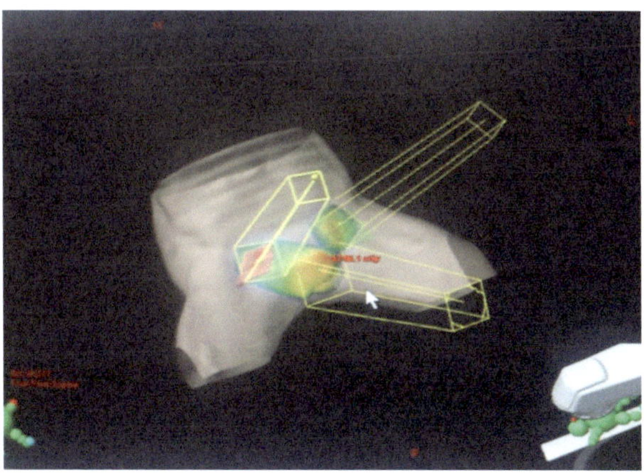

Fig. 8.8 Beam's eye view generated of tumour volume and normal structures

basic components: (1) CT scanner, (2) an interactive workstation capable of virtual simulation and (3) a mechanism for marking the beam portals on the patient's skin. The patient is scanned in the treatment position, and the CT images are transferred directly to virtual simulation workstation. The target volume and the relevant critical structures are then drawn or contoured on the CT scans, the beam geometries are optimized, and DRRs are produced for the block definition and treatment verification. Usually 65–70 cm bore size of the CT gantry can accommodate most patients and positions except extremely large patients, and some patients for breast cancer treatment, for which a larger opening of 85 cm bore is used.

The advantages of CT simulator over a conventional simulator are (1) better visualization of the treatment volumes for the portal design. (2) Since the original data set is the same, the various contoured organs and target volumes can be superimposed on the DRRs and used to create the fields both for the initial treatment and the boost volume; (3) conventional simulators have physical limitations like as many noncoplanar angles cannot be imaged. (4) DRRs for beam can be generated; their magnification adjusted and cross hairs as well as grid points projected for direct comparison with portal images.

8.4 Interventional or Image-Guided Simulation Methods

In 3D-CRT and IMRT, risk of marginal failure increases with increasing target volume conformity and normal structure sparing. There are two main reasons for occurrence of errors in the delivery of high-precision radiotherapy techniques: (1) biological and radiological uncertainty (positional or imaging) in accurately defining the clinical target volume (CTV) and (2) change in treatment geometry during treatment (due to change in body contour or target volume).

Imaging uncertainty could be because of improper or inadequate imaging or even biological factors such as infiltrative tumour or metallic artefact. In such cases more than one imaging modality such as PET + CT or MRI + CT or PET + MRI may be used and fused with simulated patient CT data [15]. Variations in treatment or positional geometry can be due to normal physiological processes such as respiration or peristalsis or patient's positioning errors on the couch. This may be accounted for by daily imaging and matching portal images and DRRs (for positional errors) or *adapting* the PTV for change in body contour during treatment or changes due to respiration or peristalsis such as by methods like active breathing control (ABC), DIBH and respiratory gating (RG). This technique in which treatment delivery takes into account these errors and changes are made accordingly is called image-guided radiotherapy (IGRT).

Active Breathing Control (ABC): This method basically aims to treat a patient during a specified part of the respiratory cycle. The theory is that there is a change in the position of the PTV during inspiration and expiration and by fixing a patient's position during the beam-on time in a certain part of the respiratory cycle, the treatment to a very limited volume could be accurately delivered. The benefit of this method is a reduced PTV as an ITV need not be created. In this method, the patient's nose is clamped, and the patient breathes through a mouthpiece with the chest strapped to a stethograph. The breathing cycle is analysed from the stethograph on the computer (based on tidal volume), and at the predetermined phase of the cycle, the clamp is tightened to "freeze" the patients breathing in that phase of the cycle during which radiation is delivered. This process takes only a few seconds, but the patient needs to be trained [16–18].

Deep Inspiration Breath-Hold Technique: In this technique, the patient is trained to maintain a state of deep inspiration through the process of treatment planning and delivery [4, 19, 20]. In DIBH, the patient is brought to approximately 100% vital capacity by slow deep breathing, followed by holding his/her breath and maintaining the same situation for a prescribed period. In this phase itself at each sitting, the various simulation and planning steps such as imaging, set-up verification and treatment are done. As in ABC, in this technique also the patient's nose is closed with a clip, and the patient breathes through a mouthpiece connected to a spirometer which is connected to a computer. Again as in ABC, the computer displays the breathing cycle, and the patient is trained to first breathe slow and then deep inspiration and expiration. The sequence usually followed for this technique is given below.

Breathing Sequence for DIBH Manoeuvre

Quiet tidal breathing → slow deep inspiration → slow deep expiration → slow deep inspiration to the maximum limit → breath hold

This technique has two advantages. Using breath-hold technique, tumour motion due to breathing is minimized or negated. Also breath hold after deep inspiration helps expand the lung to its maximum volume. This helps keep most normal lung tissue out of the target volume and hence the treatment beam, while breath hold significantly negates tumour motion caused by breathing. Hanley et al. [4] in their study reported that this technique of DIBH helped decrease the V25 (*volume of the lung receiving 25 Gy or more* [4]) of the involved lung by around 30% and was easily reproducible.

Respiratory Gating: These systems (such as the Real-time Position Management [RPM]® Respiratory Gating; Varian Medical Systems, Palo Alto, CA) allow for the acquisition of either fluoroscopic images or CT images which are synchronized with specific breathing phases such as inspiration or expiration as well as allow gated treatment (i.e. beam is delivered only during that specific breathing phase during which simulation was done) on a linear accelerator [5, 21]. This technique utilizes a video camera (charged-coupled device type) to which an infrared (IR) marker is attached. This is visualized by an IR camera mounted in the treatment room which uses the vertical motion of this IR marker on the patient's surface to trace the magnitude of movement in the breathing cycle. Two such markers are used, one on the chest and one on the abdomen; the upper one tracks the respiratory motion; the lower marker calibrates the system. There is however no single fixed range of distance by which the markers move, and in fact for the first few breathing cycles at the start of a session, the system simply tracks the movement to determine the minimum and maximum vertical position of the upper marker.

Gating During Simulation: Synchronization of fluoroscopy with the breathing is achieved. Gating threshold for the breathing waveform is selected, and those fluoroscopic images which have occurred during the selected breathing phase (called "gate interval") are reviewed, and from these images, the anatomic motion is evaluated, and the best possible or optimum gating thresholds are selected.

Gating in CT Scan: As in ABC, in this method, CT images are taken only during the selected respiratory phase identified by the IR or fluoroscopic marker. Axial images are selected, and the synchronized images are used for planning. A trace of the breathing cycle is also recorded for use during treatment delivery for calculation of beam interruption time.

Gating During Treatment: This means that the beam is "on" only during a specific phase of the respiratory cycle which is defined by a tidal volume threshold. This process differs from ABC in that the threshold volume is identified by direct imaging as explained in the preceding paragraphs. Verbal breathing instructions are also conveyed to the patient on couch.

4D-CT Scan: There is significant intra-fraction motion because of respiratory and cardiac activity especially for sites like the lung, liver, pancreas, prostate and breast. Patient motion during CT imaging can cause artefacts [22]. Generally, in these cases treatment planning CT scan is obtained under quiet breathing. But in modern helical scanners where the scanning speed can match with the tumour motion speed [23], the captured tumour position and shape can be heavily distorted because of breathing movements. Some of these problems can be reduced with the interventional techniques, such as active breathing control, DIBH, and RPM gating, so that the images are acquired at a particular breathing phase.

Four-dimensional (4D) or tumour tracking imaging is defined as acquisition of a sequence of CT image sets over consecutive segments of a breathing cycle [22]. Two devices commonly used for sensing breathing motion are air bellows or RPM respiratory gating. The air bellow system is an elastic belt worn around the abdomen that expands and contracts with respiratory motion, and it contains a pressure transducer which converts pressure changes (increasing or decreasing volume) to an electrical signal [24]. This electrical signal representing respiratory motion is displayed at the CT console, and it is interfaced with the CT scanner. CT images are obtained in synchrony with the respiratory signal. After the 4D scan is complete, the CT images are sorted according to breathing phase. Irregular breathing, particularly variations in amplitude between breathing cycles, will cause artefacts in 4D-CT images. On these 4D images, the GTV and CTV are outlined on all phases, which are then projected on the planning CT to determine internal target volume ITV [25].

8.5 Algorithm of the Simulation Process (2D and CT Simulation)

8.5.1 General Points

- The clinician must form an idea of the target volume required before the simulation process based on clinical and diagnostic mapping and staging of the disease. Simulation is not the process of identifying the target volume but a strategy for treating accurately and with near perfect reproducibility the patient on a daily basis in the most comfortable manner and which is the last complicated. It also includes decisions on the use of immobilization devices, beam-modifying devices as well as machine accessories, field sizes and shapes and beam energy.
- The field centre and the laser alignment points are tattooed or marked on the patient's skin or immobilization device to ensure correct positional representation daily during treatment.
- As explained in the simulation process earlier in the chapter, the patient is then placed in the treatment position in the X-ray or CT simulator couch, and images are taken of the fields in the treatment position. CT data in case of conformal plans are passed on to the planning system in which contouring of target volumes and normal organs is done.
- Treatment plans are designed based on these data and the DRRs, and dosimetric data is generated on basis of which plan evaluation is done.
- **Use of Contrast Material for Simulation**: Radiopaque compounds with high atomic numbers, such as iodine and barium, and low-density materials, such as air, are used to enhance radiographic contrast. These help in identifying and isolating anatomic structures and diseased tissue in radiographs and CT scans. Depending on the need, contrast material is used either during simulation or during the CT scan or both. If a contrast material with a high atomic number is present in high concentration during CT, it can give rise to artefacts that interfere with the localization of disease and normal organs. When CT scan follows a simulation, the contrast material administered during simulation may be present during the CT scan, causing artefacts. Before the administration of a contrast material, the pros and cons of its use should be considered.

Localization of the Disease in 2D Simulation: After patient is placed in the treatment position, aligned and immobilized, a tentative isocentre and the treatment field sizes are decided based on clinical information about primary and stage.

- Radiopaque catheters, wires or small metal ball bearings are taped to the patient's skin to identify anatomic landmark, diseased tissue or scar on the skin.
- A pair of orthogonal radiographs is taken, or the patient is imaged fluoroscopically. These images are reviewed for coverage of the disease based on stage and likely draining lymphatics.
- For daily reproducibility, the isocentre and maybe field border corners are tattooed on the patient's skin.

- Bony anatomic landmarks are given more importance than skin marks, especially flabby skin [26].
- The relevant beam parameters, such as gantry angles and field sizes, are recorded in the patient's chart along with the set-up depth. Photographs of the patient's set-up, obtained during the simulation, are helpful in day-to-day positioning of the patient for radiotherapy.

8.5.2 3D/CT Simulation

- CT data set in the treatment position is obtained, and a virtual simulation is carried out. DRRs are created from the CT data.
- **Patient Immobilization**: This is very essential in precision radiotherapy. The devices such as the thermoplastic mould, Alpha Cradles and vacuum-forming moulds are used. The devices should be free of large metallic pieces, which cause artefacts on CT images.
- **Patient Alignment**: After patient is placed in the treatment position on the CT couch, the anteroposterior (AP) and lateral scout (pilot) images are taken to ensure proper patient alignment. Then using alignment lasers, radiopaque markers are placed at junction of lasers for reference position for set-up verification.
- **Surface Markers**: Some areas of special interest (scars, previously treated area, skin nodules) can be highlighted with solder wire or ball bearings.
- **CT Scanning**: Superior and inferior extents are decided; if the beams are expected from noncoplanar direction, the entrance port of the beam should be within the scanned region. Smaller CT spacing and thickness are desirable for better-quality DRRs. Usually 3-mm spacing and thickness are adequate. However, if it is a large field, 5-mm spacing and thickness may be used. In some cases a combination of different spacings 3 mm or even 1 mm in the region of high definition and 5 mm in the surrounding area can be done.
- **Virtual Simulation and Isocentre Localization**: After the CT scan, virtual simulation software is used for localization. The physician outlines the gross tumour volume (GTV), clinical target volume (CTV) and planning target volume (PTV) on the CT images, and the CT simulation software automatically positions the isocentre in the middle of the target volume.
- **Isocentre Marking**: Once the isocentre location is determined, a printout is taken highlighting couch shift required to reach the isocentre from the reference set-up position. The patient couch is moved longitudinally, and the sagittal laser is shifted laterally to the location specified in the printout. Triangulation points are tattooed on the skin.

References

1. Hall EJ. Radiobiology for the radiologist. 4th ed. Philadelphia: JB Lippincott; 1994. p. 211.
2. Leibel SA, Kutcher GJ, Harrison LB, et al. Improved dose distribution for three-dimensional conformal boost treatments in carcinoma of the nasopharynx. Int J Radiat Oncol Biol Phys. 1991;20:823.

3. de Arruda FF, Puri DR, Zhung J, et al. Intensity-modulated radiation therapy for the treatment of oropharyngeal carcinoma: the Memorial Sloan-Kettering Cancer Center experience. Int J Radiat Oncol Biol Phys. 2006;64:363.
4. Hanley J, Debois MM, Mah D, et al. Deep inspiration breath-hold technique for lung tumors: the potential value of target immobilization and reduced lung density in dose escalation. Int J Radiat Oncol Biol Phys. 1999;45:603.
5. Mageras GS, Yorke E, Rosenzweig K, et al. Fluoroscopic evaluation of diaphragmatic motion reduction with respiratory gated radiotherapy system. J Appl Clin Med Phys. 2001;2:191–200.
6. Gerber RL, Marks JE, Purdy JA. The use of thermal plastics for immobilization of patients during radiotherapy. Int J Radiat Oncol Biol Phys. 1982;8:1461.
7. Goitein M. Computed tomography in planning radiation therapy. Int J Radiat Oncol Biol Phys. 1979;5:445.
8. Lichter AS, Fraass BA, van de Geijn J, et al. An overview of clinical requirements and clinical utility of computed tomography based radiotherapy treatment planning. In: Ling CC, Rogers CC, Morton RJ, editors. Computed tomography in radiation therapy. New York: Raven Press; 1983. p. 1.
9. Sherouse GW, Mosher CE, Novins K, et al. Virtual simulation: concept and implementation. In: Bruinvis IAD, van der Giessen PH, van Kleffens HJ, Wittkamper FW, editors. The use of computers in radiation therapy. Amsterdam: Elsevier Science; 1987. p. 433.
10. Sherouse GW, Bourland JD, Reynolds K, et al. Virtual simulation in the clinical setting: some practical considerations. Int J Radiat Oncol Biol Phys. 1990;19:1059.
11. Sherouse GW, Chaney EL. The portable virtual simulator. Int J Radiat Oncol Biol Phys. 1991;21:475.
12. Sherouse GW, Novins K, Chaney EL. Computation of digitally reconstructed radiographs for use in radiotherapy treatment design. Int J Radiat Oncol Biol Phys. 1990;18:651.
13. Goitein M. CT simulation: an overview. In: Jani SK, editor. CT simulation for radiotherapy. Madison: Medical Physics; 1993. p. 161.
14. Wen BC, Pennington E, Jani S. Clinical applications of CT simulators in unconventional radiation therapy techniques. In: Jani SK, editor. CT simulation for radiotherapy. Madison: Medical Physics; 1993. p. 129.
15. Chen GTY, Pelizzari CA, Hamilton RJ, et al. Image processing and integration in oncologic imaging. In: Bragg DG, Rubin P, Hricak H, editors. Oncologic imaging. 2nd ed. Philadelphia: W.B. Saunders Company; 2002. p. 92.
16. Yan D, Wong J, Vicini F, et al. Adaptive modification of treatment planning to minimize the deleterious effect of treatment setup error. Int J Radiat Oncol Biol Phys. 1997;38:197.
17. Wong JW, Sharpe MB, Jaffray DA, et al. The use of active breathing control (ABC) to reduce margin for breathing motion. Int J Radiat Oncol Biol Phys. 1999;44:911.
18. Wong JW, Yan D, Jaffray DA, et al. Interventional strategies to optimize the delivery of radiation therapy. In: Bragg DG, Rubin P, Hricak H, editors. Oncologic imaging. 2nd ed. Philadelphia: W.B. Saunders Company; 2002. p. 116.
19. Rosenzweig KE, Hanley J, Mah D, et al. The deep inspiration breath-hold technique in treatment of inoperable non-small cell lung cancer. Int J Radiat Oncol Biol Phys. 2000;48:81.
20. Mah D, Hanley J, Rosenzweig KE, et al. Technical aspects of deep inspiration breath-hold technique in the treatment of thoracic cancer. Int J Radiat Oncol Biol Phys. 2000;48:1175.
21. Ford EC, Mageras GS, Yorke E, et al. Evaluation of respiratory movement during gated radiotherapy using film and electronic portal imaging. Int J Radiat Oncol Biol Phys. 2002;52:522.
22. Keall P. 4-dimensioanl computed tomography imaging and treatment planning. Semin Radiat Oncol. 2004;14:81.
23. Jiang SB. Radiotherapy of mobile tumors. Semin Radiat Oncol. 2006;16:239.
24. Kahler PJ, Subramanian P, Yanof JH. Respiratory correlated multislice CT for radiation therapy planning: imaging and visualization methods. Medicamundi. 2005;49:34.
25. International Commission on radiation units and measurements: prescribing, recording, and reporting photon beam therapy. Supplement to report 50. Report 62Washington, DC, ICRU, 1999.
26. Khan FM. The physics of radiation therapy. 2nd ed. Baltimore: Williams & Wilkins; 1994. p. 307.

9 Planning a Patient, Deciding on the Volumes and Fields and Plan Verification

After having completed the simulation process as described in the previous chapter, the radiation oncologist must then decide on the treatment volumes, beam positions and beam parameters and along with the physicists create treatment plans and verify if the plans produced cover the targeted volume. In cases where the dose needs to be prescribed only along the central axis of the beam (e.g. treatments with a direct field, or parallel and opposed fields, and a flat beam incidence), only the SSD is required, and simple calculations for beam-on time for cobalt machines or MUs for linear accelerators are all that is required. Simple algorithms, such as Clarkson's method, are used to calculate dose distributions when standard or even customized blocks are used to shape irregular fields. Similarly methods are also available to calculate in these irregular fields, the dose to off-axis points if their coordinates and SSD are measured. In these situations, the patient shape or contour is not required.

Simple 2D treatment planning entails projecting opposed beams onto the skin overlying the target volume and checking for the coverage in an X-ray simulator. Whenever more complex plans are required such as in three- or four-field or for curved surfaces even in 2D radiation therapy planning, a single skin contour or CT scan cut taken at the point where the central axis of the beam is supposed to enter is usually enough, and then a surface contour can be prepared by using lead wire or a plaster cast.

However in the case of advanced radiation therapy techniques such as 3DCRT or IMRT/IGRT, much more complex, elaborate and precise data in the form of patient contour, body shape, body organs, electron densities, couch position, beam entry and exit volumes and beam geometry as well as tissue heterogeneities and attenuation values is required. CT scans contain all the information required for complex treatment planning and are the backbone of CT simulation and treatment planning. This chapter will deal mainly with beam definition in 2D radiotherapy and set-up verification. Conformal radiotherapy planning and verification will be dealt with separately in the next chapter.

A. Mukherji, *Basics of Planning and Management of Patients during Radiation Therapy*, https://doi.org/10.1007/978-981-10-6659-7_9

9.1 Deciding on the Treatment Volumes and Fields

Correct definition of the target volume is the necessary prerequisite for any meaningful radiotherapy treatment planning and for accurate dose reporting. Over the last three decades, radiation oncologists have moved gradually from anatomical landmark and region-based radiotherapy planning to a better image-guided treatment planning with emphasis on maximally sparing of surrounding critical normal structures. Initial guidelines towards formulation of treatment volumes were postulated by the ICRU Report number 29 [1] in the 1970s which divided volumes as treated volumes and irradiated volumes based on regular 2D square or rectangular treatment portals (Fig. 9.1).

With the advent of CT scanning and subsequently CT simulations, new guidelines for treatment volumes have been postulated which remain the bedrock for RT planning to this day. These were the ICRU Reports 50 and 62 [2, 3] which have described the various target and critical structure volumes used in modern treatment planning. These have been also revised and added to from time to time taking into account the advent of new technologies (ICRU-71, 83) and help in serving as a framework for the compilation and comparison of dosimetric and patient outcomes data. Some of the volumes described in the ICRU reports include the gross tumour volume, clinical target volume, internal target volume and planning target volume and have been defined below (Fig. 9.2).

Gross Tumour Volume (GTV): It is defined as "*the gross palpable or visible/ demonstrable extent and location of malignant growth*" (**ICRU 50,** Fig. 9.2) [2]. This volume commonly called the GTV is usually the disease volume which is clearly definable or which can be recorded and measured using imaging modalities (CT, MRI, ultrasound, etc.), diagnostic modalities (pathology and histological reports, etc.) and clinical examination.

Clinical Target Volume (CTV): It is defined as "*the tissue volume that contains a demonstrable GTV and/or sub-clinical microscopic malignant disease, which has to be eliminated. This volume thus has to be treated adequately in order to achieve*

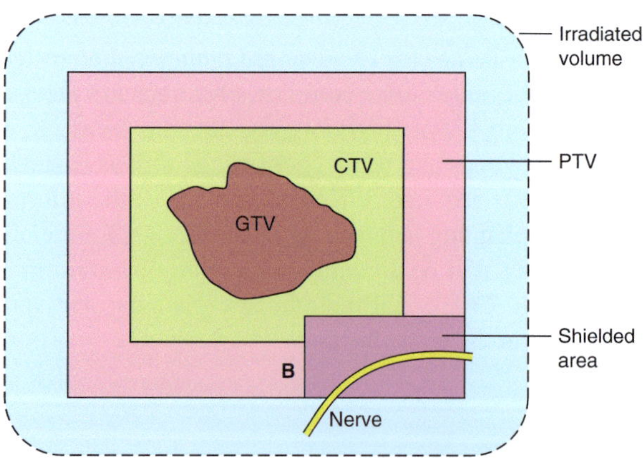

Fig. 9.1 RT volumes as per ICRU-29

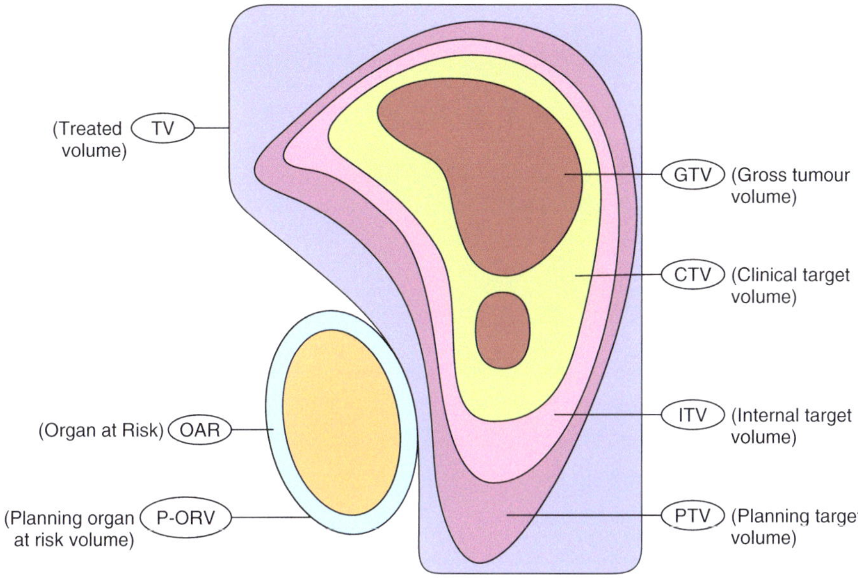

Fig. 9.2 ICRU 50 Volumes

the aim of therapy, cure or palliation" (**ICRU 50,** Fig. 9.2) [2]. Basically this refers to that volume of the primary site tissue hosting the tumour which is not overtly involved by the tumour but is a surrounding area of normal-looking tissue which may contain microscopic disease. It also includes other areas considered to be at risk such as draining lymph nodes and lymphatics likely to harbour micro-metastases and therefore which would require a significant treatment dose. Therefore the CTV is an anatomical-clinical volume which is decided by the radiation oncologist who must therefore practise utmost care in deciding how much margin to take. Many guidelines such as RTOG guidelines are available to help in determining which areas or margins should be included in the CTV especially when practising high precision radiation therapy. In 2D radiotherapy practice, the CTV is usually a fixed margin around the GTV (e.g. CTV = GTV + 1–2 cm margin), though in a few cases it may be the same as GTV (e.g. boost to the prostate gland only). While demarcating the CTV, it is important to remember the type of tumour being treated, its propensity for local spread or lymphatic involvement and whether the tumour is confined to the involved tissue planes. Blind margins should not be added as CTVs, but cognizance of tissue barriers if they have not been breached should be kept in mind. Also in advanced technology protocols, several different noncontiguous CTVs can receive different total doses (e.g. HR-CTV or IR-CTV in SIB-IMRT in head and neck cancers).

Internal Target Volume (ITV): *This is defined as the volume containing the CTV plus an internal margin* (**ICRU 62,** Fig. 9.3) [3]. An internal margin is an added margin taken around a CTV especially for tissues where there is significant organ motion (as in the lung, GIT, bladder and prostate) or in techniques

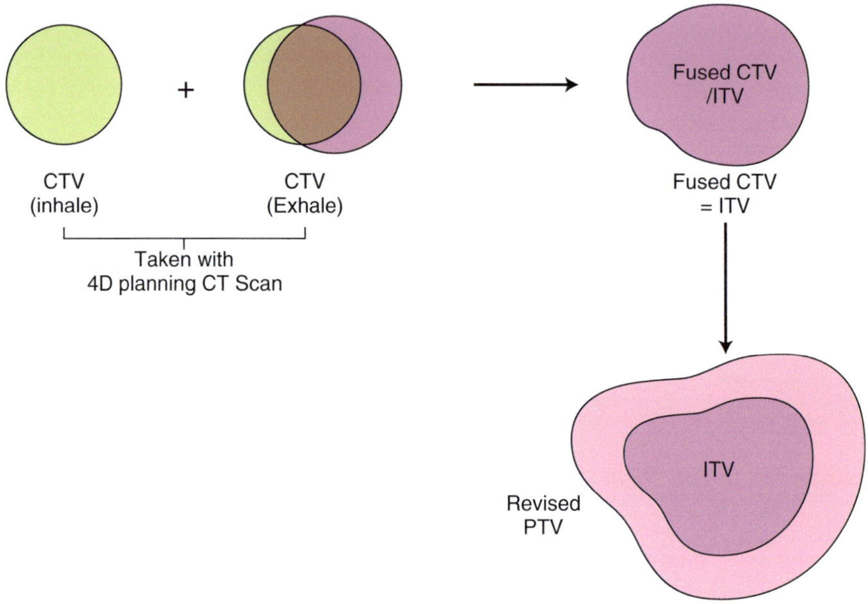

Fig. 9.3 Account for target motion; ITV & PTV

(such as IGRT) where tight margins could otherwise cause geographic miss and basically take into account variations in the size and position of CTV. As explained in Chap. 2, the ITV is calculated by simulating the patient in both phases (inspiration/expiration or bladder full/empty) and drawing the GTV accordingly to which the CTV is added. Both phase CTVs are then added together (**ICRU 62,** Fig. 9.3) [3].

Planning Target Volume (PTV): *The planning target volume is a geometrical concept, and it is defined to select appropriate beam arrangements, taking into consideration the net effect of all possible geometrical variations, in order to ensure that the prescribed dose is actually absorbed in the CTV* (**ICRU 50,** Fig. 9.2) [2]. Thus a PTV takes into account the CTV, internal target margin and further margins to account for errors or uncertainties in patient set-up, machine changes or errors and daily variations during treatment. Therefore in conventional radiotherapy, a PTV can be a CTV plus a fixed or variable margin, but in newer techniques with computerized treatment planning, the PTV can include more than one CTV (e.g. HR-CTV + LR-CTV or CTV-nodes + CTV primary). The tightness or compactness of the PTV depends on the accuracy of immobilization devices and set-up tools such as lasers. However it must be remembered that a PTV does NOT include a margin for dosimetric characteristics of a radiation beam (such as penumbral areas and build-up region), and therefore further margins may have to be incorporated during designing shields (using beam's eye view projection) as well as in treatment planning (in which the collimator opening is increased further to avoid loss of scatter component in the outer edges of the beam).

Organ at Risk (OAR): *Organ at risk is defined as an organ whose sensitivity to radiation is such that the dose received from a treatment plan may be significant compared to its tolerance, possibly requiring a change in the beam arrangement or a change in the dose* (**ICRU 50,** Fig. 9.2) [2]. Different organs have different levels of tolerance to irradiation with some organs arranged in serial-like pattern of their functional subunits, while others have a parallel distribution (covered in Chap. 21, Section D). Serial organs such as the spinal cord, brainstem, etc. have tolerance limits beyond which area maximal doses (D_{max}) could cause serious late effects, while for parallel structures the effects are dose-volume based, and D_{mean} is a better indicator of organ tolerance. Hence for structures with serial FSUs or low tolerance (e.g. eye lens during nasopharyngeal treatments), specific attention should be paid. Also while contouring it is important to contour a complete organ and not just that portion only which is within the treatment volume so as to avoid false dose-volume evaluations especially for organs whose tolerance depends on the fractionation scheme.

Treated Volume (TV): *The TV is the volume of tissue enclosed within a specific isodose envelope, with the absorbed dose specified by the radiation oncology team as appropriate to achieve tumour eradication or palliation, within the bounds of acceptable complications* (**ICRU 50,** Fig. 9.2) [2]. When prescribing a dose, the volume usually selected is the PTV, and the prescription is made for a certain volume of the PTV to be covered by a certain percentage of the dose (e.g. 95–98% dose to cover 95–98% of the PTV). However this does not mean that tissues outside the PTV will not receive any dose. In fact external beam irradiation travels through a significant amount of normal tissue before encompassing the target volume. This area outside the PTV therefore which is covered by the prescribed isodose is the treated volume, and the shape, size and position of this volume with respect to the PTV are important for the assessment of either local recurrences or late effects.

Irradiated Volume: *It is defined as the volume that receives a dose considered significant in relation to normal tissue tolerance* (e.g. 30–80% isodose surface) (**ICRU 50 & 62**) [2, 3]. This is a substantially larger volume than the treated volume and differs from it in the isodose coverage, i.e. the TV is the volume beyond the PTV covered by the prescribed isodose (usually 90–95%), and the IV is the volume of tissue receiving significant dose of irradiation (typically areas receiving more than 30–40% isodose).

Hot Spot: *It is defined as a volume >15 mm in minimum diameter outside the PTV that receives more than 105% of the specified PTV dose* (**ICRU 50 & 62**) [2, 3].

Internal Margin (IM): It is situated around CTV or organ at risk and accounts for the uncertainties in contouring of the organs and target volume and uncertainties caused by physiologic movements and/or changes of shape and size of the CTV and RV in relation to reference points (**ICRU 62**) [3].

Internal Risk Volume (IRV): *It is defined by the outer boundary of the volume of organ at risk (IRV)* (**ICRU 50 & 62**) [2, 3].

Planning Organ at Risk Volume (PORV): Following the process of contouring of OARs and target volumes, dose constraints are given for both the target volumes and the OARs. However it must be remembered that during planning there will not be sharp changes in doses between the OARs and the PTV especially if the OAR is close to the PTV. In fact, there will be a dose gradient between the OAR and the PTV which might encroach upon either volume depending upon the priority given and hence causing either overdose to OAR or underdose to PTV. Also uncertainties in the position of the OAR because of anatomical accuracy or physiological movements add to risk of wrong treatment. Therefore an added margin (usually 3–5 mm) is given around the OAR to allow for a dose gradient to occur and to cater for any variation in position of the OAR. This is especially important in serial organs.

Remaining Volume at Risk (RVR): *The RVR is the imaged volume within the patient, excluding any delineated OAR and the CTV(s), and is defined by the difference between the volume enclosed by the external contour of the patient and that of the CTVs and OARs on the slices that have been imaged* (**ICRU 62**) [3]. It is important to contour the RVR especially in techniques using homogeneous dose distribution such as IMRT because in trying to meet set constraints for the OARs, the planning system could design beams through areas which have not been contoured and cause high doses in these areas leading to severe late effects. Also drawing an RVR helps in estimating the absorbed dose in this volume and predicting the risk of carcinogenesis especially for patients expected to have a longer life span.

9.1.1 Beam Definition

Manual Beam Definition: In this technique, the physician draws the outlines for the blocks or multileaf collimators (MLCs) on the radiographs obtained during the simulation or DRRs during the CT simulation. Using the machine data table, beam-on times are calculated based on the field size, isocentre depth, extent of blocking and prescribed dose. Examples include treatment with parallel-opposed beams, four-field "box" technique and en face electron treatment.

Treatment Planning from Contours: Slice by slice location of both target volumes and surrounding normal structures is drawn by the physician on the simulation radiographs or on the treatment planning CT images. If the target volume is close to critical organs and the intent is to limit the dose to these organs during radiation therapy, it may be necessary to design suitable beam positions and arrange for customized blocks or field shaping by MLCs.

In 2D-based planning, a digitizer is then used to enter the contours into the treatment planning system. Small hard copies of the CT images can be enlarged to true size using an enlarger. The outer contour, internal organs and target volume can be projected and traced onto a paper and then digitized into the treatment planning computer. Most treatment planning systems today allow planning with the CT images.

The beams' parameters are selected by the planner and include the type of radiation, its energy, field sizes and shapes, gantry angles, collimator angles, couch angles, wedges and thickness of the bolus materials. If the planned isocentre is different from the original isocentre or if the treatment plan uses beams for which radiographs were not obtained during the first simulation, then it may be necessary to check the plan or resimulate the patient. However, if the patient was CT simulated, then it is not necessary for the patient to repeat the scan as virtual simulation can be done using the original CT data.

During the plan check, the treatment isocentre is localized according to the planner's instructions, and check films for all of the treatment beams are taken. Sometimes it is impossible to radiograph certain beams like a vertex field, and hence in such cases, a pair of orthogonal X-rays can be used for verification. The block outlines are drawn on the radiographs, and field-shaping blocks are constructed from the aperture outlines. Present available treatment machines are equipped with MLCs in which the beam apertures are digitized on a workstation based on which MLC patterns are generated by a computer programme which are transferred to the treatment machine.

Image Registration: The process of image registration (also called fusion) is based on the definition of the transformation of an image from one modality to another and results in the alignment of the two image data sets. This process brings into spatial registration the different imaging modalities providing a much better clinical awareness and "tumour mapping". High-resolution CT images used in modern radiotherapy planning provide excellent visualization of bony structures, while MR images give detailed soft tissue information. Sometimes abnormalities not visible on the CT scans can be clearly seen on the MR studies, while functional images such as SPECT and PET provide physiological imaging, i.e. they show metabolically active areas in a scan. But these studies do not contain enough anatomic information, and therefore they are often performed along with a CT scan to provide both anatomical and physiological imaging (Fig. 9.4a, b). Some of the basic techniques are:

1. **Point-Based Registration**: In this method either externally placed point landmarks or internal anatomic landmarks on both primary and secondary data sets are used to match image superimposition. The registration process can be carried out automatically, manually or semi-automatically.
2. **Interactive Registration**: In this method, the two image sets are overlaid using different colour in different images: axial, sagittal and coronal. The planner manipulates the secondary image set to best match the primary set. Rotation and translation controls are available.
3. **Contour Matching Registration**: In this method, the contours that can be identified on both image set are drawn, and then the software automatically manipulates the studies using multiple image shifts and rotations until the best registration between the two data sets is found.
4. **Combining Option**: Once the two image sets are registered, fusing the two can generate a third data set. This is usually the way to deal with combined anatomic-functional studies from sources such as CT or MR and PET or SPECT. Commercially available combined units can obtain CT and PET in the same treatment position, and thus no specific registration process is required.

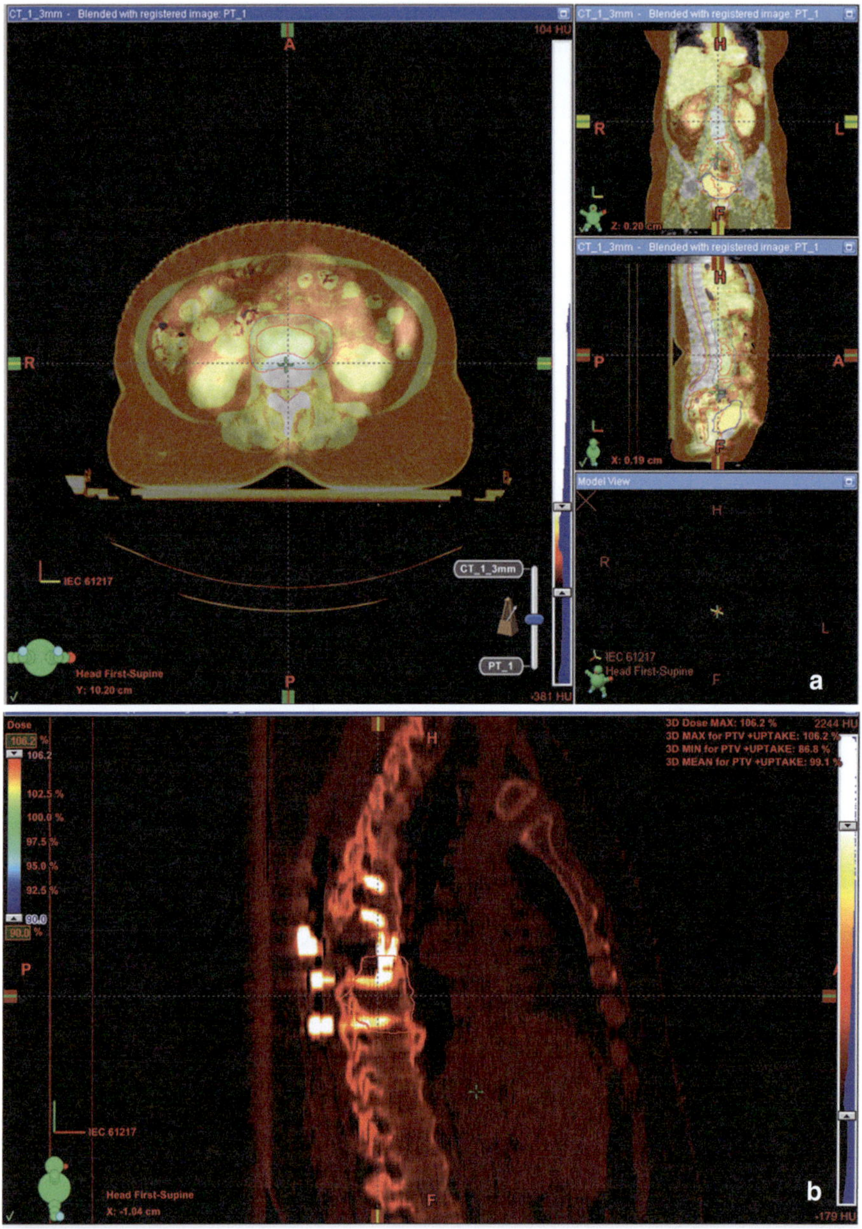

Fig. 9.4 (**a**) Both anatomical and physiological imaging by PET-CT simulation. (**b**) Both anatomical and physiological imaging by PET-CT simulation

CT-Based 3D Planning: Three-dimensional treatment planning systems use CT scans for treatment planning [4–7]. These systems provide more flexibility in treatment planning and accurate dose calculations. Studies comparing the 3D plans with the two-dimensional (2D) plans have found that the 3D plans can offer better target coverage and reduced dose to normal tissues [8]. In 3D treatment planning as described in Chap. 8, after CT simulation, data is transferred to the planning system, and the various target and critical structures are contoured. After contouring, these structures can be viewed from the BEV, and the planner can select the beams to cover target volumes while sparing surrounding tissues. The CT Hounsfield units being proportional to the electron density of the body tissue allow dose calculations for the plans using the CT numbers to correct for tissue inhomogeneities. Planning with noncoplanar beams is easier on a 3D treatment planning system. For a 3D plan, if the isocentre is moved or if there are treatment beams for which no radiographs were initially taken, a plan check or resimulation is carried out to obtain a complete set of radiographs. However, if the DRRs are used instead of the radiographs, there is generally no need to bring the patient back.

Selection of Isocentre: The isocentre is the point where the central axes of all beams used in treatment intersect and is generally the point to which the dose is prescribed in conventional radiotherapy, though in IMRT or IGRT, wherein the aim is to have in a built-in inhomogeneity in dose distribution, the dose is prescribed to a volume. Therefore in conventional radiotherapy, this ICRU reference point or the isocentre varies with different combinations of beams used:

- **Single beam**: In this type of arrangement, the isocentre lies on the central axis of the beam in the centre of the PTV.
- **Parallel-opposed equally weighted beams**: The target volume in this case is the entire interparietal distance between the two treated surfaces, and the isocentre lies on the central axis halfway between the beam entry points.
- **Parallel-opposed unequally weighted beams**: The target volume again in this case also is the entire interparietal distance between the two treated surfaces. However because of unequally weighted beams, the isocentre gets pushed towards the side with lower beam weightage and lies on the central axis near or at the centre of the target volume.
- **Other intersecting beams**: The point at the intersection of the central axes inside the target volume if the weightage of all beams is equal.

Surface Dose: Megavoltage external beam irradiation is characteristically **skin sparing**, while orthovoltage and lower energies (superficial X-rays) do not exhibit this phenomenon. This means that the dose at or just below the skin/irradiated surface is less than the maximal build-up dose, which occurs at a fixed depth (D_{max}) below the skin or irradiated surface. This depth at which the maximal dose occurs depends on the beam energy and field size and is directly proportional to the size of the field while inversely proportional to the beam energy. This is because a larger field size will have more backscatter adding to the surface dose, while higher beam energy will mean more forward scatter and hence a deeper build-up region as well as less backscatter. Therefore a surface dose represents a dose on the irradiated surface which is made up of a combination of photons scattered from the collimators, air, etc.; photons backscattered from the patient; and high-energy electrons produced by photon interactions with air and any shielding structures before hitting the surface. Typically for a 10×10 cm^2 field, the surface dose is estimated to be about 30% of D_{max} for a cobalt beam, 15% for a 6 MV X-ray beam and 10% for an 18 MV

X-ray beam. The surface dose is usually measured using thin window parallel-plate ionization chambers for both chamber polarities, and the average reading between the positive and negative polarities is counted as the surface dose.

Build-Up Region: This phenomenon is also a characteristic of megavoltage beam radiotherapy and is associated with the property of skin sparing in these beams. As explained in "surface dose" part in the preceding paragraph, ***a build-up region refers to that depth of tissue just below the irradiated surface where there is an increase in the dose delivered but which has yet not reached the maximal dose or Dmax***. Basically what is happening in this region is that the incident photon beam results in the release of energetic secondary charged particles (electrons and positrons) which however have a definite range. Due to photon-tissue electron collisions, kinetic energy is released into the tissue (KERMA) which results in a certain amount of absorbed dose in the tissue which increases with depth. This collision KERMA is thus negated by the absorbed dose, and till the depth that this is not completely negated, the secondary electrons keep moving deeper. The depth at which the absorbed dose is comparable with the collision KERMA and Coulomb-photon equilibrium or CPE is eventually reached. This occurs at D_{max} which is supposed to be the range of the secondary charged particles.

Depth of Maximum Dose (D_{max}): As explained in the two preceding paragraphs, photon beams after penetrating the irradiated surface travel through a depth of tissue before depositing the maximum absorbed dose. This is called the D_{max}, and its depth is mainly dependent on the incident photon beam energy and to a much lesser extent on the field size. This D_{max} can vary from 0 in case of superficial X-rays to as high as 5 cm for megavoltage beams greater than 21 MV (Table 9.1).

Exit Dose: This refers to that component of the delivered dose that is measured at the beam exit point. Photon beams do not have a definite range unlike charged particles, and a portion of the incident beam always exits the opposite surface of the patient. It must be also remembered that at this exit point, the actual measured dose is less than the extrapolated dose based on isodose charts because of the loss of scatter contribution to the beam which has exited the body.

9.1.2 Beam Profile

- **The central region** of a beam is the region extending from the central axis to just short of the geometric field edges by 1–1.5 cm. This geometric field edge is usually indicated over the treated surface by the optical field lights and refers to the area covered by the 50% isodose. Various machine-related factors affect the dose profile across this region. In the case of cobalt-60 machine, the dose profile is affected by inverse square dose fall-off and increased phantom thickness for

Table 9.1 Depth of maximum beam dose from various photon beam treatment machines

Machine	Orthovoltage	Cobalt-60	LINAC	LINAC	LINAC	LINAC	LINAC
Energy	250–500 kV	1.3 MV	4 MV	6 MV	10 MV	18 MV	25 MV
Depth dose (cm)	Surface	0.5 cm	1.0 cm	1.5 cm	2.5 cm	3.5 cm	5 cm

off-axis points. In case of linear accelerators, the dose profile is affected by the electron energies of electrons, atomic numbers (and hence electron densities) of the target and flattening filter and field shape.

- **The penumbral region** is the edge of the beam, and in this region, rapid changes in dose is seen which depends on scatter from the collimators, the source size and any lateral electronic disequilibrium. This dose fall-off around the geometric beam edge is sigmoid in shape and has three components. Near the collimator jaws, there is some amount of transmission through the jaws which can affect the edge dose. This is called **transmission penumbra**. There is also a penumbral area caused by the finite size of the source in a cobalt machine, and this is called the **geometric penumbra**. This is not a significant issue in the linear accelerators. Finally a component of the dose at the edge of the beam is due to scatter wherein the component of scatter from area outside beam is absent leading to decreased point doses, and this is called the **scatter penumbra**. ***The total penumbra is the sum of all these three components and is called the physical penumbra***, and it is dependent on factors like beam energy, source size, SSD, source to collimator distance and depth in phantom.
- **Umbra** is the region outside the defined beam edge which is far away from the field edges. The dose in this region is generally low and results from radiation transmitted through the collimator and head shielding.

9.1.3 Beam Characteristics from Commonly Used Photon Beam Machines (Table 9.2)

9.1.4 Use of Beam Modifiers

Sometimes simple positioning of beams around the target volume may result in either inadequate coverage because of variability of the patient's anatomy resulting in either "missing tissue" or in oblique beam incidence. In such cases, various devices are used to alter beam characteristics especially percentage depth dose coverage to cover the target volume.

Table 9.2 Commonly used therapy machines are the cobalt-60 and linear accelerators

Machine	SSD (cm)	D_{max} (cm)	PDD at 10 cm (percent depth dose)	Remarks
Cobalt-60	80	0.5	55	Beam edge not well defined at penumbra due to larger source size
4-MV X-ray	80	1–1.2	61	Smaller penumbra and also horns (beam intensity off-axis) due to flattening filter design of about 14%
6-MV X-ray	100	1.5	67	Small penumbra and horns due to flattening filter design of about 9%
18-MV X-ray	100	3–3.5	80	Small penumbra and horns due to flattening filter design of about 5%; higher exit dose compared to entry dose

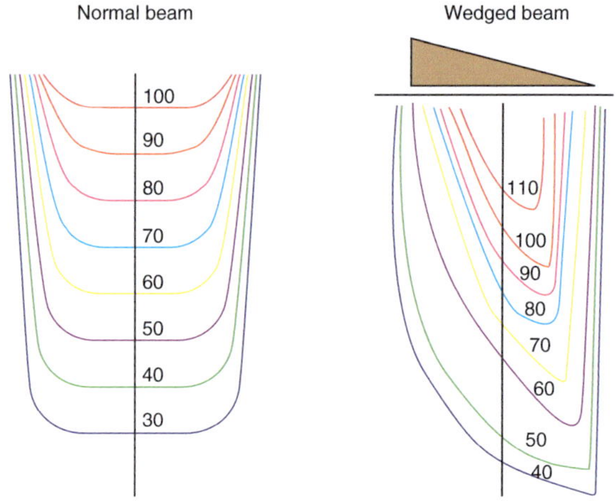

Fig. 9.5 Depth dose distribution due to insertion of wedge

Wedge Filters: The most commonly used types of wedge filters in present radiation oncology practice are the manual wedge, the motorized wedge and the dynamic wedge. Physical or manual wedges were the earliest form of wedges used and consist of angled pieces of lead, tungsten or steel which are placed manually in the beam just before treatment delivery so as to *turn the isodoses through an angle* and thus create a homogeneous dose distribution over the target volume. This wedge is shaped like a triangle in its cross section with a thick end called the heel and a thinner end called the toe; this creates a differential in the dose attenuation across the wedge with more attenuation beyond the heel and less attenuation below the toe. This leads to a turning or tilt of the isodose lines towards the heel (Fig. 9.5). This beam modifier is used wherever the irradiated surface is at an angle with the incident beam (where there is supposed "tissue deficit") as otherwise in the area where there is tissue deficit, there would be less beam attenuation and hence more penetration. The heel of the wedge is positioned opposite the area of "tissue deficit". A motorized wedge is similar to a manual wedge in shape and design except for the fact that it is incorporated into the treatment head of the LINAC and is remotely controlled. A dynamic wedge produces the same wedged intensity gradient by having one jaw close gradually while the beam is on.

The basic principle of use of wedge is its ability to turn the isodose lines through an angle thereby creating required dose distribution. This is called ***hinge angle***. A *Wedge angle is defined as the angle between the 50% isodose line and the perpendicular to the beam central axis*. The optimal wedge angle is calculated as 90° – 1/2 (hinge angle). *The wedge factor is defined as the ratio of dose at a specified depth (usually D_{max}) on the central axis with the wedge in the beam to the dose under the same conditions without the wedge.* Since there is beam attenuation while travelling through the wedge which will depend on the beam energy and field size, this wedge factor is used as a correction factor while calculating treatment time or monitor units. Wedges are therefore most commonly used:

- To compensate for an angled surface or missing tissue as in nasopharyngeal, laryngeal, breast tangential or maxillary treatments where wedges are used to compensate for decreased thickness anteriorly or to obtain homogeneous dose distribution between two beams at right angles to each other.
- Wedged beams are also useful in the treatment of lesions where two beams are placed at an angle to get a homogeneous dose distribution.

Bolus: Many times it is not advantageous to have skin sparing during irradiation such as in head and neck treatments where nodes reach the subcutaneous plane or in treatment of superficial lesions. In such cases the isodose needs to be pulled to the skin or subcutaneous tissue, and to do this, a tissue-equivalent material has to be placed in contact with the skin. This is called a bolus. ***The basic principle is to negate the skin-sparing effect of megavoltage photon beams by introducing a tissue density comparable material before the skin***. For a bolus, a layer of uniform thickness (0.5–1.5 cm) material is used which matches the contour of the skin surface (Fig. 9.6) while at the same time providing for a perpendicular surface to the incident beam. This results in pulling the isodoses more superficially as the bolus now acts as the build-up region, while the skin and subcutaneous tissue now get the required isodose coverage. Commonly used materials for making bolus include wax, saline or rice bags. Wax is easily available, cheap, tissue-equivalent and malleable when heated and can match the patient's contour. Bolus is also used as a compensator in tissue extremities to account for lack of scatter to achieve reasonable dose coverage.

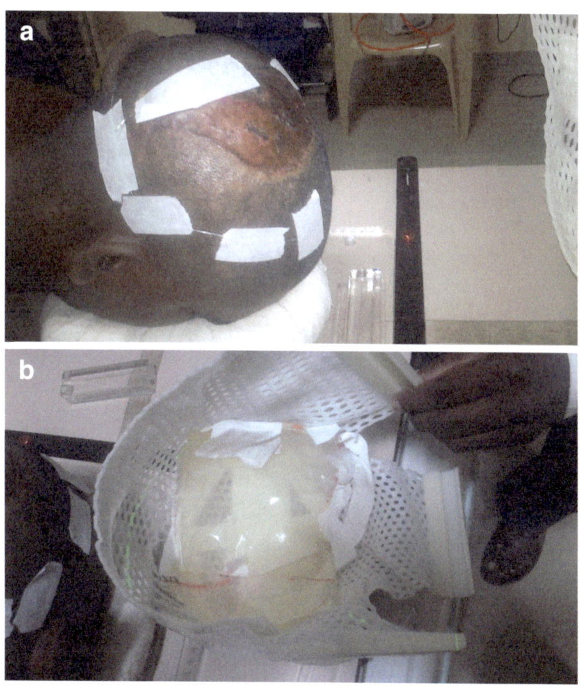

Fig. 9.6 (**a**, **b**) Use of bolus to achieve skin surface dosing

Compensating Filters: A compensating filter is similar to a bolus in design but is used to cause beam attenuation in areas where there is "tissue deficit", and basically it functions as the missing tissue that would have otherwise caused beam attenuation. The objective is to achieve a homogeneous dose distribution like a bolus **but does not cause a loss of skin sparing**. Compensating filters are usually made of metals such as lead or tungsten which are compact. They are usually placed at the level of the shield tray on the treatment unit head (*unlike the bolus which is placed on the treatment surface*) and cause beam attenuation without the secondary electrons reaching the irradiated tissue and therefore no loss of skin sparing. The dimensions of the compensator are scaled in length and width by the ratio of SSD to the distance from the source to the compensator (Fig. 9.7a–c). As in wedges, so also in tissue compensator, because of beam attenuation through the compensator, there is reduction in output which needs to be measured and accounted for in MU/time calculations.

Bolus vs. Compensator: Preparing and using compensating filters instead of bolus is a more tedious and time-consuming planning operation; and it is difficult to account for it in estimating dose distributions unless dosimetric studies have been done for different beam profiles using a tissue compensator from which tables could be prepared. Boluses however are considered part of the patient contour, and further dosimetry is not required. But skin-sparing preservation is a big advantage with compensator compared to bolus limiting the uses of bolus.

Corrections for Contour Irregularities: In 2D radiotherapy planning, beam dosimetric data are usually generated by applying irradiation to a regular water phantom which provides for a flat incident surface and homogeneous internal electron density. But when this beam data has to be applied to a patient, corrections for surface irregularity as well as tissue inhomogeneities have to be made so as to achieve actual dose coverage. Various methods used for correction of dose calculation in 2D radiotherapy for applying phantom-derived beam data to patient contours include:

- **Isodose shift method**: This is a simple method and can be used for planning on a manual contour. In this method, the isodose lines are first charted as they would otherwise appear if the contour surface was uniform with no tissue deficit and no tissue inhomogeneities. On these isodose lines, new gridlines are drawn parallel to the central axis of the beam so that ideally they should match the isodose lines. However because of tissue deficit (or excess in view of inhomogeneities), there is a difference between the SSD along a gridline and the ideal SSD on the central axis. To correct for this tissue mismatch, for each gridline, the overlaid isodose distribution is shifted up (or down) such that the corrected ideal SSD matches the gridline SSD, and the corrected depth dose can be calculated by this movement up or down along the central axis read directly from the overlaid distribution. Factors which determine the magnitude of these isodose shift factors for the different types of tissue or for the various tissue-inhomogeneity interface types (air-lung, bone-tissue, etc.) are predetermined and are energy dependent but not affected by field size.

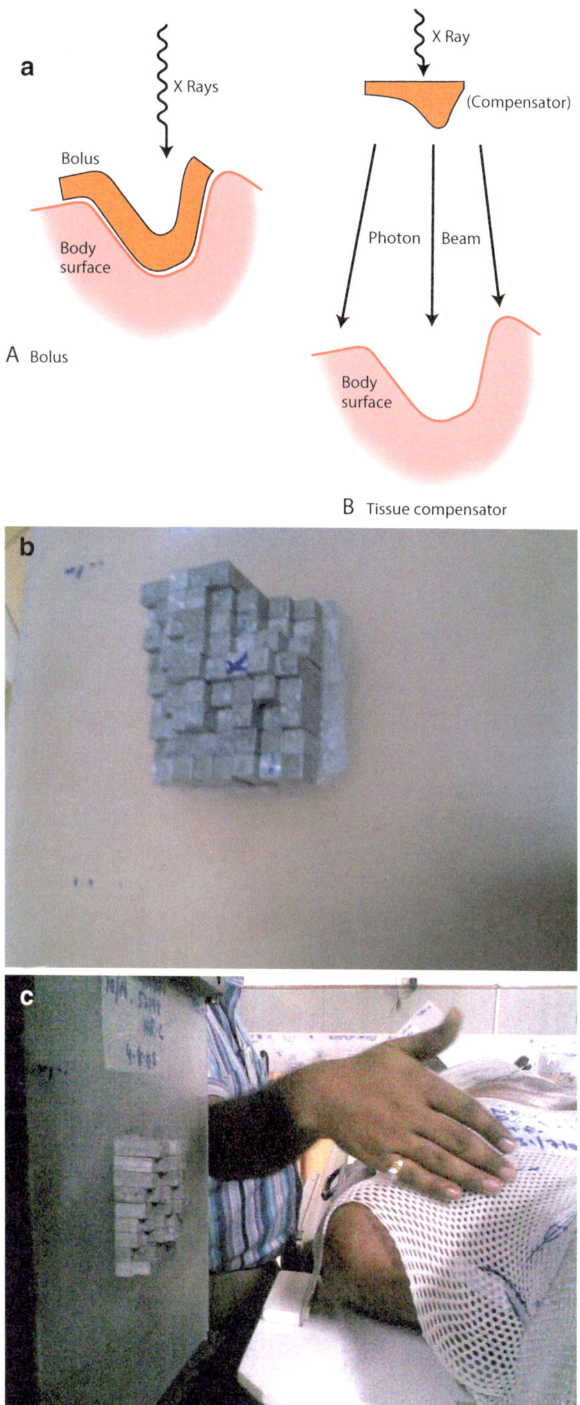

Fig. 9.7 (**a**) Principle of use of compensator to account for "missing tissue". (**b**) Compensator to account for "missing tissue". (**c**) Actual compensator being used

Examples of correction factor in the case of a 4 MV photon beam are air cavity → (−)0.6, lung → (−)0.4 and hard bone → (+)0.5. In this example, the minus sign denotes shift of the isodose curves away from the surface towards the treatment head. The net isodose shift can be calculated by multiplying the thickness of inhomogeneity with the predetermined inhomogeneity factor for that given tissue.

- **Effective attenuation coefficient method**: Another method for applying contour or patient-based corrections to isodose distributions is by using attenuation factors for *missing or extra tissue*. This correction is called effective attenuation coefficient and is calculated as an exponential function "exp($-\mu x$)", where x represents the magnitude of extra or missing tissue above the calculation point and μ is the beam energy-dependent linear attenuation coefficient of tissue. These factors are usually precalculated and available as graphs or tables and used for treatment time calculation. They are dependent on field size and SSD.
- **TAR method**: A tissue-air ratio (TAR) correction method is also based on relative beam attenuation in air compared to tissue and making use of correction factors. Additionally this method also takes into account depth of the calculation point and the field size. It is basically the ratio of the dose through tissue compared to that through air and is a measure of the dose attenuation through tissue.

Beam's Eye View (BEV): Beam's eye view (BEV) is a projection on to a supposed or virtual X-ray film or patient surface, the beam axes, contoured target volume and field boundaries. BEVs can be superimposed on a DRR to obtain a simulation film based on which changes in field shape or beam position could be affected with respect to the patient's anatomy seen on the DRR and matched with the outlined target as well as critical organ volumes projected by the BEV (Fig. 9.8). The importance of BEV lies in the ability to subsequently view the treatment beams as they would be incident on the patient surface, to evaluate target volume coverage and normal structure sparing as well as for feasibility of beam positions.

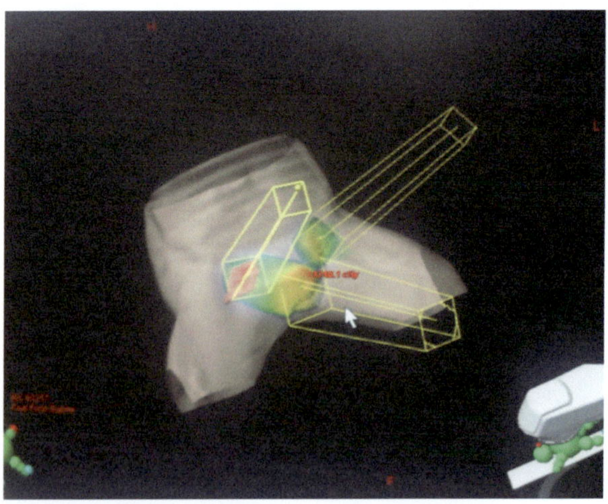

Fig. 9.8 BEV showing target volume and normal structures

9.2 Beam Combinations and Clinical Application

Once the target and normal volumes have been decided and beams have been placed and verified, the planner then has to decide if the combination of beams is the desired one or further adjustments are required. The planner also has to decide if a single or multiple, planar, noncoplanar or rotational fields are to be used and what weightages have to be given to each beam and where would be the point of dose prescription. Once all these decisions are made, the planner then prescribes the dose schedule, evaluates whether planned objectives have been met, verifies the plan for feasibility and delivers treatment after verification of set-up.

Treatments with photon beams using only a single beam are generally not commonly used. The main indications for such single beam treatment include superficial skin or subcutaneous tissue lesions wherein the target volume coverage can be enclosed within 5 cm [where it can deliver a reasonably uniform dose to the target (±5%) with a low maximum dose outside the target (<110%)], or in case of palliative irradiation. Deep-seated lesions are better treated with a combination of beams as single beams will result in a higher dose near the entrance than at prescription depth (Fig. 9.9) [9].

9.2.1 Weighting and Normalization

- **Normalization** of a beam refers to the point on the central axis of the beam or the isodose-covered volume or the target dose volume which is selected for prescription of the desired dose. This means, for example, if the target volume is covered by the 95% isodose line, then beam is "normalized" to that isodose, meaning that volume of irradiated tissue enclosed in the 95% isodose line will get 100% dose. This may mean that this 95% isodose is now normalized to full

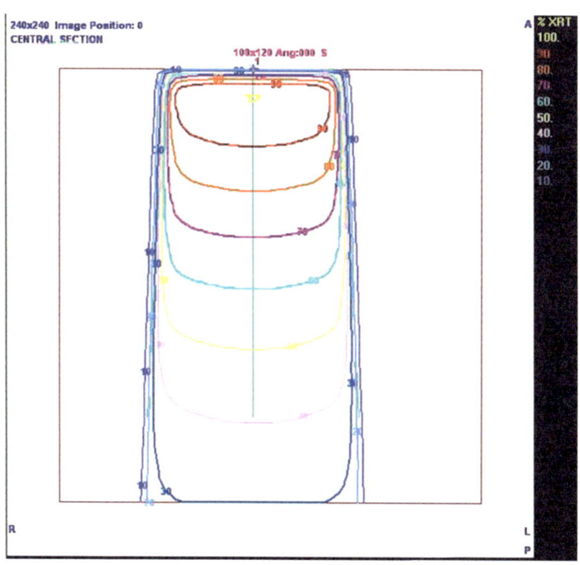

Fig. 9.9 Isodose lines seen with single direct field

dose and the otherwise 100% isodose line will get more than 100% dose. Similarly other combinations can be used such as "normalizing to target mean", i.e. the mean dose in the target volume is the prescribed dose. Similarly other combinations are used in normalization such as 95% volume getting 95% dose, prescribing dose to D_{max}, etc. If normalization during therapy with more than one beam is not done, the dose distributions are presented as multiples of prescribed dose by adding the dose as 100% for each beam (for which care has to be taken during prescribing the dose), and hot spots may occur.

- **Beam weighting** refers to the relative contribution of each beam towards the total prescribed dose in the target volume, and this is applied at the normalization point for the given beam. This is one of the methods of achieving a desired dose distribution especially if the target volume is skewed in location, i.e. the target volume is not located midway between the beams but may be nearer to one or more beams than the others. If the beams are "unweighted", this means that the relative contribution of each beam to the total target dose is the same (i.e. if 200 cGy is prescribed for a three-field technique, then each beam provides 66.7 cGy to the target volume). However sometimes to get a good volume coverage by the prescribed dose, "differential weighting" is used such as 3:2 for unilateral tonsillar fossa treatments or mantle field.

9.2.2 Fixing the Gantry Isocentre: SSD or SAD?

After having immobilized the patient on the couch and decided on the fields, the next important point is to decide where the gantry or the treatment beam isocentre would lie. This is important both for set-up verification and daily treatment reproducibility. An SSD (source-to-skin constant distance) treatment is one in which the field is projected onto the patient's skin after setting up the patient at a fixed distance from the gantry head (usually 80 cm for cobalt machines and 100 cm for 6–15 MV LINACS). This same distance between the source and the patient's skin is maintained for all beams used. On the other hand in SAD technique, the gantry is set up to an isocentre lying inside the target volume (where all the treatment beams intersect), and the machine can be simply rotated to each treatment angle after setting up the isocentre. The SSD technique scores over the SAD technique in simplicity of technique with higher percent depth dose compared to SAD as well as less beam divergence. But the biggest advantage of an SAD technique is that all fields can be set at a single time to an isocentre lying inside the tumour; the gantry rotated accordingly to the various angles for beam set-up.

9.2.3 Parallel-Opposed Beams

As we have seen in the section earlier on single beam treatments, a major disadvantage is proper coverage of deep-seated tumours by the required dose without causing very high-dose depositions in superficial tissues. This problem can be solved by using multiple beam treatments. In this, the most commonly used combination is

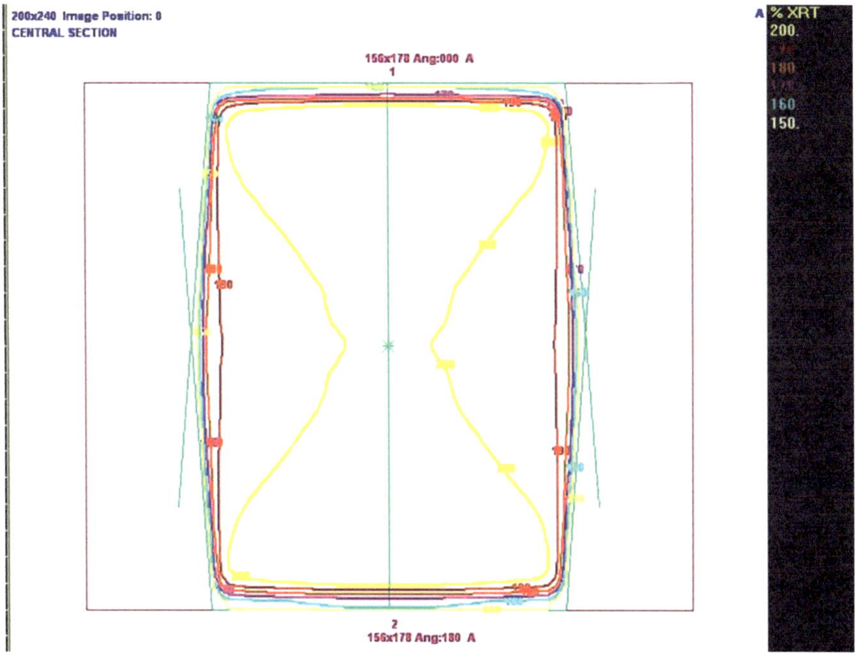

Fig. 9.10 Isodose lines seen with parallel opposed beams

the use of two beams delivered opposed to each other from either side of the patient's body segment. These are called parallel-opposed beams, and they help overcome the issue of high superficial dose by compensating for the decrease in the depth dose of one beam by the contribution from the opposing beam resulting in an almost uniform distribution in the depth of the irradiated volume (Fig. 9.10). The energy of the beams used in this type of combination depends on the separation between the two irradiated surfaces. In cases where this separations is less (<10 cm), low-energy beams (of 4–6 MV) are used so as to obtain a relatively homogeneous dose distribution between the irradiated surfaces and a less dose build-up gap. On the other hand, where the interparietal separation is more than 20 cm, higher energies (>15 MV) are used to allow for a homogeneous distribution while limiting any significant hot spot at D_{max} locations. Sites such as the lung, extremities, pelvis as well as head and neck can be treated with parallel-opposed beams.

9.2.4 Multiple Coplanar Beams

Multiple coplanar beams can also be planned using a 2D approach on a single plane, but their use entails a higher dose in the beam intersection region. Common field arrangements include:

- **Wedge pair**: Two beams with wedges are used to achieve a homogeneous dose distribution inside an otherwise trapezoid or diamond-shaped irradiated area which, if treated without wedges, would have resulted in very high doses in the inner part of the volume (at the intersection of both beams) and low doses at the periphery of the area. This is useful in superficial lesions with angled surfaces (e.g. maxillary sinus, laryngeal or thyroid lesions). The principle of using such wedged beams has been explained in the section on wedges (Fig. 9.11a).

- **Four-field techniques**: In the classical ***four-field*** technique, there are two pairs of parallel-opposed beams incident in such a way that each is at a right angle to its neighbouring beam, and this arrangement produces a box-shaped region of tissue receiving the prescribed dose (Fig. 9.11b). This type of beam geometry is helpful in areas where the opposing surfaces are relatively parallel and the region to be irradiated lies sufficiently deep or is near or at the centre of the inter-surface distance such as in the pelvis (for cancers of the prostate, bladder or uterus). There is another similar arrangement of beams called four-field ***crossfire***, in which the angle between each beam is less than 90° and resultant irradiated volume takes the shape of a diamond (Fig. 9.11c). This technique is used if more anteroposterior coverage is required rather than lateral extension or some critical normal structure is present lateral to the target volume which requires sparing from beam portal.

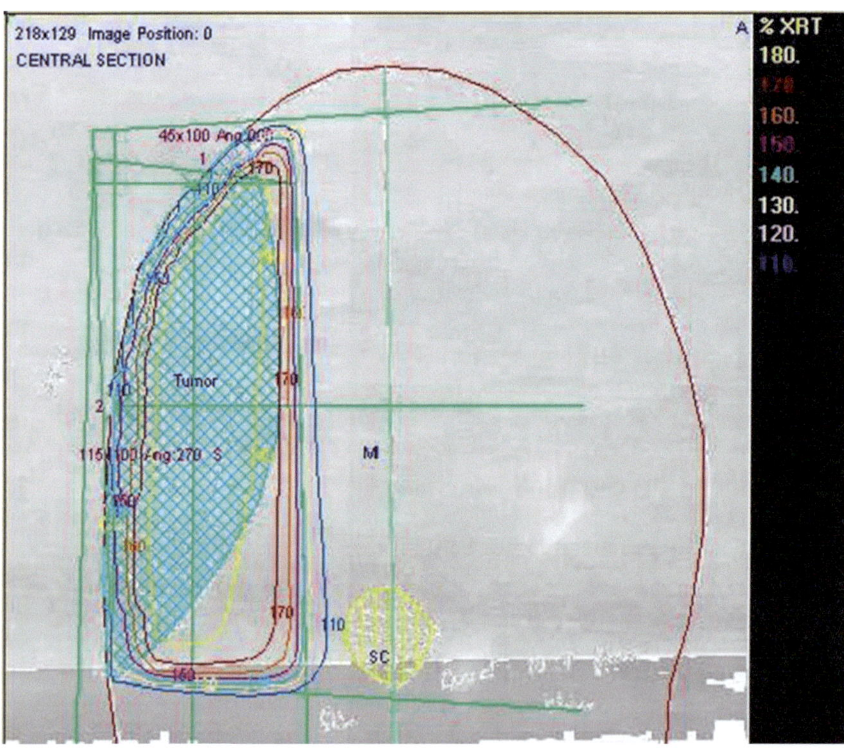

Fig. 9.11 (**a**) Isodose lines seen with wedged pair beams. (**b**) Isodose lines seen with four-field box technique. (**c**) Isodose lines seen with four-field crossfire. (**d**) Isodose lines seen with three-field box

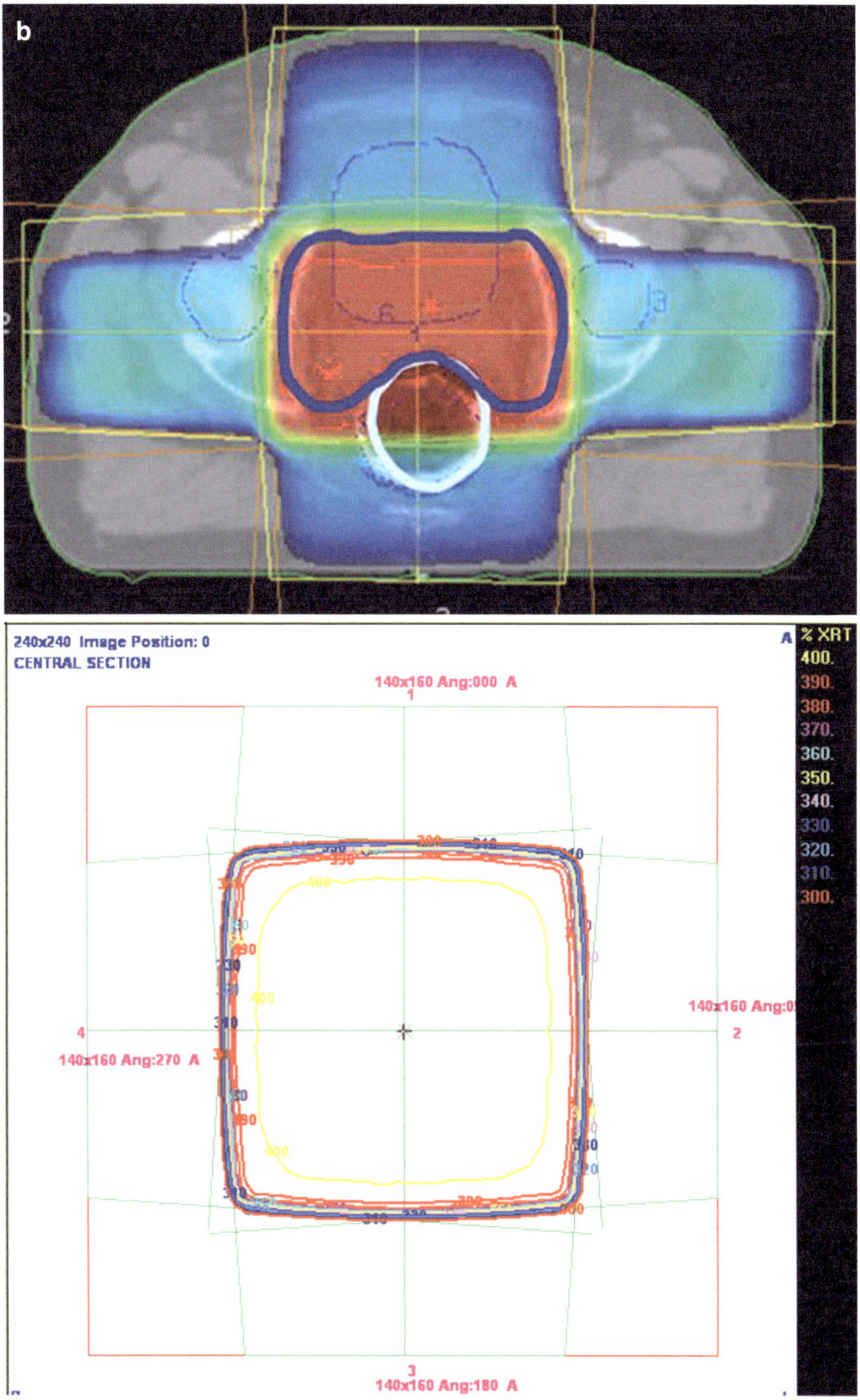

Fig. 9.11 (continued)

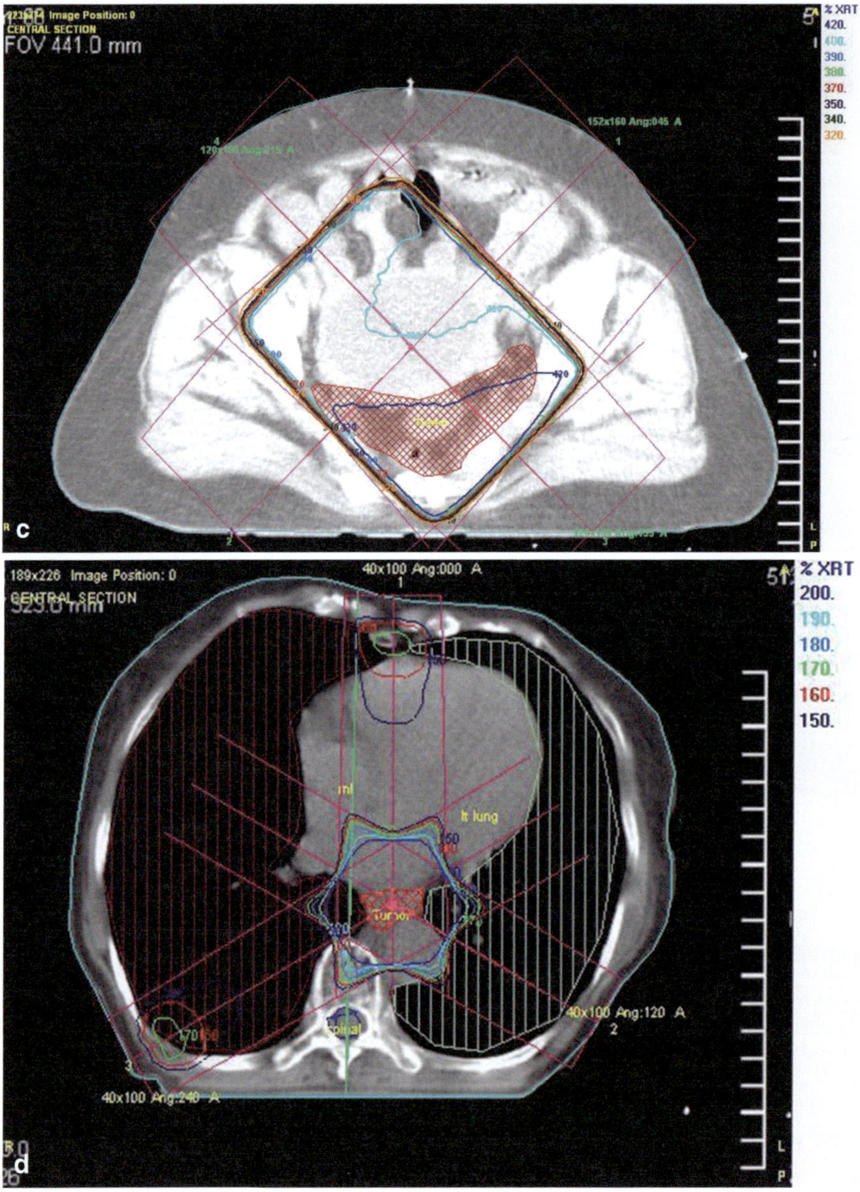

Fig. 9.11 (continued)

- **Three-field box**: This technique is similar to the four-field technique and is generally preferred in areas which are closer to the surface or where the tumour is located in area with lot of surrounding critical structures and thus to avoid more beams passing through these tissues such as in the rectum, oesophagus or in some cases lung. Wedges are used in the two beams which are angulated at each other to compensate for the dose gradient in the third beam (Fig. 9.11d).

- **Multiple fields**: Three or more sets of opposing beams are used sometimes, especially for large irregular target volumes resulting in a complicated dose distribution and spreading of low and intermediate isodose area over a larger tissue volume. This leads to sparing of more sparing of tissues surrounding the target volume. These techniques are used in GI tumours like the stomach or pancreas head in centres where 3D-CRT is not available. The fields are usually complicated and may require blocks. Equivalent square field sizes may have to be determined to calculate beam-on times, or computerized calculations would be required.

9.2.5 Rotational Techniques

In this type of treatment, the centre of the target volume is the isocentre or the point at which all the treatment beams converge. The difference between this technique and those with multiple beams is that as the gantry head moves through an angle range, the beam is continuously "on" and dose is being delivered to the target volume. Therefore in a way, this can be thought of as an infinite number of beams at succeeding angles delivered continuously. This technique because of such higher degrees of freedom (because of *infinite number of beams*) produces a much better dose conformity with less steep dose gradient at beam edges. However in this technique a larger volume of normal tissue receives low- to intermediate-dose irradiation. This technique is used in sites such as the prostate, bladder, head and neck as well as CNS/pituitary lesions. The treatment planning system calculates the number of MUs per unit time for the range of angles prescribed from the average TAR/TMR in these angles.

9.2.6 Multiple Noncoplanar Beams

Usually patients receive their irradiation with coplanar beams, i.e. the beams move around a single axis. Sometimes this is not suitable to get a required dose distribution or to avoid entry or exit doses to important structures. In such cases, the beams can be positioned in a noncoplanar distribution, i.e. the axis of movement of the gantry head will be different. This type of arrangement is frequently used in treating CNS tumours as well as in providing direct perineal irradiation. However in planning such beam arrangements, it is important to ensure that the axis of gantry rotation is freely available to prevent any collision between the gantry and patient/couch. Also the exit planes of these beams should be designed such that there is no exit through the length of the body to decrease whole body integral dose (e.g. true vertex beams are not used as the exit beam is through the whole body). This type of beam arrangement is used frequently in sites like the brain as well as the head and neck where the target volume is surrounded by critical structures. In special machines, these noncoplanar beams are used along with beam intensity modulation, highly localized and identified target volume and continuous gantry rotation or independent robotic arms, along with high doses per fraction which have led to the emergence of the concept of radiosurgery or stereotactic radiation therapy.

9.2.7 Field Matching

This term denotes arranging adjoining treatment fields in such a way that there is no overlap of dose distribution in the treated at prescribed depth. Usually matching between various adjoining fields is done at the skin because it is easy to do so. However because treatment beams are always divergent, the field width may increase at the prescribed depth causing overlap of dose. This can be avoided by following certain protocols such as calculating beam divergence at depth or matching the beams at depth, using specific isodoses for beam matching (e.g. 50% isodose) or using predetermined gap junctions.

Plan Check or Resimulation: Planning complex fields may require moving the isocentre, change of treatment beams or adjusting gantry angles, field sizes and other beam parameters. If the isocentre has been changed or beams have been used for which the radiographs were not taken during initial simulation, the patient is brought back to the simulator for a resimulation. The patient is set up in the treatment position, and the original isocentre is verified radiographically. The isocentre is then shifted as per the plan, and all the required X-rays are taken with the appropriate gantry angles and field sizes. If Cerrobend (a low-temperature melting alloy) blocks are used for the treatment, the blocks are fabricated based on the aperture outlines. Before the patient's treatment, either double-exposure localization port films are obtained or portal verification films are taken on the first day of the treatment. Portal verification is discussed in a later section. These films are compared with the corresponding simulation radiographs. The placement of the radiation fields and aperture shapes is verified. In 3D planning volumetric CT data are used with patient simulated by CT scan in treatment position. The advantage here is that even for beam or isocentre shifts, fresh simulation scans need not be taken, unless the treatment position itself is changed.

In some cases, a DRR can be constructed, but it is not feasible to obtain a simulation radiograph (e.g. it is impossible to radiograph a vertex field). In such cases, one of the orthogonal films can be used for verification of the aperture shape. An anterior simulation radiograph can be used to draw the block shape for a vertex field. The orthogonal pair of films verifies the treatment isocentre, and the aperture shape is verified on the anterior localization port film. This film is just for verification; the beam pointing in the vertex direction delivers the actual treatment.

Transfer of Treatment Information to the Therapy Machine: The information needed for patient's treatment produced during the simulation, treatment planning and plan check include positioning, immobilization and tattoo marks on the skin for setting the isocentre. These are then documented in the patient's chart. Any special immobilization device used is recorded as also the ***position of the isocentre or beam entry point*** in case of 2D planning or the simulation isocentre set-up indices on ***x, y and z axes*** in case of 3D planning. For each treatment beam, all necessary parameters like type of radiation; the beam energy; the beam-on time; the couch angle; the gantry angle; the collimator angle; the collimator jaw settings; the presence of a field-shaping block; if a wedge is used, its angle and orientation; the presence of a tissue compensator; and the type of bolus and its thickness are recorded. For the treatment machines equipped with MLCs, the MLCs, rather than the Cerrobend blocks, define field shapes, and their configuration for each beam is either designed on a treatment planning computer or a dedicated workstation. The information about the MLC leaf settings is transferred to the therapy machine's MLC computer. On each day of the treatment, the aperture shape is defined by the MLC.

In modern dicom connected computer-controlled therapy machines, treatment plans are directly transferred from the treatment planning computer to the treatment machine's computer [10]. Even in these set-ups, it is necessary to conduct a check set-up and delivery before therapy to ensure that all beam positions and MLC patterns are achievable. During this *virtual treatment*, the patient is placed in the therapy position, and all set-up and beam delivery instructions are followed through without actually delivering the radiation dose, to ensure that the set-up does not cause a collision between the machine and couch during movement.

9.3 Treatment Verification

On the basis of instructions generated during the simulation and treatment planning, the patient is placed in the treatment position. To verify the correctness of the set-up, the patient is imaged directly on the treatment machine with the shielding blocks or MLCs in place. This process is carried out before treatment and confirms that the patient is set up correctly and the shielding blocks are protecting the normal structures as planned. Also it documents the patient's position for future reference. Frequent treatment verification has been shown to reduce localization errors [11]. Various methods for set-up verification include:

1. **Portal Imaging with Films**: High-energy therapy beams are used for portal radiographs. These could be either portal localization images or portal verification images. The quality of these images is generally poor compared with that of simulation radiographs, because of the high energy and hence high penetration of the beam.
2. **Portal Localization**: A portal film is obtained by exposing a radiographic film in a specially designed cassette with a metal screen. Only a fraction of the treatment beam-on time is used for the exposure. Droege and Bjarngard [12] investigated the screen-film combinations for portal imaging. The purpose of the front metal screen is to prevent the electrons generated within the patient from reaching the film and to generate electrons for image production. The purpose of the high atomic number back screen is to serve as an intensifier and to provide additional film exposure. The use of a back screen results in higher speed but with a slight reduction in resolution. To expose a portal localization film, a double-exposure technique is used. The first exposure is given with the treatment field size and shielding blocks in place. For the second exposure, a graticule tray replaces the blocks and an open field is used. The resulting image contains the image of the shaping block and the surrounding anatomic structures and grid points that serve

as the cross hairs and scale for measurement. These films are compared with the simulation films to verify the treatment port shape and its location with respect to the patient's anatomy.

3. **Portal Verification**: For portal verification, a slow film with or without a screen is used. In this method the film is exposed to the exit beam for the duration of the treatment. Here also the front metal screen is used to stop the electrons generated within the patient from reaching the film and to produce electrons for the radiographic image. The second metallic back screen is not used; instead, a plastic backing is used to provide support for the film and to eliminate artefacts from backscattered radiation. These radiographs image only the treatment area; the surrounding anatomic structures are not imaged.
4. **Electronic Portal Imaging**: For electronic portal imaging, instead of a film, an electronic portal imaging device (EPID) is placed in the exit beam to produce the image which are then displayed on a video screen. Boyer et al. [13] and Antonuk [14] have reviewed the existing EPIDs. EPIDs produce images almost instantaneously and store the images digitally on a computer [15] which are then compared with the simulation films to determine the set-up differences [16]. The patient can be monitored throughout the treatment, and motion during the therapy can be detected. EPIDs can either be video based [17] where after the exiting photon beam strikes the metal plate coated with phosphorous material to produce fluorescence, a video camera and computer combination digitally record the resulting light and display the images on a video monitor or they can be used a matrix of liquid ion chambers as detectors [18, 19] where an organic liquid serves as the ionizing medium between the electrodes. The ionization current in each chamber is measured with a current-to-voltage converting electrometer. An analog-to-digital converter, providing the intensity information for the pixel corresponding to the ionization chamber, then digitizes the collected charge.

   In many modern treatment machines, active matrix flat-panel imagers (AMFPIs) are available for portal imaging [14, 20] which consist of ~1-mm-thick glass substrate on which thin-film electronic circuits are placed which are created through a series of semiconductor processing steps. This solid state technology creates compact detectors that can be easily mounted on therapy accelerator and have a high degree of image quality. Also these detectors are highly radio resistant.
5. **On-board imager and cone beam**: MV portal imaging available with most modern linear accelerators and used for portal imaging however results in poor quality images because of high penetration of the MV beams and low tissue contrast [13]. This was overcome by the addition of a kV source and imager to a LINAC (Jaffray et al.) [21] which generates high-resolution soft tissue images of the patient at the time of treatment for the purpose of guiding therapy and reducing uncertainties. The combined system consists of medical accelerator and two imaging systems (MV and kV). In addition to the improved image quality of the kV imaging, the dose delivered during kV exposure is significantly lower compared to dose for MV imaging and allows for more frequent imaging and acquisition of images to improve treatment precision [21].

This on-board imaging (OBI) system provides three imaging modes: (1) 2D radiographic acquisition, (2) fluoroscopic image acquisition and (3) 3D cone beam computed tomography (CBCT). After the patient has been set up on the couch in treatment position, an orthogonal pair of kV radiographs (kV-kV imaging) is obtained and matched with corresponding reference image DRRs. Using this tool, the couch set-up correction can be checked with simulation images and any changes corrected for and downloaded to the treatment machine. The fluoroscopic mode can be used to monitor the breathing motion and to verify the gating threshold of the RPM system to account for the respiratory motion.

During CBCT, the gantry rotates around the patient while acquiring hundreds (~700) of low-dose radiographs. From these projections, axial CT images are reconstructed. The advantage of a cone beam CT scan compared to normal spiral CT is that in a single rotation, the imager can cover the entire treatment volume and hence the patient set-up position need not be disturbed. This helps in image-guided treatment delivery (Fig. 9.12). Image acquisition modes can be either full fan or half fan where full fan is used for small anatomical size sites like the brain and half fan for larger field sizes. An accessory called a bowtie filter is placed in front of the kV beam to attenuate the edges of the kV beam. This filter reduces

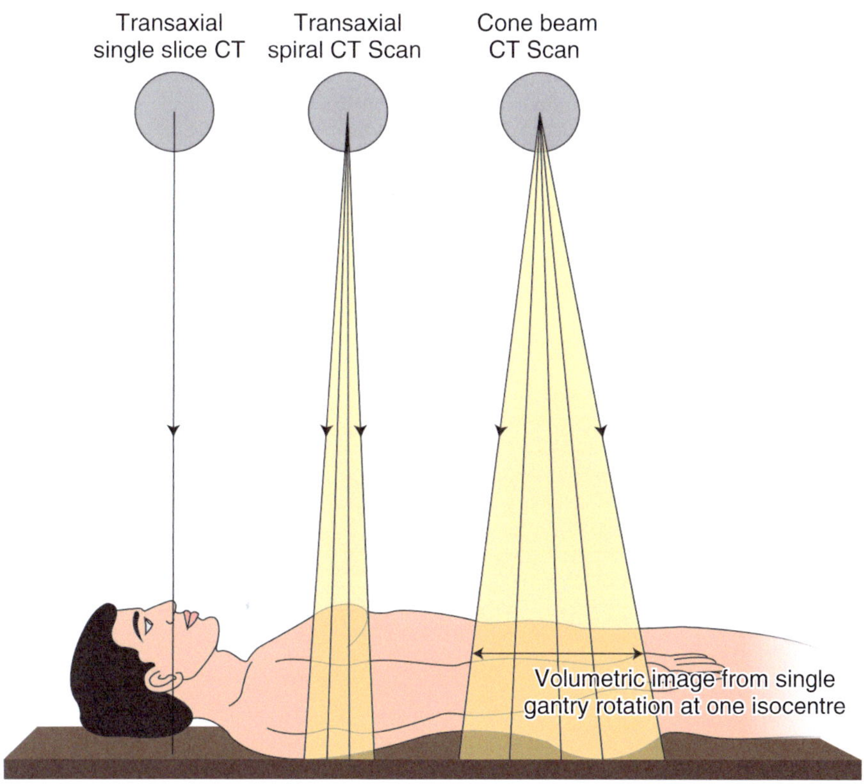

Fig. 9.12 Advantage of cone beam CT in OBI

the skin dose, allows larger X-ray technique without saturating the detector and reduces X-ray scatter and the effect of charge trapping in the detector [22].

After the CBCT images are acquired, these are transferred to the OBI application to be compared with the corresponding planning CT and anatomic contours. The patient's positioning is analysed on the two sets using 3D match. Based on the match, the couch shift parameters are determined and downloaded to the linear accelerator. The couch can be moved remotely to correct the patient set-up.

References

1. International Commission on Radiation Units and Measurements, (ICRU). Prescribing, recording, and reporting photon beam therapy. International Commission on Radiation Units and Measurements, ICRU Report 29, ICRU, Bethesda; 1978.
2. International Commission on Radiation Units and Measurements, (ICRU). Prescribing, recording, and reporting photon beam therapy. International Commission on Radiation Units and Measurements, ICRU Report 50, ICRU, Bethesda; 1993.
3. International Commission on Radiation Units and Measurements, (ICRU). Prescribing, recording, and reporting photon beam therapy (Supplement to ICRU Report 50). ICRU Report 62, ICRU, Bethesda; 1999.
4. Purdy JA, Wong JW, Harms WB, et al. Three dimensional treatment planning system. In: IAD B, van der Giessen PH, van Kleffens HJ, Wittkamper FW, editors. The use of computers in radiation therapy. Amsterdam: Elsevier Science; 1987. p. 277.
5. Mohan R, Barest G, Brewster L, et al. A comprehensive three-dimensional radiation treatment planning system. Int J Radiat Oncol Biol Phys. 1988;15:481.
6. Sailer SL, Chaney EL, Rosenman JG, et al. Treatment planning at the University of North Carolina at Chapel Hill. Semin Radiat Oncol. 1992;2:267.
7. Photon Treatment Planning Collaborative Working Group. State-of-the-art of external photon beam radiation treatment planning. Int J Radiat Oncol Biol Phys. 1991;21:9.
8. Armstrong JG, Burman C, Leibel S, et al. Conformal three-dimensional treatment planning may improve the therapeutic ratio of high dose radiation therapy for lung cancer. Int J Radiat Oncol Biol Phys. 1993;26:685.
9. International Commission on Radiation Units and Measurements. Measurement of absorbed dose measured in a phantom irradiated by a single beam of X or gamma rays. ICRU Report 23, ICRU, Bethesda; 1973.
10. Mageras GS, Podmaniczky KC, Mohan R. A model for computer-controlled delivery of 3-D conformal treatments. Med Phys. 1992;19:945.
11. Marks JE, Haus AG, Sutton HG, et al. The value of frequent treatment verification films in reducing localization error in the irradiation of complex fields. Cancer. 1976;37:2755.
12. Droege RT, Bjarngard BE. Influence of metal screens on contrast in megavoltage x-ray imaging. Med Phys. 1979;6:487.
13. Boyer AL, Antonuk L, Fenster A, et al. A review of electronic portal imaging devices (EPIDs). Med Phys. 1992;19:1.
14. Antonuk LE. Electronic portal imaging devices: a review and historical perspective of contemporary technologies and research. Phys Med Biol. 2002;47:R31.
15. Leszczynski KW, Shalev S, Ryder S. A study of efficacy of digital enhancement of on-line portal images. Med Phys. 1992;19:999.
16. Bijhold J, Gilhuijs GA, van Herk M. Automatic verification of radiation field shape using digital portal images. Med Phys. 1992;19:1007.
17. Munro P, Rawlinson JA, Fenster A. A digital fluoroscopic imaging device for radiotherapy localization. Int J Radiat Oncol Biol Phys. 1990;18:641.

18. Van Herk M, Meertens H. A digital imaging system for portal verification. In: Bruinvis IAD, van der Giessen PH, van Kleffens HJ, Wittkamper FW, editors. The use of computers in radiation therapy. Amsterdam: Elsevier Science; 1987. p. 371.
19. Meertens H, van Herk M, Bijhold J, et al. First clinical experience with a newly developed electronic portal imaging device. Int J Radiat Oncol Biol Phys. 1990;18:1173.
20. Antonuk LE, El-Mohri Y, Jee KW. Active matrix flat-panel imagers (AMFPIs) for electronic portal imaging. In: Hazel JD, Boyer AL, editors. Imaging in radiation therapy; American Association of Physicists in Medicine 1998 Summer School Proceedings. Madison: University of Wisconsin; 1998. p. 371.
21. Jaffray DA, Drake DG, Moreau M, et al. A radiographic and tomographic imaging system integrated into a medical linear accelerator for localization of bone and soft-tissue targets. Int J Radiat Oncol Biol Phys. 1999;45:773.
22. Yoo S, Kim GY, Hammoud R, et al. A quality assurance program for the on-board imager. Med Phys. 2006;33:4431.

10 Conformal Radiotherapy: Simulation and Contouring

10.1 Principles of Conformal Radiotherapy

In conventional radiotherapy, patient receives radiotherapy from either a single or a few beams. The radiation portal from each beam is manually drawn on the projected two-dimensional (2D) images, taken from a simulator. ***Conformal radiotherapy is different in design and delivery from conventional radiotherapy in the essential use of a CT scan configured for treatment planning to define tumour volume and shape treatment portals and in the use of beam shaping devices called multileaf collimators to obtain desired portal shapes to achieve critical organ sparing*** (Fig. 10.1a–c). Thus basically in conformal radiotherapy, the field is checked by CT scans, target volumes and OARs defined and beams positioned.

In 2DRT, all beams are aimed at a single point called the isocentre which is a representation of the point of intersection of the axis of rotation of the linear accelerator gantry head, the collimator assembly and the treatment couch. In case of conformal techniques like 3D-CRT and IMRT, planning the isocentre may not indicate the geometric centre of the tumour, and usually it reflects a point on the patient's anatomy in the treated area which is used as a marker for initial beam set-up. After planning CT is done with patient immobilized in treatment position, the treatment tumour volumes and normal organs are drawn or contoured on the CT images, and the radiation portals are then shaped to match the target volume and avoid as far as possible surrounding normal structures. Thus conformal therapy compared to conventional irradiation treatment planning involves complex processes of complete immobilization, beam shaping and achieving desired dose distribution by selection of beam directions with or without fluence modulation based on three-dimensional reconstruction from a simulation CT of the patient. These images are then projected forward as if in a beam's eye view (BEV) format and permit selection of beam directions with better avoidance of normal tissues (Fig. 10.2). Once this is done, computer-aided algorithms help in dose calculation and meeting plan objectives.

A. Mukherji, *Basics of Planning and Management of Patients during Radiation Therapy*, https://doi.org/10.1007/978-981-10-6659-7_10

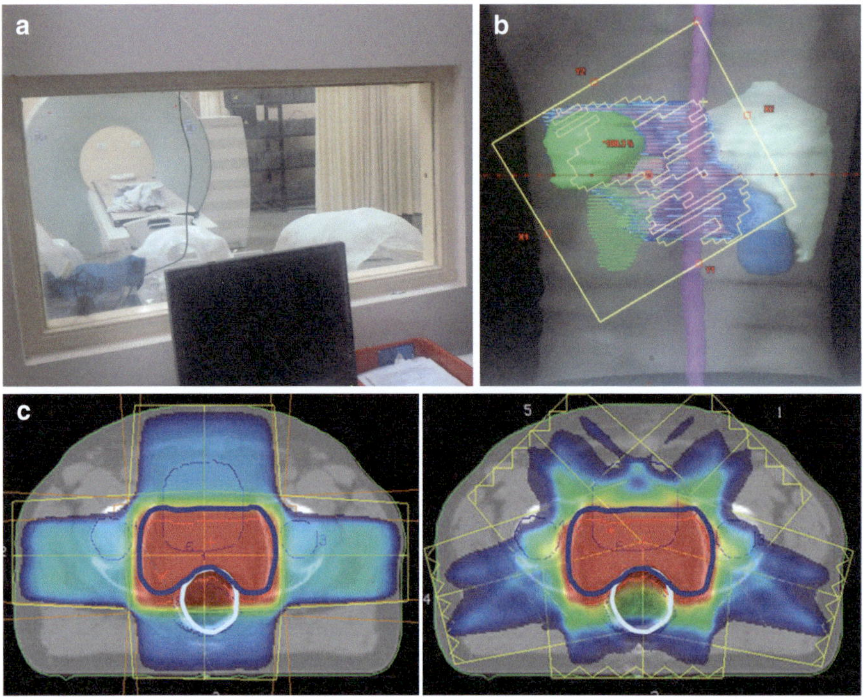

Fig. 10.1 (**a**) Console of a planning CT simulator used to define tumor volume and design treatment portals. (**b**) Use of planning CT to define tumor volume and design treatment portals. (**c**) Change in target coverage with 3DCRT and IMRT

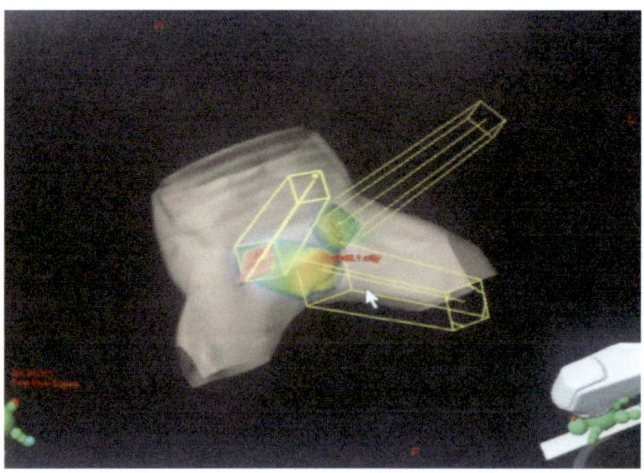

Fig. 10.2 Beam's eye view generated of tumor volume and normal structures

10.2 Treatment Process

The treatment planning steps broadly for both IMRT and 3D-CRT are similar with identical imaging and simulation in both techniques. IMRT is different compared to 3D-CRT only in plan optimization. The treatment planning process begins with "treatment simulation", which is done by taking a CT scan of the immobilized patient (by required device as explained in Chap. 8) in the treatment position and applying fiducial markers for identifying the targeted volume and isocentre. The obtained simulation images are then matched with the diagnostic MRI, PET or any functional imaging studies taken so as to define the target volume which has to be irradiated as well as identify and mark surrounding critical normal structures and tissue volumes to which dose avoidance needs to be done.

10.3 General Principles

The first step is decision of treatment position and simulation in that position. Proper immobilization device selection is a very important factor in the planning process and a must for an exact reproduction of the patient's position during simulation to aid precise treatment delivery as explained in Chap. 8. After simulation is done, the CT scan images of the patient are then transferred to a planning system following which the radiation oncologist then draws (or contours) using specialized software the various required target volumes as well as identifies and labels the surrounding normal critical organs and tissues. MRI, PET or PET/CT images taken during the initial diagnostic and staging work-up process can be used to identify extent of tumour and decide on the target volumes and can be merged with planning CT images to provide better soft tissue details or physiologic information. This entire process is called **contouring**, and once this is done, the radiation oncologist then provides a set of target volume and avoidance tissue *dose constraints* so as to achieve the desired prescription doses based on dose-volume cut-off limits to the contoured target and normal tissue volumes. After this, the physicists use these prescribed dose constraints in various permutations and computational algorithms by manual or computer-aided software using principles of beam direction, weightage and beam shaping and using beam modifiers as well as varying beam intensities to prepare a treatment plan which can be practically applied and which can optimally satisfy the given dose constraints.

In case of 3D-CRT planning, each beam direction, shape, weightage as well as intensity is manually applied by the physicist in consultation with the oncologist according to their experience. Once these objectives have been specified, the treatment planning software is used for estimating and assessing the resultant dose distribution. This dose distribution obtained is then assessed to see if the initial planning objectives and tissue constraints have been achieved; and if not, then the whole process is redone. In 3D-CRT, however, optimization refers to only adjusting beam angles, weightage, use of beam accessories like wedges or shape change with MLCs or even a slight change in intensity using field-in-field technique. Hence true optimization of dose distribution in the 3D-CRT process is limited in scope and does not include tine intense dose-volume calculations as well as beam intensity and beam positioning modulations seen in IMRT. This type of optimization is also called ***forward planning*** (FP).

In IMRT, there is variation of the radiation intensity or fluence within each beam. Basically this means that through computerized-aided algorithms, the number of electrons passing through unit area of the beam per unit time is varied across the cross section of the beam leading to creation of hundreds of ***pencil beamlets*** in a given field with varied dose distribution. The resulting accretion of the intensity modulations across all these beamlets results in a higher dose to the tumour with sparing of surrounding normal tissue. This intensity modulation can be achieved by the use of multileaf collimators (MLCs) which can alter a beam intensity profile across its width by programmed movements into or away from the middle of the portal or the use of multiple static beams which can be preprogrammed by computer for various shape alterations by MLCs or even continuous beam shape conformality by MLCs as the gantry moves in an arc. IMRT uses computerized iteration of radiation beams in which the computer performs a large number of iterations based on dose-volume criteria for various targets given by the oncologist [1]. After dose calculation, the radiation oncologist evaluates the plan with respect to dose constraints by analyzing prepared dose-volume histograms (DVHs) of the achieved dose distribution. If the achieved distribution matches or satisfies the initial planning constraints and is physically achievable on the patient, then such a plan is accepted, and the beam data and patient set-up coordinates as well as portal images and DRRs are then transferred to the linear accelerator and patient's treatment proceeds. During such high precision treatment, it is vital that the physicists perform regular and periodic dosimetric and quality assurance verification to verify accuracy and functionality of equipment and treatment plans.

10.4 Patient Set-Up, Immobilization and Simulation

Patient set-up and reproducibility are very important in conformal radiotherapy because reducing errors in patient set-up is essential in view of improved conformity of the dose distribution and tighter margins. Achieving reduction of errors in positioning and dose delivery is even more critical in IMRT since these plans have very sharp-dose gradients at the tumour volume, and normal tissue interfaces and any error can lead to either overdose to a critical structure or underdose the target volume [2].

Along with patient immobilizing verification with image guidance is done to ensure precise reproducibility of the patient's position and ensure accurate delivery. The first step is to acquire a treatment planning CT scan and is called CT simulation. CT simulation is performed with a spiral or helical CT scanner with volumetric data acquisition, laser localization system similar to treatment machine and a high-speed graphic workstation that emulates a treatment planning computer. The laser localization system permits marking the treatment isocentre with fiduciaries on the patient's skin, which is used for setting up the patient on treatment couch and as reference point for shift to planned treatment isocentre for the entire treatment. The CT image set is obtained with the patient in the treatment position on a flat couch which is geometrically identical to the couch on which the patient will be treated. In case of treatment of organs with significant motion like the lungs and liver, new CT scanners are capable of acquiring 4D-CT images, and digitally reconstructed fluoroscopy from 4D-CT allow radiation oncologists to measure the magnitude of the organ motion in any direction. If CT images are acquired in synchronization with the breathing cycle, the cine mode of CT images can be constructed into multiple breathing phases. To synchronize the CT acquisition with the patient's breathing cycle, a breathing sensor, either a belt attached to the patient's chest (stethograph) or an infrared sensor placed on the patient's chest, is needed.

In PET/CT simulation, a CT scan and a PET scanner are placed sequentially, and the patient is scanned by both lying on the same couch top in same position, after which the two images are transferred both as fused and separate images. The advantage of PET/CT simulation is that both the anatomical and physiological images are obtained, and the tumour mass as well as biologically active tumour can be identified. Direct PET/CT simulation avoids the additional planning CT acquisition and reduces the potential errors during image registration if a PET scan is done separately or in a nontreatment position [3]. For some cancer sites, MRI provides much better soft tissue contrast than CT images. MRI simulation can be desirable for reasons similar to the desirability of PET/CT. MRI scanners used in radiotherapy are open MRI simulators designed to set up the patient in the desired treatment position with the required immobilization device fastened on to the patient. The MRI scanner table can move longitudinally along a set of rails mounted on the floor and laterally on an orthogonal set of rails built in the couch. Vertical movement is by using a composite flat top with hard foam spacers beneath the patient. A set of three triangulation lasers (centre and laterals) is used for patient's positioning. Chen and colleagues [4] reported their clinical implementation using a 0.23-tesla (T) open MRI scanner in prostate cancer patients. They reported that with a low magnetic field of less than 0.5 T, the distortion caused by the inhomogeneity of the magnetic fields increases as the patient size increases. In spite of the reported advantages of MRI in soft tissue delineation and therefore in proper target volume contouring as well as avoidance of errors, the use of MRI for radiotherapy simulation and planning is still as a supplement to CT-based patient simulation rather than as a standalone technique because of several reasons. These include present designs of MRI simulators and their imposed limits on the use of patient immobilization devices and treatment positions, long imaging time and high possibility of patient developing claustrophobia, absence of bone signal which would prevent generating DRRs to compare with portal images for set-up verifications and a lack of electron density information for correcting dose calculation in cases where there is extensive tissue heterogeneity. In addition, accuracy of an MRI image can be significantly affected by geometrical artefacts and distortions which would then affect the accuracy of the treatment.

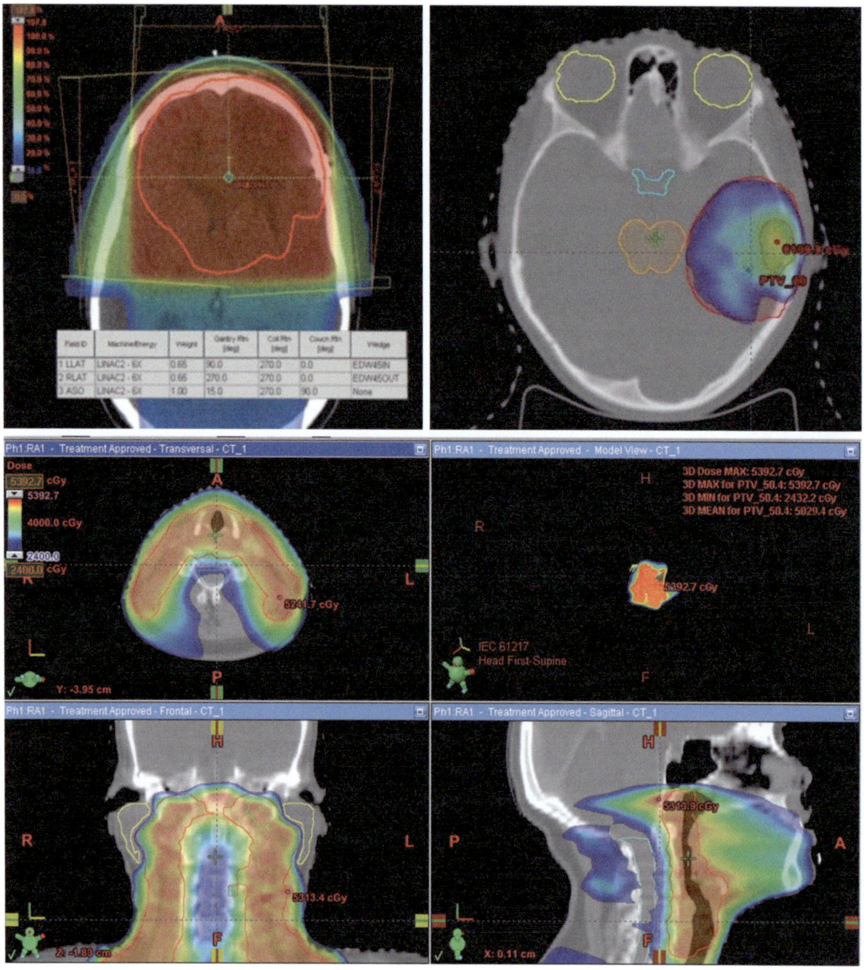

Fig. 10.3 Treatment planning using CT images

In most present planning systems, patient images can be acquired with both CT and MRI; target and normal tissue contouring especially in soft tissues is done by the MRI images which are then extrapolated onto the CT scan and checked for any distortion. Treatment planning is then done using the CT scan images (Fig. 10.3).

10.5 Contouring of Treatment Volume and Critical Organs

Treatment volumes in conformal radiotherapy are defined according to the ICRU Reports 50 and 62 as described in Chap. 9 [5, 6] with the gross target volume (GTV) defined as tumour extent identified by clinical examination and imaging; the clinical target volume (CTV) is the GTV along with areas at risk of microscopic extension of disease; and the planning target volume (PTV) is the CTV expanded to include set-up errors, patient motion, alignment errors and other uncertainties. In case of tumour motion, internal tumour volume includes magnitude of movement of the tumour.

The manual delineation of these target volumes and normal structures has to be done on each CT slice after which a 3D image is created by the computer. This process is time consuming and subject to large variations among users with some studies reporting as much as 25–30% variation. The Radiation Therapy Oncology Group and many other groups have tried to establish a consensus to minimize these variations, and many institutions use the RTOG contouring guidelines for target and normal tissue delineation [7, 8]. Many treatment planning systems now have software tools for automatic delineation of tissue structures, but these are presently only accurate for outlining external body contours and internal contours of very high contrast like the bone, lung and air cavities. Deformable image registration algorithms [9–12] have also been developed which permit the planner to map contours from a template case to a patient case with a similar tumour stage and site but different anatomic features. The deformable image registration tools are also useful for adaptive planning in patients with anatomic changes during radiotherapy. However the critical initial event is the correct identification of the GTV in which the human element plays a vital role. It is for this reason that MRI and PET images can also be factored in as they can provide useful information regarding soft tissue delineation between tumour and surrounding normal soft tissue (MRI) or between biologically active tumour tissue and rest of tumour mass (PET).

Contouring Principles: Contouring of target volumes and normal tissue structures is one of the most important sections of modern radiotherapy practice, and one that has been subjected to extensive research. Innovations in modern radiotherapy technology has enabled delivering a higher dose to the marked out target volumes with studies reporting improved local disease control and at the same time restricting as far as possible dose to surrounding critical structures by techniques such as IMRT or VMAT, thus possibly decreasing treatment morbidity. However these techniques are technology intensive and success of therapy depends on proper delineation of target volumes, proper correction of set-up and treatment delivery uncertainties in addition to extensive and regular quality control steps. These techniques therefore require optimal imaging modalities as well as proper dose prescription and plan evaluation with recommended dose-volume constraints. Checklists have to be prepared for each step of treatment planning so that in this complex technique with many repeating steps, no step is missed which could lead to serious consequences for the treated patient.

For patient simulation, contouring and treatment planning, contrast enhanced CT scanning is preferred by most planning systems as it allows dose calculation with corrections for tissue density inhomogeneity. Using contrast helps differentiating better between normal tissues and tumours. In addition to an initial imaging, it is also advisable to correct volumes during therapy with fresh simulation to conform the GTV to any tumour regression or change in patient's body contours. Also, there is a role for PET-based imaging using both FDG as well as hypoxic tissue markers for targeting biological pathways for radiation response (e.g. proliferation, hypoxia) [13]; the clinician can then identify and sub-volumes which would require additional dosage [14].

With modulated beam radiation therapy (IMRT/VMAT/tomotherapy), it is possible to obtain very highly conformal dose distributions for both target volumes coverage and critical organ sparing with the treated area shaped by contoured target and hence could be of almost any shape. It becomes therefore very important to ensure that there is a correct delineation of both target and organ at risk volumes, which should therefore be based on standard contouring atlases, recommendations or guidelines. Since these techniques involve contiguous areas of high and low doses, margins and contouring principles based on 2D planning would result in large areas of normal tissues getting significant dosage and would afford no benefit of dose sparing to normal tissues. On the other hand, restricting the target volumes with very close and tight margins and not allowing for physiological organ motion or set-up uncertainties would result in catastrophic geographic misses and would result in loss of any clinical benefit from using conformal dose delivery and dose escalation.

The first step in contouring is in the correct identification of the target volumes which is done through fusion of relevant imaging modalities (CECT/MR/PET) and the CT simulation image. The initial gross tumour volume (GTV) is defined. This GTV might be the only GTV to which an initial bigger margin for clinical target volume (CTV1) and planning target volume (PTV1) is added, followed by a smaller CTV2 and PTV2 for boost dose to the gross disease only. In many cases where chemotherapy has been given as in lymphomas and paediatric solid tumours, a pre-chemo and post-chemo GTV may need to be drawn. Similarly after surgery, a pre-op GTV and a post-op CTV2 (tumour bed) might be required for differential dose prescription. This is especially relevant in primary CNS tumours where different MR sequences are used to identify the GTV1 and GTV2 (T2 FLAIR for GTV1 and T1 for GTV2). Also in head and neck cancers, PET-based contouring helps in identifying areas requiring higher doses and guides boost therapy. In case of organs where there is significant internal motion, either inspiratory and expiratory CT images are taken and fused to obtain an ITV from the combined CTV, or the simulation is done in specific respiratory phase, contours are drawn accordingly and treatment is delivered in that phase also.

An accurate delineation of the tumour volume and critical organs is even more important in IMRT than in 3D-CRT because with inverse planning (IP) optimization these delineated contours are used for providing priorities in beam angle, target and normal tissue constraints to the computer optimization algorithm. Thus it is often necessary with inverse treatment planning in IMRT to contour many more normal tissues near or around the PTV that would not normally be contoured for 3D-CRT treatment planning. This is because once constraints have been given to the system for the contoured structures, other organs or structures which have not been contoured or constraints not provided may lie in regions receiving higher dose as the planning system tries to optimize both beam path placement as well as fluence patterns and avoids or tries to conform to the provided constraints while pushing higher doses through areas not delineated. For example, in a head and neck case, in addition to the commonly contoured structures in 3D-CRT planning like spinal cord and brainstem, it may also be necessary to contour the parotid glands, optic structures, the oral cavity, the mandible and inner ears; otherwise the optimization process will ignore these organs and deposit large doses to these volumes to meet dose constraints placed on other structures (Fig. 10.4).

A basic principle in IMRT/VMAT is that if an organ or volume is not delineated, it is not recognized by the planning system and no dose constraints can apply to it. Therefore it is extremely essential that the organs at risk (OARs) be correctly contoured and labelled as a first step in the contouring and beam placement process. In this regard, it would be useful to introduce the concept of "parallel" and "serial" organs as well as functional subunits (FSUs). This concept has been explained in more details in Chap. 21 Section D. Basically according to this concept, there are organs which have their FSUs in parallel units so that even if a few are damaged by

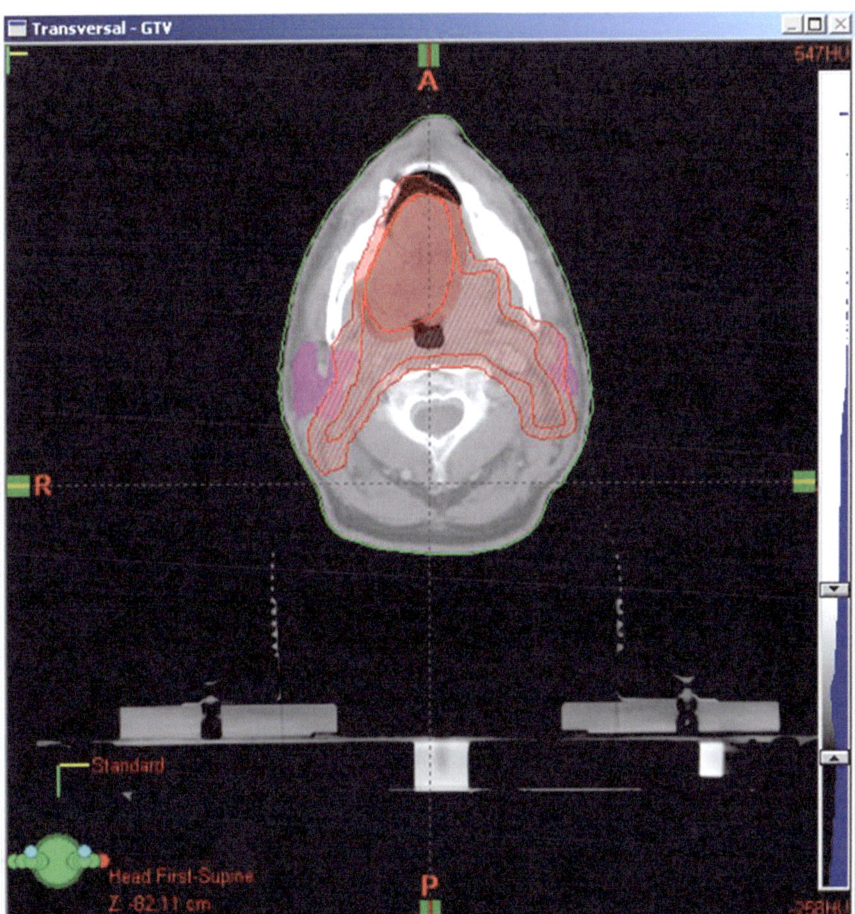

Fig. 10.4 Contouring of target volumes and OARs

irradiation, other units can take over their function provided the number of damaged units remain limited to organ tolerance limits. In organs with FSUs arranged serially one after another, loss of function of even one unit could affect the functions of those following the damaged unit. Therefore in both serial and parallel structures, the initial contouring should include the entire organ so that the dose to the entire FSU could be assessed. Additionally in serial organ, a planning organ at risk volume (PRV) should be contoured around the OAR so that a dose gradient can be created. Also the irradiated volume would include a large volume of normal connective or mucosal tissue which may not be a part of the CTV or any specific OAR. This volume of tissue expected to receive significant irradiation should also be delineated and named as remaining volume at risk (RVR). Identifying and applying dose-volume constraints to the RVR helps avoid high-dose regions outside CTV; and this dose could be used to assess risk of late effects, such as tissue fibrosis or carcinogenesis.

In case of soft tissue margins for CTV, the surrounding mucosa and structures have to be first delineated as OARs (e.g. parotids, mandible, oral mucosa, spinal cord, larynx, trachea, etc. for head and neck tumour). As a rule, one should draw all structures in their entirety to allow for correct dose-volume calculations. Based on tumour biology, margins are given by (a) adding to GTV through various “margin enhancement” tools in the planning system or (b) where such margin expansion is not possible (like neck nodes in head and neck cancers), Boolean operations are used to add various structures at risk to the fused GTV as a CTV. The CTV is then expanded to achieve the PTV by adding a margin for uncertainties. However one should remember at all times that while expanding target volumes to achieve CTV/PTV, one should not cross natural tissue boundaries which have not been breached by the tumour.

In cases where there is significant organ motion due to respiration, two CT simulations are done – one in inspiration and one in expiration. Two CTVs are drawn – an inspiratory and expiratory CTV which are then fused together to form the ITV (internal target volume). To this added a margin for uncertainties for getting a PTV. Also in cases where part of the PTV is overlapping with an OAR (e.g. PTVneck with parotid or PTVbrain with brainstem), the area of overlap should be first assessed whether the GTV itself is encroaching into the overlap area. Then priority for dose constraint has to be decided, whether it should be given for PTV (in case of parotid) or for brainstem (in case of brain tumours) in case the overlap is just because of PTV expansion. In case priority is given to PTV, then this overlap area will get much higher dose than the dose constraint for the rest of the OAR, skewing the DVH for that OAR and perhaps giving a false impression of a bad plan. In such cases, the overlap area has to be taken as separate structure, dose constraint followed for rest of OAR and final result obtained from the average of volume weighted median values of OAR free of overlap and that within overlap. For example, if 65% of parotid is out of PTV and 35% in overlap area, then plan should be generated where the 65% free parotid receives median dose of 26 Gy; and the overlap area receives at least 90% of dose prescribed to PTV (about 46 Gy). The final median dose would be [{26 Gy (×0.65) + 46 Gy (×0.35)}/2]. On the other hand if the priority is for the OAR, then the D_{max} of the PTV in the overlap area also has to conform to D_{max} of the OAR. For example, in cases of the CTV involving brainstem, the PTV is given constraints so that the D_{max} receives less than primary constraint (54 Gy), and point dose in overlap is less than secondary constraint (less than 1% receives less than 60Gy) [15]. Also in IMRT, it has to be remembered that there is up to a 10% loss of skin sparing with the use of beams which can enter tangentially as decided by the computer-aided algorithm and by the thermoplastic mask immobilization. This can be partially offset by contouring all target volumes 1–2 mm short of the skin, unless there is infiltration of the skin itself by tumour. This will allow up to 20–30% decrease in dose to the skin and sparing skin of higher grade reactions.

PET-Based Contouring: Once each organ at risk has been delineated along with the "planning organ at risk volume (PORV)" for serial structures, the GTV has to be correctly identified. Many centres now use PET-based contouring to identify (a) an anatomical GTV which comprises the anatomically visible tumour volume and (b) a biological target volume which is the physiologically active tumour identified using PET-based imaging which is separately contoured along with regular GTV (Figs. 10.5 and 10.6). Later a composite GTV is delineated based on the fusion of

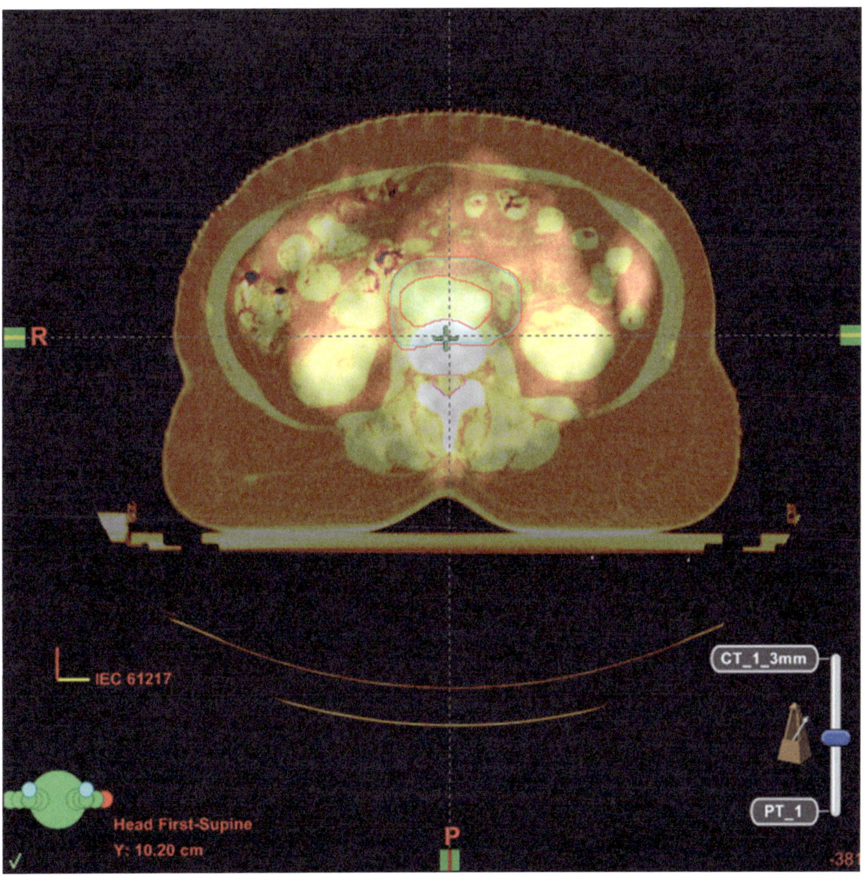

Fig. 10.5 PET based GTV contouring

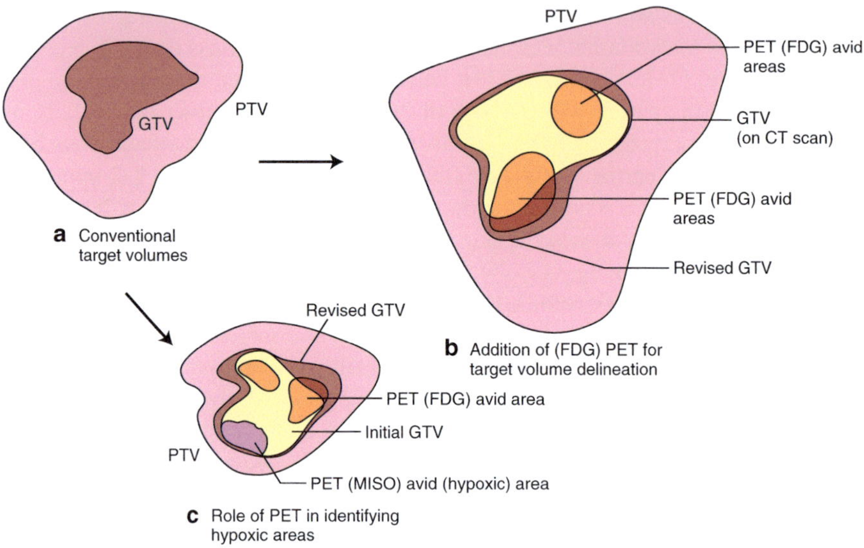

Fig. 10.6 Functional target volumes

the above two as well as grossly identified nodes (**fused GTV = GTV-T + biological GTV + GTV-N**). Once the GTV has been delineated, based on the disease site, stage and natural history, a clinical target volume is drawn. This includes the surrounding normal tissue expected to be at risk for subclinical disease as well regional nodes at risk for occult metastases.

10.6 Selection of Treatment Beams

Once the target volumes and the normal structures have been contoured, the system generates three-dimensional images for the whole body with the volumes contoured. Based on these beam placements, beam's eye view (BEV) images and digitally reconstructed radiographs (DRRs) are generated. Clinically, selection of beams is based on a combination of the treating physician's experience, protocols being followed, institutional experience and patient load as well as patient-specific anatomy.

3D-CRT: Beam orientations are chosen by observing the patient in BEV from various beam directions and selecting those directions for which the PTV appears to be best separated from the normal tissues [16, 17] (Fig. 10.2). Based on the planner's own experience, beams are place at various angles and dose distribution noted. This is a trial-and-error method in which a few iterations can be checked and the final beam placement angles and beam weightages chosen depending on the plan objectives being met. Both anatomical and dosimetric tolerances of the target and involved organs are taken into account for guiding the beam placement process.

IMRT: In general, IMRT fields with large fluctuations in intensity require higher velocities and accelerations of MLC leaves during beam delivery. Selection of optimum beam directions is often more critical when treating PTVs with a complex shape or where there is minimal separation between the PTV and a critical normal structure. Carefully selecting optimum beam directions in IMRT may also reduce the complexity of intensity profiles (i.e. the magnitude of intensity gradients within the field), thus improving delivery accuracy and efficiency. BEVD (beam's eye view-based dosimetry) objectively evaluates how good the beam placement is, and it has shown that the incorporation of the BEVD score in IMRT planning can improve selection of beam configuration [18–20].

Having explained the process of simulation, identification of various volumes and set-up of beams, we shall further examine the treatment planning and plan verification process in conformal radiotherapy.

10.7 Treatment Planning

Forward Planning: Forward treatment planning involves manual selection by the planner of the number of beams, their directions and shapes, inclusion or exclusion of dynamic wedges and the relative weightings of each beam shape. The computer then calculates the resultant dose distributions from these beam parameters. This is fundamentally different than inverse planning (IP) in which the human treatment planner specifies the desired dose constraints, and the computer calculates the required beam intensities and shapes to best meet the specified dose constraints. If the resultant dose distribution does not meet pre-planning objectives or is not physically achievable, the planner adjusts the beam intensities (or weights) and or field shapes and directions, and then the computer again calculate the dose distribution. This process, called manual optimization, is repeated by the planner until a dose distribution is obtained which satisfies the pre-planning delineated volume dose constraints and is physically achievable. The disadvantage of this method is the large amount of time taken; restriction of the quality of the plan as manually a large number of iterations may not be possible which the computer undertakes during optimization for IP. The advantage of FP is in its ability to produce a simple plan with a small-dose variation inside the tumour volume [21, 22]. In a study of treatment plans for breast irradiation, Mayo and colleagues [23] compared 3D-CRT plans with wedges to FP-IMRT, IP-IMRT and a hybrid of open fields and some IP fields. This study reported that the tangent-only IMRT plans, created with an IP method, resulted in the worst dose homogeneity inside the breast, the worst maximum dose outside the target and 2.3 times more monitor units (MUs) than the FP-IMRT plans.

10.8 Inverse Planning

Principle: Inverse planning as a technique in the treatment planning process was introduced by Brahme in 1988 [24]. In this technique, it is the computerized planning system which starts the optimization algorithm. The planner defines the beam directions, irradiated volumes, various contoured structures and their specific dose constraints as "priorities". The computer optimization algorithm starts this process of optimization by dividing each beam into many small "beamlets" and then sequentially through a process of permutations and combinations alters the beamlet intensities until a dose distribution is achieved which best conforms to the planned dose objectives. The next step in this process is to check the physical viability of this dose distribution; in which again the obtained optimized beam intensity distribution is correlated with the sequence of MLC leaf motions, beam positions as well as gantry positions that could achieve it most efficiently.

Optimization Priority: The first step in starting an IMRT planning process is the specification of the dose-volume constraints of both the target volumes and all organs at risk. The prescribed dose to the target, specified tolerance doses to normal tissues and weighting factors that reflect the importance of each tissue are designated as the constraints. A typical dose-volume constraint is described as *no more than q% of the particular organ may receive a dose greater than d.* These constraints can be:

- Mean or median doses (D_{mean}/D50).
- Dose received by 2 cm^3 vol (D2cm^3) or D1% (dose to 1% of volume) usually signifying maximum dose received by a volume (D_{max}).
- Maximal coverage of volume by dose prescribed (D95 or D98: meaning dose received by 95 or 98% volume).
- Volume receiving "*x*" dose usually 20 Gy in lung (V20) or V50, i.e. volume receiving 50 Gy.
- In case of brachytherapy; V90, V150 and V200 signify volumes receiving 90%, 150% and 200% of prescribed dose.

Thus dose constraints are the prescribed dose and allowable dose inhomogeneities to the PTV plus the dose limits to various sensitive structures, specified by the treatment planner to the IP computer system. For each volume also multiple such points can be defined with different penalties assigned to each point. DVH-type constraints, rather than a single dose limit, can also be assigned to the PTV. Once these constraints have been defined, the physicist then allots a priority number to the target volume. This can depend on shape, size of target as well as distance from normal structures and expected dose gradient. This priority or cost function is a mathematical definition of the "goodness" of a treatment plan, and the computer optimization algorithm attempts to minimize the cost function as it adjusts the beam weights from one iteration to the next. Objective functions (OFs) can be based on biologic criteria [25, 26] but are more often based on dose criteria [27–29]. The table below shows a typical priority setting for an IMRT plan based on ranges provided for doses and volumes (Table 10.1):

The numerical value of a dose-based OF is calculated from weighted average of the differences between delivered and prescribed doses for every voxel in every tissue defined in the treatment plan (i.e. the PTV plus all normal tissues for which a dose constraint has been specified) [27, 29, 30]. In the above table, for example, the PTV has been allowed a maximal point dose of 160 cGy extra from prescribed dose, while the lower limit expected to cover 95% of the volume has been prescribed a

Table 10.1 A typical priority distribution giving optimization objectives to the computer for dose distribution computation

Organ	Volume	Dose (cGy)	Priority
Kidney_Rt	Upper: 105%	2400	240
	Upper: 90%	2000	245
	Lower: 50%	1750	230
Spinal cord	Upper: 100%	4000	200
PTV	Upper: 102%	5200	250
	Mean: 50%	5040	240
	Lower: 95%	4750	250

dose of 4750 cGy. This means that the computer will try to generate plans which will deliver 4750 cGy to 95% of PTV and at same time restrict maximal PTV dose to below 5200 cGy – mean kidney dose to below 1750 cGy and maximal spinal cord dose to below 4000 cGy. Automation of the weighting factors in IP has been reported by Xing and colleagues [31]. The resultant treatment plan depends on the specification of these constraints. Extremely relaxed or restrictive constraints may lead computer optimization to produce an inferior plan. In particular, if specified dose constraints are physically impossible, the resultant inverse plan may be worse than a conventional plan.

To specify realistic dose constraints, users need to learn the relationship between the dose constraints and the resulting dose distributions for the specific IP system they are using and have familiarity with basic radiation dosimetric concepts. This learning process is one of trial and error, and once the treatment planner has gained this experience, it is possible to develop disease-specific templates as starting-point dose constraints for commonly treated tumour sites such as the prostate [32, 33], nasopharynx [34] and oropharynx [35].

10.9 Multileaf Collimators

Multileaf collimators or MLCs are specialized collimators used in conformal radiotherapy in addition to the primary and/or secondary collimators and help in:

(a) Field shaping and conforming, with these irregular fields, can be shaped as per beam's eye view of the target volume.
(b) Creating fluence variation across the beam or modulating the beam, by movement of the MLC across the field completely or partially according to a computer-optimized pattern, it can modulate the fluence across the beam.
(c) Acting as beam modifying devices especially as dynamic wedges; again by their planned movements across the beam, these MLCs can create a wedge effect.

The MLC can be installed within the accelerator gantry head either above the upper set of secondary collimator jaws or below the lower set of secondary collimator jaws as a tertiary collimator (Fig. 10.7). In commercially available designs from

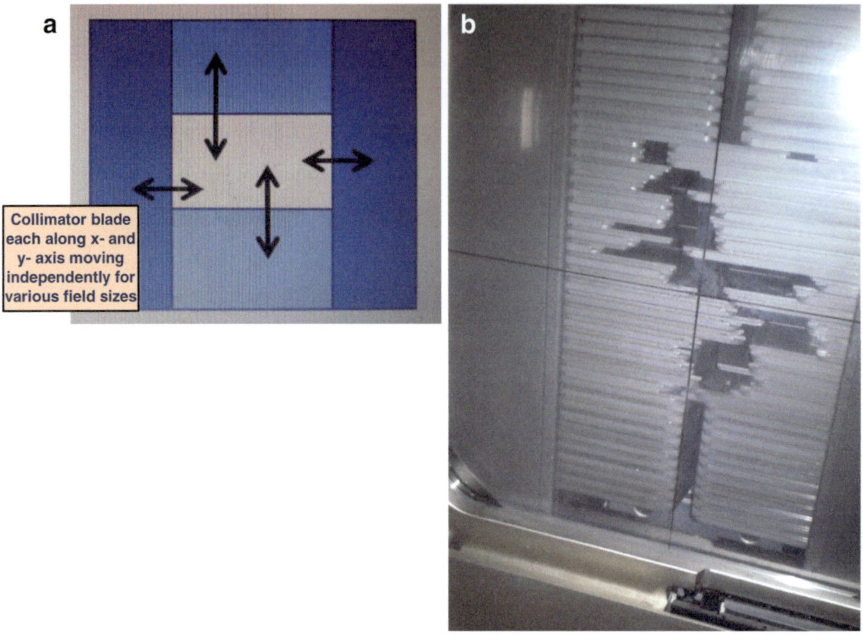

Fig. 10.7 Standard collimators and MLCs. (**a**) Standard collimators showing axis of blade movement for each of the collimator blades. (**b**) MLCs

the three major manufacturing companies, MLCs can replace the upper (Y) jaws and are augmented with an additional 3-cm thick Y jaw to reduce the radiation leakage from the MLC (Elekta) or can completely replace the lower (X) jaws (Seimens) or even can function as a tertiary collimator located below in addition to the conventional X and Y secondary collimators (Varian).

If MLCs are placed below both sets of secondary collimators, it is closer to the patient and improves the geometric penumbra but results in a physically larger device with less clearance between the MLC and the patient. If the MLC is above the secondary collimators, there is a poorer geometric penumbra, but MLC design is smaller and lighter with increased physical clearance between the accelerator head and the patient. Radiation leakage and transmission across the MLCs is minimized by reducing gaps between leaves by allowing adjacent leaves to slide smoothly across each other by cutting tongues and grooves into the sides of the leaves. In an MLC, one leaf has a side with a projected portion called the tongue, while the adjacent leaf has a corresponding depression called the groove. The two leaves lie adjacent to each other in such a way that the tongue of one leaf slides within the groove of the adjacent leaf; this is called ***tongue-and-groove effect*** (Fig. 10.8). This design reduces radiation leakage, but it also complicates treatment planning dose calculations because the transmission through any leaf depends on whether the beam passes through the tongue, the centre or the groove portion of the leaf. Thus two MLC shapes fit snugly into each other [36].

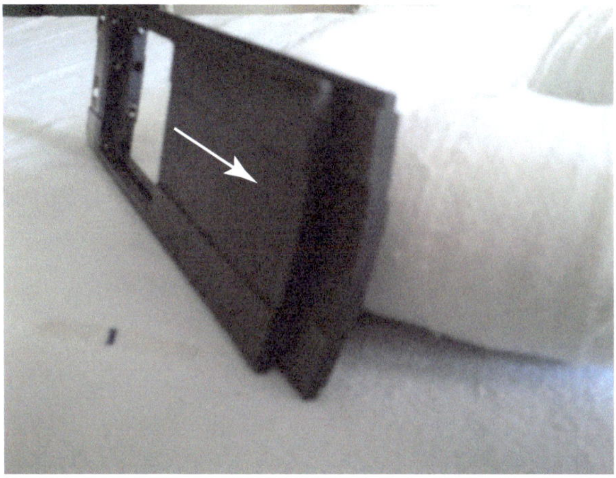

Fig. 10.8 MLCs with tongue and groove design (*arrow*)

Focussing of the MLC leaves to match beam divergence also has to be factored in during dose calculation. The width of each MLC leaf is designed to be slightly narrower at the side of the leaf facing the radiation source than that facing the patient. MLCs focused only in the *Y* direction are called single-focused MLCs while those focused in both *x*- and *y*-axes are called double-focused MLCs. Focussing of the MLC along *y*-axis is simpler with MLC being somewhat aligned like the secondary collimator with respect to the beam profile; but in case of focusing along *x*-axis, where the MLC has to move with leaf position, the divergence angle at the end of each leaf must be equal to the arc tangent of the ratio of the leaf position divided by the distance of the MLC from the source. This can be achieved by having the leaves move along a spherical surface centred at the radiation source.

The MLC leaves are made of tungsten alloy, and the leaf thickness is often referred to as the physical thickness. The leaf width is the width projected at the isocentre. The maximum possible field size for a single IMRT treatment field is a function of the number of leaves, projected leaf width and the distance that a leaf can travel past the field centre.

Generation of Leaf Motion Files: An optimum plan which matches all given constraints is still an abstract algorithm. To actualize this algorithm, two important conditions have to be fulfilled. One is the generation of actual leaf sequences for the multileaf collimator which would deliver the planned dos distribution, and the other is beam sequences or the gantry positions. These two conditions are the physical "actualities" which would ensure that the planned patient set-up and dose distribution can be actually achieved on the treatment couch.

Leaf sequencing is done by a computer-generated algorithm in the planning system that translates the beam intensity pattern produced by the IP system into an instruction set describing how to move the MLC leaves during beam delivery. There are thousands of possible sequences of leaf motions which can produce the desired intensity pattern, and depending on the delivery method, algorithms can minimize

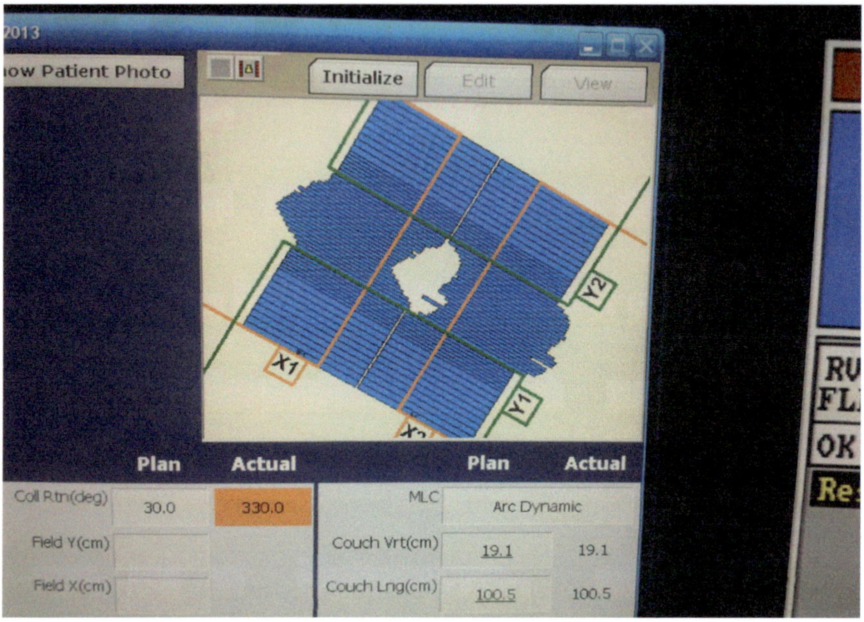

Fig. 10.9 Leaf movement of MLCs

the number of segments, the number of total MUs, the leaf travel distance and the total delivery time [37–40]. Leaf sequencing and dose delivery in an IMRT plan can be either *dynamic* or *static field*. Dynamic MLC dose delivery or also called sliding window technique delivers a constant intensity profile, where the leaf sequences keep changing to achieve planned fluence modulation during the entire time beam is "on". On the other hand, in static delivery (also called step-and-shoot), the gantry moves to each treatment position, leaf sequences changed as per position and plan and dose delivered; after which gantry is set to next position by the therapist.

The process of leaf sequencing [40] divides the intensity distributions into a number of one-dimensional "beamlet intensity profiles", with each pair of leaves accounting for a dose profile. Figure 10.9 shows the effect of leaf movement on the dose profile and delivery in sliding window IMRT. In this as the beam is turned on, both leaves of the multileaf collimator (MLC) move at different speeds at different points across the field. A point begins to receive irradiation when one leaf of the MLC moves past it opening the MLC sequence and continues to receive radiation until the other leaf blocks the beam. Thus by controlling the speed and pattern of movement of these leaves and therefore the "beam-on time" which is the time taken by each half of the MLC (right and left leaf), various patterns or distributions of fluence or beam intensity are obtained for all such points in the beam. The cumulative of these varying intensities across the beam is the basis of beam modulation.

Thus extrapolating the above principle for the multiple leaf pairs present in the gantry head, any desired intensity-modulation pattern can be produced with designed sequences of leaf positions. In the leaf sequences, each leaf pair delivers a different intensity profile, and hence the speed of each leaf and its position is individually controlled. For maximum efficiency to enable shortest treatment times, it is necessary to be able to move all leaves simultaneously and requires both leaf-speed modulation and dose-rate modulation. But in practice, not all desired intensity profiles are exactly achievable because of the constraints on leaf motion imposed by the design of the MLC and the clinical dose rate of the machine.

10.10 Static Versus Dynamic Multileaf Collimator Delivery

In ***static MLC-based IMRT***, the intensity pattern which is aimed for is achieved by breaking down the beam modulation sequence into a large number of segments either manually or with a computer program depending on whether the system used is forward or inverse planning; and the total numbers of these segments is in direct proportion to the field shape, size and complexity of treatment. During treatment delivery, treatment parameters associated with each segment are recorded and verified. The advantages of static or step-and-shoot IMRT are its simplicity of operation, nonnecessity to control the individual leaf speeds or delivery dose rate; intensity patterns for each field can be independently verified in case of treatment interruption, with fewer MUs required compared with DMLC delivery [41]. Disadvantages of static IMRT include a higher treatment time with its attendant problems of patient discomfort, lesser machine turnover time as well as higher risk of delivery error and a restriction in the available degrees of plan optimization iterations because of discrete segments utilized which may not be significant in routine cases but could cause a compromise in dose distribution for very complex cases.

In ***dynamic MLC delivery*** as explained before, the MLC leaves constantly move and change their opening-closing patterns even during radiation delivery which happens guided by a computer-generated algorithm. The advantage of this technique is that the varying or modulation of the intensity pattern occurs smoothly during treatment delivery thus ensuring a shorter treatment time, without repeatedly entering treatment room to reset the gantry angle and set-up verification, thus providing for less situation for creating errors. But this is achieved at a cost of extremely complex delivery mechanisms of leaf-speed and dose-rate modulation with very high wear and tear and an absolute necessity for accurate, regular and complex quality assurance to ensure there is absolute control of individual leaf speeds and avoiding any error in the calibration of leaf positions and gantry movements which could otherwise result in significant errors in delivered doses.

10.11 Delivery of Intensity-Modulated Treatment

Delivery of an FP 3D-CRT field is very similar to conventional treatment delivery except that plans often require an increased number of treatment fields. IMRT can be also delivered without use of computer-controlled MLCs. In this method, custom-designed 3D physical compensators are fabricated using a computer-controlled milling machine to cut either the compensator itself or a negative mold of the compensator to be filled with Cerrobend. This technique results in physical hardening of the beam, with increased scattered radiation, as well as skin doses and doses outside the field. But this method is technically capable of delivering dose distributions comparable to MLC-based beam delivery systems [42, 43].

IMRT delivered by using a computer-controlled MLC is more commonly followed and can be either by multiple static fields (called the step-and-shoot or sometimes the static field technique), dynamic fields (the sliding window technique) or by continuous arc therapy. All of these require computer-controlled MLCs, but while in arc and dynamic field, there is continuous movement of MLC leaves, while the radiation beam is on; in the step-and-shoot technique, after the dose from the first subfield is delivered, the beam is turned off, the field shape is reset by the MLC, the second incremental dose is delivered, and so on. Tomotherapy is another technique wherein a rotating fan beam is intensity-modulated with a bimodal MLC (each leaf pair has only two positions – completely open or completely closed). In a tomotherapy machine, a 6-MV fan beam X-ray source rotates around the patient, modulated by the opening and closing of MLC leaf pairs as a binary movement. Simultaneous with the beam rotation and MLC leaf movements, the treatment couch moves through the treatment gantry donut to facilitate 3D dose delivery. The small 6-MV photon fan beam rotates around the patient in synchrony with a translating treatment couch. Thus, the patient is treated with a spiral fan beam.

Intensity-Modulated Arc or Volumetric Arc Therapy: With gradual increase in experience in planning IMRTs, it was noted that there was an increase in the dose conformity when the number of fields used were increased as a higher number of fields provided for higher degrees of freedom of dose delivery and beam modulation but at the cost of increasing treatment times, complexity of treatments and integral body dose. A volumetric arc therapy with fluence modulation delivered with a conventional linear accelerator was proposed by Cedric Yu and colleagues in 1995 [44] and is called intensity-modulated arc therapy (IMAT). In this method, intensity-modulated beams are delivered continuously in an arc around the isocentre and are equivalent to multiple closely spaced beams delivering IMRT. A key feature of this type of intensity-modulated therapy is the continuous change in leaf positions with gantry angle to produce the shaped fields. Arc-based radiotherapy techniques are supposed to deliver the prescribed radiation dose to the target volume at the same time that the gantry is continuously revolving around the area to be treated with beam centre fixed at an isocentre and the MLC leaves continuously changing their patterns to achieve the planned beam modulation without any interruption of beam delivery. In these systems, there is variation during treatment delivery of both the dose rate and gantry speed yielding a greater degree of freedom for generation of conformal dose distribution. The resultant advantage of arc therapy over IMRT is a better coverage of target volume achieved with much shorter treatment time and reduction of MUs, which has the potential to reduce the probability of secondary cancer induced by increased total body dose.

The increased flexibility of iterations for dose distributions in an arc therapy plan is not always practically possible as there may be restrictions on some MLC leaf positions because the continuous gantry rotational movements may not allow certain MLC position changes. This limitation in the benefit of using arc therapy can be overcome by using multiple arcs either in coplanar or noncoplanar setting; however, this is again at a cost of an increased treatment time with its associated risk of increased error of delivery. Additionally in arc therapy, the optimization process of dynamic gantry motion is done by a random sampling of gantry directions and MLC leaf positions which are basically an estimate of the gantry angle and MLC pattern at a certain time point during treatment delivery; and multiple such samples are taken to approximate a continuous gantry and MLC motion. These samples are optimized at 5°–10° gantry angle increments with MLC leaf positions variation of up to 2–4 cm and could result in increased dose computation errors, because a sampling of 1° and 0.5 cm for gantry rotation and MLC leaf motions, respectively, could result in up to 5% of the volume receiving a dose error of around 3%. Ma and colleagues have recently proposed an IMAT IP algorithm with incorporation of BEVD information [45]. Instead of setting the initial weight of a beam arbitrarily, precomputed BEVD is adopted as the initial weight of the corresponding beam. The BEVD-guided optimization significantly improves the computational efficiency and the plan quality.

Direct Aperture-Based Optimization (DAO): Standard pixel-based or fluence-based inverse optimization usually creates complex IMRT plans, prolonging the treatment time and increasing the number of MUs [46]. This increase in the number of monitor units or the beam-on time would as a result cause increased leakage and scattered radiation adversely affecting the accuracy of treatment delivery [47]. Additionally the increased integral body dose caused by a larger volume of the body receiving smaller doses may result in a higher risk of development of radiation-induced secondary malignancies as has been reported in many studies that changing from 3D-CRT to an IMRT treatment plan nearly doubled occurrence of secondary cancers at 10 years from 1 to 1.75% [48]. During leaf sequencing, the computer program may generate many subfields to avoid significant deviation from the initially optimized plan. The use of these subfields in IMRT plans significantly reduces overall efficiency and may introduce additional dosimetric errors. Various techniques such as increasing number of leaf sequencers [40, 48–51] and the use of smoothing filters to eliminate unnecessary noise inside the intensity profiles [52, 53] have been tried but with limited success in an attempt to simplify IMRT plans and to improve delivery and irradiation efficiency.

A technique called direct aperture optimization (DAO) is now used, especially in arc IMRT, in which there is a single step optimization process to account for both contoured volume priorities and optimizing leaf positions rather than the initial algorithm of prioritizing weights given to contoured structures followed by leaf sequencing and optimization. This process is computer software controlled and directly optimizes both priorities and leaf positions with a predetermined number of MLC shapes for each beam [54–56]. In a study, Shepard and colleagues [55] reported that there was significant reduction of both the number of segments and the number of MUs with DAO compared to two-step traditional method, and highly conformal IMRT plans with five or less apertures per beam angle were obtained.

Ludlum and Xia [57] compared pixel-based two-step optimization and direct aperture-based one-step optimization. They reported that direct aperture-based one-step optimization resulted in improved plan quality, compared with pixel-based two-step optimization in IMRT plans similar in complexity, and concluded that one-step DAO is more effective in simplifying IMRT plans, reducing errors and treatment times. In day-to-day use, DAO is usually used in arc IMRT.

Dose Calculation Algorithms: A few considerations are kept in mind during dose calculation for an IMRT plan.

1. In 3D-CRT treatments, dose calculation is by conventional methods taking into consideration beam shapes, treatment depths, beam weightages and the use of any beam modifying devices.
2. During IMRT treatment delivery, only a portion of the entire field is exposed at any given time. Therefore the total beam-on time (or MUs) required can be two to four times longer than for conventional treatments [46].
3. The more complex the intensity modulation, the more are the MUs required.
4. Factors such as variable-beam transmission through rounded leaf ends or through tongues and grooves of the MLCs must be more accurately accounted for with IMRT.
5. Overall leakage through MLC leaves can also amount to several percent of the total IMRT dose compared to less than 1% for conventional treatments.
6. The variable field sizes during IMRT beam delivery can also complicate calculation of the output factor because of the effect of the collimator scatter is more marked compared to conventional treatment [58].

The Monte Carlo (MC) method can provide the most accurate dose calculation but has a lengthy computation time and requires faster computer speed. This method was developed at Memorial Sloan-Kettering Cancer Center [59] and entails calculation of pencil beams or dose kernels to describe the transport of photons and electrons in homogeneous and inhomogeneous media. In this dose model, inhomogeneity effects are accounted for by the method of equivalent path length, and pencil-beam convolution is used only as a correction factor to explain any variation of intensity relative to a flat, uniform field [59]. But this method may not be accurate with extremely high inhomogeneities like an air-tissue interface in lung tissue.

Planning Aims for IMRT: The aims for planning an intensity-modulated dose delivery include:

- Defining the dose in the PTV including the build-up region if PTV extends outside the body contour
- To limit dose to the critical normal structures contoured within the prescribed parameters
- Prioritize between any overlapping volumes and conflicting absorbed dose objectives
- Taking care of any unexpected region of the remaining volume at risk (RVR) receiving a high dose

After the beam angles have been optimized and dose constraints put as objective functions for dose optimization, the computer algorithm works out a set of beam angles and intensity-modulation patterns to best achieve the dose constraints. This is then viewed by the planner in the form of DVHs and dose colour washes or isodose lines. However in many situations, the classical optimal-dose patterns seen for IMRT may be difficult to achieve, especially in cases when the CTV-to-PTV margin reaches the skin surface. In such a situation, a part of the PTV can extend into the build-up region of incident photon beams or even into the surrounding air (so-called in-air PTV). This commonly occurs in treatment of the head and neck cancers with neck nodes where clear spatial separation between the superficial extent of the node and the skin/thermoplastic mask may be sometimes difficult or may be too close for steep dose gradients.

PTV-in-Air and Dose in Build-Up Region: An important consideration during the demarcation of the PTV is the extent of the PTV volume which is outside the body contour, i.e. the PTV-in-air. This is frequently caused by adding a defined margin to the CTV even when the CTV is close to the skin (e.g. in breast or head and neck patients). While theoretically this is correct because the PTV is basically a margin added to the CTV to account for set-up errors or positional changes during treatment, this situation could lead to a problem in dose calculation. This is because most algorithms in treatment planning systems cannot accurately calculate this dose in the "PTV-in-air" or build-up region in the regions of the PTV close to or outside the patient's outline causing erroneous readings. As a result there is increased dose inhomogeneity if standard constraints are used resulting in very high D_{max} in this area or at junctional area if maintenance of coverage is tried for 95–98% of prescribed dose. On the other hand, if the D_{max} is brought down to less than 105%, then it is seen that the PTV coverage goes down to 90–92% of prescribed dose. Removing the part of this PTV-in-air or creating a calculation PTV (PTVevl) by limiting it within the skin by cropping the volume of PTV outside skin can avoid optimizing of absorbed dose in air. But this creates a situation of false "skin sparing" and can lead to underdosing areas involved by the tumour just below the skin especially in head and neck cancers where frequently in advanced cases dose is planned to be "flashed" on skin. If this under-dosage of the target volume affects even the CTV, then it is clinically unacceptable and a bolus needs to be applied. However if the under-dosage in this junctional or build-up area below the skin is clinically acceptable (i.e. there is no risk of missing microscopic or gross tumour) but there is risk of dose variability because of positional errors, the PTV can be further divided into various sub-volumes (SVs) and that particular sub-volume of PTV which is in the build-up area can have a more relaxed dose-volume constraint, while higher coverage of dose for other sub-volumes can be indicated. Finally if it is accepted by the clinician, the physicist could relax dose constraints for the entire PTV volume to avoid a high D_{max}. But the main fault in this method is that the lower coverage can occur over any part of the PTV and not necessarily in build-up region, and this would negate all benefits of inverse planned treatments if high-dose coverage is not achievable.

PTV and OAR/PORV Overlap: As explained before in the section on contouring, a PORV is usually added to an OAR and especially a serial-type OAR to allow for a dose gradient to occur between an adjacent PTV and the OAR and at the same time meet OAR constraints. This prevents large differences in dose constraints between the PTV and adjacent OAR which would otherwise have led to either a decreased dose in PTV or high dose in OAR. However sometimes it is not unusual to have the PTV extend inside the PORV of the OAR, or the two separate PTVs overlapping at some point, such as in the PTV and parotid volume interface where overlapping can occur. This can lead to a conflict in the dose optimization process where different volumes with different constraints are overlapping. One way of solving this issue can be by further dividing the two adjacent volumes into subdivisions of each without the overlapping part and the overlapped area as a separate sub-volume. New constraints could then be given individually to each subdivision. Another method used is to choose priority of one volume over the other in the overlapped area and relax the dose constraints according to the volume priority chosen. This is done to either control the dose deficit in the overlapped PTV area or decrease the extra dose in the overlapped OAR area or even both. It is also possible to apply both of the above methods in the same planning process, but it is important to decide beforehand the priority ranking while deciding objective functions (OFs).

PTV and RVR: A basic rule of IMRT planning is that the computer recognizes only those areas which have been demarcated and for which dose constraints have been decided. Any other tissue even if anatomically or physiologically important will not be recognized. During the process of beam definition and dose distribution, the computer will therefore only recognize areas with constraints which have been so delineated while it will use the non-demarcated areas to deliver doses required to achieve the desired dose distribution. This can result in areas such as the back of the neck which while not having any defined structure with dose constraint receiving high doses. This can lead to severe postirradiation effects such as tissue fibrosis or even skin breakdown. This can be prevented by designating these undefined areas as the RVR or ***remaining volume at risk***. This volume is also considered an additional structure, and a dose constraint is defined for this area (usually 50–70% of prescribed dose). The main aim in defining this volume and prescribing a constraint for it is to avoid beam hot spots in this volume.

Plan Evaluation and Improvement: After a treatment plan has been generated, it has to be then evaluated to assess if it meets all the constraints provided. For this knowledge of dose tolerance and the limiting volume that is safe for each organ has to be factored. For example, a volume of more than 20 Gy for a healthy lung was found to be associated with increased incidence of pneumonitis [60, 61]. A mean dose of more than 26 Gy [62, 63] to the parotid glands is associated with the xerostomia. The tools used for plan evaluation are similar for 3D-CRT and IMRT. This section gives a general view of the evaluation process and will be covered in detail in Chap. 6 subsequently. Evaluation tools include:

- 2D dose distributions superimposed on CT images (dose isodoses or dose colour washes)
- 3D volumetric or dose distribution colour-washes overlaid on the PTV and critical organs.

- Structure-specific DVHs and structure-specific endpoints such as mean and maximal doses as well as dose-volume cut-offs
- Biologic indices like equivalent uniform dose (EUD) [64, 65], a tumour control probability (TCP) or a normal tissue complication probability (NTCP) [66–69]

3D-CRT Plan Evaluation: The plan derived is evaluated based on the field placement, beam weightages, use of any beam modifying devices, dose distribution inside target volume and critical normal structures, dose volume histograms as well as beam's eye view of target volume. Any deficiencies present are identified and corrected as far as possible. The effort-intensive nature of this approach limits the practical number of iterations of evaluation and alteration.

IMRT Plan Evaluation: In IMRT plans, inspection of the intensity profiles is often useful for evaluating an individual beam's contribution to the dose distribution. Inspection of beam intensity distributions can be made using an "observer's view" or by the projection of "isointensity" lines on a BEV. This inspection can prevent gross mistakes such as unintended tumour volume accidentally depicted on the planning CT, which a computer would faithfully treat as a part of the tumour volume. As described above, plan evaluations can be done either ***biologically*** with estimation of TCP or NTCP or EUD or ***physically*** with DVH or evaluating dose washes or dose statistics.

Improving an unacceptable IMRT plan can be difficult as one usually does not know whether the deficiency is because of inappropriately chosen beams, dose volume constraints or penalties. Also in inverse planning, the relationship between changes made to dose constraints and the resultant changes to the ensuing dose distribution are difficult to predict. Sometimes plan changes cannot be possible even by repeated iterations to even reviewed constraints and techniques such as converting a region of high dose to a structure and then giving fresh dose constraints to that structure might result in better dose distribution.

Similarly, dividing normal tissues into areas expected to receive higher doses such as those lying next to or within PTV and giving less stringent dose constraints than have been assigned to the rest of the structure may permit the optimization algorithm to find a better plan. These methods are used because DVH-based OFs do not take into account the spatial distribution of "hot" or "cold" dose regions.

Verification of IMRT Plans: Verification of IMRT treatment plans entails use of independent MU and fluence map calculations for assurance of IMRT delivery [70–72]. In a computer-based approach, instead of using an ionization chamber or radiographic films to actually perform the dosimetric measurements, the treatment is simulated on a computer, and dosimetric quantities, such as the spatial doses or fluence maps, are calculated.

In a general algorithm developed by the Stanford group [71] for fluence map calculation, the software first takes into account the MLC leaf sequence obtained for generating a dose distribution which is then used to generate a fluence pattern called a map. This generated "fluence map" is compared with the desired fluence pattern obtained from the TPS. Thus the basic idea of this test is to obtain standardized leaf sequences which are used to obtain desired fluence patterns and can help simplify therapy by eliminating the need to do a QA for every treatment field.

References

1. Xing L, et al. Physics of intensity modulated radiation therapy. In: Mundt AJ, Roeske JC, editors. Intensity modulated radiation therapy: a clinical perspective. Hamilton & London: BC Decker Inc.; 2005. p. 20–52.
2. Xing L, et al. Dosimetric effects of patient displacement and collimator and gantry angle misalignment on intensity modulated radiation therapy. Radiother Oncol. 2000;56:97–108.
3. Hwang AB, et al. Can positron emission tomography (PET) or PET/computed tomography (CT) acquired in a nontreatment position be accurately registered to a head-and-neck radiotherapy planning CT? Int J Radiat Oncol Biol Phys. 2009;73(2):578–84.
4. Chen L, et al. MRI-based treatment planning for radiotherapy: dosimetric verification for prostate IMRT. Int J Radiat Oncol Biol Phys. 2004;60(2):636–47.
5. International Commission on Radiation Units and Measurements, (ICRU). Prescribing, recording, and reporting photon beam therapy. International Com-mission on Radiation Units and Measurements, ICRU Report 50, ICRU, Bethesda; 1993.
6. International Commission on Radiation Units and Measurements, (ICRU). Prescribing, recording, and reporting photon beam therapy (Supplement to ICRU Report 50). ICRU Report 62, ICRU, Bethesda; 1999.
7. Myerson RJ, et al. Elective clinical target volumes for conformal therapy in anorectal cancer: a Radiation Therapy Oncology Group consensus panel contouring atlas. Int J Radiat Oncol Biol Phys. 2008;74(3):824–30.
8. Gregoire V, et al. CT-based delineation of lymph node levels and related CTVs in the node-negative neck: DAHANCA, EORTC, GORTEC, NCIC, RTOG consensus guidelines. Radiother Oncol. 2003;69(3):227–36.
9. Chao M, et al. Automated contour mapping with a regional deformable model. Int J Radiat Oncol Biol Phys. 2008;70:5599–608.
10. Chao M, et al. Automated contour mapping using sparse volume sampling for 4D radiation therapy. Med Phys. 2007;34:4023–9.
11. Kashani R, et al. Objective assessment of deformable image registration in radiotherapy: a multi-institution study. Med Phys. 2008;35(12):5944–53.
12. Wang H, et al. Implementation and validation of a three-dimensional deformable registration algorithm for targeted prostate cancer radiotherapy. Int J Radiat Oncol Biol Phys. 2005;61(3):725–35.
13. Ling CC, Humm J, Larson S, et al. Towards multidimensional radiotherapy (MD-CRT): biological imaging and biological conformality. Int J Radiat Oncol Biol Phys. 2000;47:551–60.
14. Frank SJ, Chao KS, Schwartz DL, et al. Technology insight: PET and PET/CT in head and neck tumor staging and radiation therapy planning. Nat Clin Pract Oncol. 2005;2:526–33.
15. Bentzen SM, Constine LS, Deasy JO, Eisbruch A, Jackson A, Marks LB, Ten Haken RK, Yorke ED. Quantitative analyses of normal tissue effects in the clinic (QUANTEC): an introduction to the scientific issues. Int J Radiat Oncol Biol Phys. 2010;76:S36–41.
16. Goitein M, et al. Multidimensional treatment planning. II: beam's eye view, back projection and projection through CT sections. Int J Radiat Oncol Biol Phys. 1983;9:789–97.
17. McShan DL, Fraass BA, Lichter AS. Full integration of the beam's eye view concept into computerized treatment planning. Int J Radiat Oncol Biol Phys. 1990;18:1485–94.
18. Pugachev A, et al. Role of beam orientation optimization in intensity-modulated radiation therapy. Int J Radiat Oncol Biol Phys. 2001;50(2):551–60.
19. Pugachev A, Xing L. Computer assisted beam orientation selection in IMRT. Phys Med Biol. 2001;46:2467–76.
20. Schreibmann E, Xing L. Dose-volume based ranking of incident beam direction and its utility in facilitating IMRT beam placement. Int J Radiat Oncol Biol Phys. 2005;63(2):584–93.
21. Vicini FA, et al. Optimizing breast cancer treatment efficacy with intensity-modulated radiotherapy. Int J Radiat Oncol Biol Phys. 2002;54(5):1336–44.

22. Kestin LL, et al. Intensity modulation to improve dose uniformity with tangential breast radiotherapy: initial clinical experience. Int J Radiat Oncol Biol Phys. 2000;48(5):1559–68.
23. Mayo CS, Urie MM, Fitzgerald TJ. Hybrid IMRT plans—concurrently treating conventional and IMRT beams for improved breast irradiation and reduced planning time. Int J Radiat Oncol Biol Phys. 2005;61(3):922–32.
24. Brahme A. Optimization of stationary and moving beam radiation therapy techniques. Radiother Oncol. 1988;12:129–40.
25. Bortfeld T, et al. Physical vs. biological objectives for treatment plan optimization. Radiother Oncol. 1996;40(2):185–7.
26. Brahme A. Optimized radiation therapy based on radiobiological objectives. Semin Radiat Oncol. 1999;9(1):35–47.
27. Bortfeld T. Optimized planning using physical objectives and constraints. Semin Radiat Oncol. 1999;9(1):20–34.
28. Shou Z, et al. Quantitation of the a priori dosimetric capabilities of spatial points in inverse planning and its significant implication in defining IMRT solution space. Phys Med Biol. 2005;50(7):1469–82.
29. Xing L, Chen GTY. Iterative algorithms for inverse treatment planning. Phys Med Biol. 1996;41(2):2107–23.
30. Webb S. Intensity-modulated radiation therapy. Series in Medical Physics. Bristol and Philadelphia: Institute of Physics Publishing; 2000.
31. Xing L, et al. Optimization of importance factors in inverse planning. Phys Med Biol. 1999;44(10):2525–36.
32. Chan LW, et al. Proposed rectal dose constraints for patients undergoing definitive whole pelvic radiotherapy for clinically localized prostate cancer. Int J Radiat Oncol Biol Phys. 2008;72(1):69–77.
33. Odrazka K, et al. Comparison of rectal dose-volume constraints for IMRT prostate treatment planning. Phys Med. 2005;21(4):129–35.
34. Xia P, et al. A study of planning dose constraints for treatment of nasopharyngeal carcinoma using a commercial inverse treatment planning system. Int J Radiat Oncol Biol Phys. 2004;59(3):886–96.
35. Hunt MA, et al. Geometric factors influencing dosimetric sparing of the parotid glands using IMRT. Int J Radiat Oncol Biol Phys. 2006;66(1):296–304.
36. Sykes JR, Williams PC. An experimental investigation of the tongue and groove effect for the Philips multileaf collimator. Phys Med Biol. 1998;43(10):3157–65.
37. Bortfeld TR, et al. X-ray field compensation with multileaf collimators. Int J Radiat Oncol Biol Phys. 1994;28(3):723–30.
38. Galvin JM, Chen XG, Smith RM. Combining multileaf fields to modulate fluence distributions. Int J Radiat Oncol Biol Phys. 1993;27(3):697–705.
39. Spirou SV, Chen-Shou C. Generation of arbitrary intensity profiles by combining the scanning beam with dynamic multileaf collimation. Med Phys. 1996;23(1):1–8.
40. Xia P, Verhey LJ. Multileaf collimator leaf sequencing algorithm for intensity modulated beams with multiple static segments. Med Phys. 1998;25(8):1424–34.
41. Chui CS, et al. Delivery of intensity-modulated radiation therapy with a conventional multileaf collimator: comparison of dynamic and segmental methods. Med Phys. 2001;28(12):2441–29.
42. Chang SX, et al. Compensators: an alternative IMRT delivery technique. J Appl Clin Med Phys. 2004;5(3):15–36.
43. Chang SX, et al. A comparison of different intensity modulation treatment techniques for tangential breast irradiation. Int J Radiat Oncol Biol Phys. 1999;45(5):1305–14.
44. Yu CX, et al. A method for implementing dynamic photon beam intensity modulation using independent jaws and a multileaf collimator. Phys Med Biol. 1995;40(5):769–87.
45. Ma Y, et al. Beam's-eye-view dosimetrics guided inverse planning for aperture modulated arc therapy. Int J Radiat Oncol Biol Phys. 2009;75:1587–95.

46. Galvin JM, et al. Implementing IMRT in clinical practice: a joint document of the American Society for Therapeutic Radiology and Oncology and the American Association of Physicists in Medicine. Int J Radiat Oncol Biol Phys. 2004;58(5):1616–34.
47. Mohan RA, et al. The impact of fluctuations in intensity patterns on the number of monitor units and the quality and accuracy of intensity modulated radiotherapy. Med Phys. 2000;27(6):1226–37.
48. Hall EJ, Wuu CS. Radiation-induced second cancers: the impact of 3D-CRT and IMRT. Int J Radiat Oncol Biol Phys. 2003;56(1):83–8.
49. Crooks SM, et al. Minimizing delivery time and monitor units in static IMRT by leaf-sequencing. Phys Med Biol. 2002;47(17):3105–16.
50. Langer M, Thai V, Papiez L. Improved leaf sequencing reduces segments or monitor units needed to deliver IMRT using multileaf collimators. Med Phys. 2001;28(12):2450–8.
51. Siebers JV, et al. Incorporating multi-leaf collimator leaf sequencing into iterative IMRT optimization. Med Phys. 2002;29(6):952–9.
52. Chui C-S, et al. A simplified intensity modulated radiation therapy technique for the breast. Med Phys. 2002;29(4):522–9.
53. Sun X, Xia P. A new smoothing procedure to reduce delivery segments for static MLC-based IMRT planning. Med Phys. 2004;31(5):1158–65.
54. Bedford JL, Webb S. Constrained segment shapes in direct-aperture optimization for step-and-shoot IMRT. Med Phys. 2006;33(4):944–58.
55. Shepard DM, et al. Direct aperture optimization: a turnkey solution for step-and-shoot IMRT. Med Phys. 2002;29:1007–18.
56. Van Asselen B, et al. Intensity-modulated radiotherapy of breast cancer using direct aperture optimization. Radiother Oncol. 2006;79(2):162–9.
57. Ludlum E, Xia P. Comparison of IMRT planning with two-step and one-step optimization: a way to simplify IMRT. Phys Med Biol. 2008;53(3):807–21.
58. Wang X, et al. Dosimetric verification of intensity-modulated fields. Med Phys. 1996;23(3):317–27.
59. Chen-Shou C, LoSasso T, Spirou S. Dose calculation for photon beams with intensity modulation generated by dynamic jaw or multileaf collimations. Med Phys. 1994;21(8):1237–44.
60. Jin H, et al. Dose-volume thresholds and smoking status for the risk of treatment-related pneumonitis in inoperable non-small cell lung cancer treated with definitive radiotherapy. Radiother Oncol. 2008;91(3):427–32.
61. Yom SS, et al. Initial evaluation of treatment-related pneumonitis in advanced-stage non-small-cell lung cancer patients treated with concurrent chemotherapy and intensity-modulated radiotherapy. Int J Radiat Oncol Biol Phys. 2007;68(1):94–102.
62. Murdoch-Kinch CA, et al. Dose-effect relationships for the submandibular salivary glands and implications for their sparing by intensity modulated radiotherapy. Int J Radiat Oncol Biol Phys. 2008;72(2):373–82.
63. Eisbruch A, et al. Xerostomia and its predictors following parotid-sparing irradiation of head-and-neck cancer. Int J Radiat Oncol Biol Phys. 2001;50(3):695–704.
64. Niemierko A. Reporting and analyzing dose distributions: a concept of equivalent uniform dose. Med Phys. 1997;24(1):103–10.
65. Park CS, et al. Method to account for dose fractionation in analysis of IMRT plans: modified equivalent uniform dose. Int J Radiat Oncol Biol Phys. 2005;62(3):925–32.
66. Lyman JT. Complication probability as assessed from dose volume histograms. Radiat Res. 1985;8:104–13.
67. Kutcher GJ, et al. Histogram reduction method for calculating complication probabilities for three-dimensional treatment planning evaluations. Int J Radiat Oncol Biol Phys. 1991;21(1):137–46.
68. Burman C, et al. Fitting of normal tissue tolerance data to an analytic function. Int J Radiat Oncol Biol Phys. 1991;21(1):123–35.

69. Kutcher GJ, Burman C. Calculation of complication probability factors for non-uniform normal tissue irradiation: the effective volume method. Int J Radiat Oncol Biol Phys. 1989;16(6):1623–30.
70. Kung J, Chen G. A monitor unit verification calculation in intensity modulated radiotherapy as a dosimetric quality assurance. Med Phys. 2000;27:2226–30.
71. Beavis A, et al. Slide and shoot: a new method for MLC delivery of IMRT. The use of computers in radiation therapy. Heidelberg: Springer; 2000.
72. Yang Y, et al. Independent dosimetric calculation with inclusion of head scatter and MLC transmission for IMRT. Med Phys. 2003;30:2937–47.

11 Prescribing a Radiotherapy Schedule and Dose Fractionation

11.1 Dose Specification

Once a patient has been positioned and simulated, the treatment intent, extent, schedule as well as the dose to be delivered have to be prescribed in a clearly defined format according to standard reporting principles. This would help in proper plan evaluation and delivery as well as allow for collection, study and comparison of results. The International Commission for Radiation Units (ICRU) has over the last two decades come out with various reports for determining parameters for dose prescription, measurement, analysis and delivery. These include the ICRU Reports 50, 62 and 83 for 3D-CRT and IMRT and more recently the ICRU91 for SBRT/SRT. These parameters are the minimum dose to the target volume as determined from a planning system dose colour wash, isodose distributions or even a dose-volume histogram (DVH), maximum dose inside target volume as well as maximum dose in treated area, mean target volume dose, as well as other endpoints such conformity and homogeneity indices, etc.

It is necessary to identify first the **ICRU reference point** as this point usually represents the delivered dose. This ICRU reference point is generally located in that part of the treated volume where the dose can be calculated accurately and should be clear and unambiguous with no source of inhomogeneities or requirement for corrections such as in a build-up region or areas with sharp dose gradients. Finally it is also very pertinent that this point should lie in an area which is clinically relevant such as in the central part of the PTV and not over some distant landmark or target volume edge so as to minimize couch shift [1]. Generally the isocentre, which is the point of intersection of all the treating beams, is recommended as the ICRU reference point.

According to ICRU 50 and 62, dose reporting was done with the following: volumes GTV, CTV, ITV, TV, IR, OAR, PRV and PTV; doses with D_{max}, D_{min}, D_{median} and CI; dose at ICRU reference point; dose at centre of PTV; and dose near central axis of beam.

A. Mukherji, *Basics of Planning and Management of Patients during Radiation Therapy*, https://doi.org/10.1007/978-981-10-6659-7_11

In ICRU 83, the following changes have been made – D98%, D2% and D50% instead of D_{max}/D_{min} or D_{median}, RVR added to volumes, ICRU reference point not used as volume-based dose statistics, and calculated effect of tissue inhomogeneities and HI (homogeneity index calculated). ICRU 83 also reports dose to small volume of water not tissue [2].

11.2 Therapeutic Ratio

Cancer cure is not always free of cost but may come at the cost of normal tissue damage, and the basic aim of radiotherapy is to deliver accurately the maximum possible dose to tumour with maximum possible sparing of surrounding normal tissue. Various factors have an effect on how a patient will respond to a course of irradiation. These include variables such as the dose given both the total dose and the daily dose, the volume of tissue irradiated and the patient's inherent responsiveness or radiosensitivity as well as factors such as the patient's age, medical condition, the absence or presence of other diseases which may confound or influence the radiotherapy and any drugs being concurrently taken by the patient. Hence, there may be situations where in additional dose or dose escalation or even the full radical dose required may not be delivered because of the patient's inability to tolerate radiation (patient developing severe acute or late effects) or may be having a co-morbid condition limiting the dose that be safely delivered. The dose of radiation can also be affected by the treatment technique with more modern and precise methods (IMRT, SBRT, etc.) being able to deliver higher target volume doses with less normal tissue sequelae. Finally it is not just the dose and the patient's medical condition which affects the dose of irradiation tolerated. The nutritional status, family, mental strength as well as relief of symptoms all have an effect on the radiation dose tolerated and hence the treatment response.

The effectiveness of any radiotherapy dose or schedule is determined by its *therapeutic ratio. This is usually defined as the ratio of the tumour control probability (TCP) to the normal tissue complication probability (NTCP)* [3]. To know whether a treatment schedule can produce better overall tumour control outcomes and to predict acute and late normal tissue damage, these two determinants play the key role (Fig. 11.1). All constraints used for treatment planning are based on the models utilizing these two factors. Addition to or change in the prevailing condition of any of the factors whether patient-related such as medical condition, regime related such as dose fractionation or use of chemo- or biological agents or even technique related such as use of conformal or precise irradiation methods (IMRT, IGRT, SBRT) could shift the therapeutic ratio, and it is therefore necessary to ensure that any change occurring to this ration is an improvement (whether increased TCP with same or less NTCP or decreased NTCP with same or more TCP).

All irradiation treatments are associated with some extent of normal tissue damage, and the challenge is to limit this damage to within the tissue tolerance limits and keep this damage reversible so that both the structure and functioning of the tissue are repaired over the next few weeks or months. This tissue damage is also called radiation sequelae or radiation-induced toxicities and depending on the extent of tissue damaged is graded in its severity (will be covered in Section D). The sequence of appearance of these effects is also named accordingly with effects seen

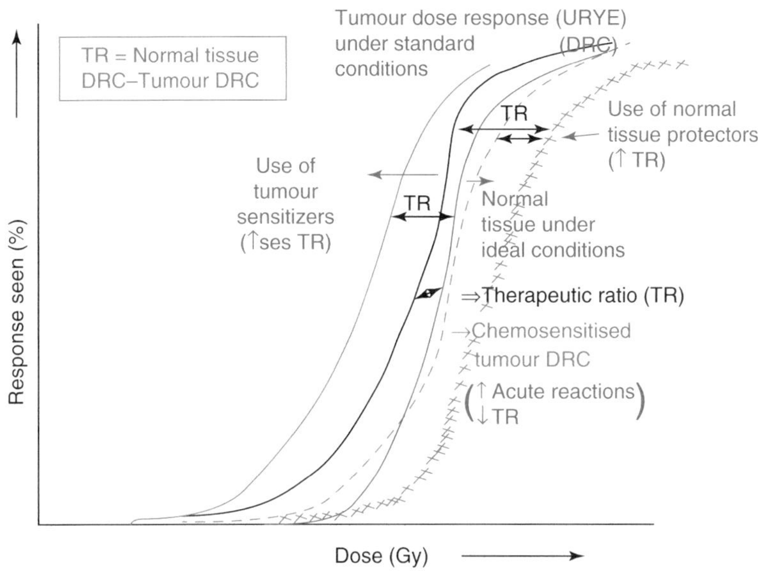

Fig. 11.1 Therapeutic ratio with effect of TCP and NTCP

within 6 months of irradiation called acute and those after 6 months called late (see Chap. 21). Expression of radiation-induced effects also depends on the genetic make-up of the individual with some people showing more effects at lower doses, while others are able to tolerate higher doses of irradiation. In addition, there are many conditions which can predispose an individual to abnormal radiation sensitivity such as ataxia telangiectasia, Fanconi's anaemia and Bloom's syndrome; and these occur mainly because of aberrations in the repair of DNA damage caused by ionizing radiation and which subsequently cause dysregulations in cell physiology, signalling and synthesis of components. Large-scale loss of function or structure could lead to extensive cell death in tissues seen in the form of atrophy or necrosis as in the bone, nerves or brain. Late damage also depends on the hierarchical organization (functional subunits or FSUs) of the irradiated tissue at risk – whether the cells are serial in arrangement (e.g. spinal cord) or parallel (e.g. liver).

11.3 Organs at Risk

The ICRU defines OAR as those normal tissues which lie adjacent to tumours and may therefore be included within treated volumes, with a risk that the radiation may impair their normal functioning [1]. Preparation of a treatment plan involves contouring on a CT scan or simulation radiographs of the tumour and its potential extensions as well as the OARs and a margin around them called the PRV (planning organ at risk volume as described in Chap. 3). Dose limits for organs at risk depend on their functional organization. In case of organs which are arranged in a parallel fashion, dose constraints take into account the total volume of the organ irradiated and the mean dose in that volume. Tissue or organs which are arranged in a serial structure such as the spinal cord or brainstem are delineated during contouring and provided as explained before with an additional margin (the PORV) so that the dose variation occurs outside the structure. In these serial organs, the constraint is given to a maximal point dose cut-off beyond which serious late effects are expected to occur. Here the volume is not that important; it is the D_{max} which is more important.

For some tumours, the radiation oncologist is fortunate to have a treatment plan wherein the PTV can be treated to the required dose while the accepted tolerance doses to normal tissues are not exceeded. But this is usually not the case and many times there may be overlap between PTV and PRV. In such situations, the clinician may need to make a choice between dose escalations to the PTV or complete sparing of PRV. In such times priority for the tissue or target volume is decided based on the tumour type and its likely behaviour, the type of OAR involved (whether serial or parallel FSUs) and how an individual patient would tolerate the dose. If we were to illustrate this with examples, exceeding the point D_{max} for the spinal cord or brainstem may result in irreversible neural damage, but irradiating the deep lobe of the parotid or exceeding lens dose while covering the dose constraint for PTV will result in sequelae, but these can be managed. Similarly one kidney can be irradiated to higher dose if the other one is functioning normally, but not if it is functionally damaged by co-existing conditions such as hypertension or diabetes.

11.4 Tolerance Doses

Even though various radiobiological models had been put forward to explain the necessity of dose fractionation in radiotherapy, there had been a lack of consensual guidelines for dose prescription, both for target volumes and organs at risk. The ICRU reports 50 and 62 provided description of the various treatment volumes which have been upgraded subsequently and added to for IMRT (ICRU 83) and SBRT (ICRU91). Dose tolerances and constraints used in clinical practice were however systematically put forward for the first time by Emami et al. [4]. These were however not based on trials and experimental data but arrived at by consensus and often extrapolated from laboratory or animal studies or older techniques and technology. These initial Emami tables provided probabilities of developing serious adverse effects with respect to dose delivered to specified volumes for parallel organs and maximal point doses for serial organs. These probabilities were described as either $TD_{5/5}$ or $TD_{50/5}$ which meant either a 5% or a 50% risk of developing serious toxicity at 5 years on exceeding the prescribed doses for these values. However, these values were given during the era of 2D radiotherapy when the dose rates across the field were uniform. In the present era with a focus on planned dose inhomogeneity and fluence variation across the beam, these values may not make much sense [5]. But even then these tables help in guiding and predicting dose-related sequelae and/or probability of reactions and are still helpful in planning and evaluating radiation therapy.

The availability of computers and CT scans has brought new changes in radiotherapy dose prescription. Doses are no longer prescribed to a point; doses are now prescribed to a volume and within the same tissue, or organ-differing volumes can have different dose prescriptions. CT-based planning allows for a more holistic appreciation of the dose distribution for a particular arrangement of beams, and this is presented in the form of a dose-volume histogram which is basically a graphical presentation of correlating doses and volumes of various organs in a two-dimensional (x- and y-axis) presentation. The shape and area under the DVH curve are used to assess the dose-volume distributions for the delineated organs for each set of beam arrangements. A DVH basically can be read for either volume of tissue (of each specific organ) "*V*" receiving a particular dose "*d*", i.e. *Vd*, or as dose "*D*" received by a particular volume of tissue "*v*", i.e. *Dv*. For example, PTV-D98 means dose received by 98% of the PTV, while lung V20 means volume of the lung receiving 20 Gy or more. Along with these values, a DVH also helps calculating the mean, median doses, point dose maximum, etc.

Thus a DVH can give an idea about the dose distribution, but it does not provide a predictive value for acute or late effects. These depend on the dose, fraction size and treatment duration as well as tissue type. As explained in Chap. 7, the most commonly followed model for radiobiological assessment is the LQ model, and based on this, the concept of BED was developed by Withers and colleagues [6] to compare different dose schedules to the same structure for an equivalent total dose. BED is based on the correlation between the number of fractions, fraction size and linear quadratic value for late effects. It is calculated as:

$$\mathrm{BED}=\left\{n\times d\left[1+d/(\alpha/\beta)\right]\right\}-\left[(0.693\times T)/(\alpha\times Tp)\right]$$

In the above formula:

n stands for number of treatments.
d is the dose per fraction.
T is the total treatment time.
α/β is the LQ coefficient and differs for different tissues and tumours.
It is usually 3 Gy for late effects and 8–10 Gy for early effects and many tumour tissues. However, some tumours have lower α/β values such as in the breast (about 3) and prostate (1.5–3). In addition, values for Tp (potential doubling time) and α (linear component of cell killing) are taken from published data for each tumour.

Various unequal or inhomogeneous dose schedules can be compared or reported by the concept of **equivalent uniform dose (EUD)**, according to which any two dose distributions are equivalent if they cause the same radiobiological effect. Since the last decade of the last century, radiation treatment planning has followed the consensus guidelines laid down by Emami et al. (1991) [4] with record to normal tissue and organ tolerance limits to therapeutic irradiation. These values were however devised in an era of mainly 2D radiotherapy and with a sizeable number of centres practicing 3D-CRT. However beam intensity modulation was not then frequently practiced. In the present era of widespread IMRT/VMAT, fresh guidelines have been framed to decide tissue tolerances to intensity-modulated beams. In recent years, there has been a joint effort by the radiation oncologists and physicist (ASTRO and AAPM), called Quantitative Analyses of Normal Tissue Effects in the Clinic (QUANTEC), to update Emami et al. using models for normal tissue complication (Bentzen et al., 2010) [5] for most treatment sites with the use of IMRT and has led to a reassessment of tissue tolerances. Chao et al. reported in 2001 that in head and neck patients treated with IMRT, about 17–30% had grade 2 xerostomia compared to 75% of patients receiving non-IMRT radiotherapy [7]. In 2013 and in a fresh update in 2017, Bahman Emami has come out with fresh dose constraints for IMRT as well as SBRT planning based on differing fractionation schedules and α/β values in various tissues [8].

11.5 Treatment Scheduling

Over the last few decades, it has been the general practice among radiation oncologists to prescribe curative radiotherapy in daily fraction sizes of 1.8–2.0 Gy for 5 days a week for a total of 5–8 weeks depending on the total dose required. Subsequently schedules have been designed which treat continuously, more than once daily throughout or part of the course with lower fraction sizes or schedules which have higher fraction sizes (various schedules given in Table 11.1). As has been explained in Chap. 7, the benefit of dose fractionation is in the selective targeting of tumour tissues over normal tissues (both acute and late-reacting ones) because of their different repair potentials by taking advantage of differences between the cell survivals of late-responding tissues (low α/β ratio and fraction size sensitivity), cell survivals of early-responding tissues (high α/β ratio but better cell repair during fraction intervals) and the survival of typical tumours (with higher α/β ratios but decreased cell repair).

Therefore when lower fraction sizes (either conventional size of 1.8–2.0 Gy or even lower of 1.2–1.6 Gy) are used at interval more than reparative time of the acutely reacting tissue, late-responding tissue is spared, while tumour tissue suffers damage. Damage to acutely reacting tissue is theoretically minimized by obeying tissue repair constraints. This allows for a favourable therapeutic ratio. Also designing a treatment schedule has to take into account the effect of cell repopulation which in most tissues is expected after 4–5 weeks into the schedule. Late-responding tissues are not affected by treatment duration, only the fraction size, and this can suitably modified to minimize both late toxicities and avoid repopulation [9]. However excess shortening the treatment time cannot be done as it has to account for reoxygenation of hypoxic cells during therapy (needs fractionation) and allow for repair of acute-responding tissues as well as avoid as far as possible repopulation. Basically it means that the regime should not be too short like CHART which will increase acute effects or too long as in standard fractionation which will allow repopulation.

Table 11.1 Different fractionation schedules followed in radiotherapy practice and their effects

S. no.	Fractionation type	Rationale for fractionation	Description of schedule	Acute reactions	Late reactions	Effect on tumour
1.	Conventional fractionation	Fractionated therapy to try and achieve tumour cell kill and allow normal tissues to repair damage in between doses	1.8–2 Gy once daily 5 days per week for 5–7 weeks	–	–	–
2.	Hyperfractionation	Tumours are tissues with high turnover rate and resemble acutely reacting tissues; hence need for multiple smaller daily fractions to take into account redistribution	2–3 daily fractions of 1.2–1.6 Gy; increased total dose; same treatment time	Increased	May be increased	Increased cell kill
3.	Accelerated fractionation	Dose fraction same as conventional, treatment time decreased – 6 days per week treatment to counter repopulation	1.8–2 Gy per day; 6 days per week	Increased	May or may not increase	Increased tumour cell kill
4.	Continuous hyperfractionated accelerated fractionation (CHART)	Small fraction sizes with continuous treatment; accounts for redistribution and repopulation; estimates treatment will be over before reactions set in	1.2 Gy per fraction three times per day for 12 continuous days (54 Gy/36 #/12 days)	Increased	Decreased	Increased tumour cell kill
5.	Concomitant boost	Conventional fractionated therapy for first 4 weeks followed by addition of a second daily fraction of lower dose to take into account repopulation and decrease overall treatment time	1.8 Gy per fraction 5 days a week for first 4 weeks; then 1.5 Gy per fraction added for next 2 weeks as second daily fraction 6 h later; 54 Gy/30 #/6 weeks +18 Gy in 12 # as second daily fraction from week 5 and 6; total dose 72 Gy	May increase	Decrease	Increased tumour cell kill

(continued)

Table 11.1 (continued)

S. no.	Fractionation type	Rationale for fractionation	Description of schedule	Acute reactions	Late reactions	Effect on tumour
6.	Hypofractionation	In less radiosensitive tissues, palliative intent cases or in small volumes of tissues. Aim for ablating tumour cells	Palliative intent: 30 Gy in 10 # or 8 Gy single #; stereotactic body radiotherapy: 15 Gy in 4 #; or in melanomas: 30 Gy in 6 fractions twice weekly over 3 weeks	Same	If total dose increased, then increased else same	May or not
7.	Split course	Bulky tumours with large proportion in hypoxic areas benefit by disease debulking; if tumour responds well, second part of treatment given by regular fractionation	Large laryngeal tumours: 35 Gy in 15 # followed 2–3 weeks gap; if tumour responds then further 20 Gy in 10 #	Same	May increase	Inferior cell kill
8.	Simultaneous integrated boost (SIB)	Simultaneous hyper- and hypoconventional fractions to different volumes at same times to decrease overall treatment with greater cell kill but with however more acute effects and slightly more late effects	PTV divided into two or more regions each of which is planned to a different dose with different fraction sizes but in same overall treatment time. For example, high-risk PTV (HR-PTV) receives 2.2 Gy per fraction, and low-risk PTV (LR-PTV) receives 2 Gy per fraction both over 30 fractions to a dose of 60 and 66 Gy, respectively	Increased	May or may not increase	Increased cell kill

S. no.	Fraction-ation type	Rationale for fractionation	Description of schedule	Acute reactions	Late reactions	Effect on tumour
9.	Ablative doses: SRT/ SBRT	Hypofractionated dose schedules to a tightly defined target volume with precise dose delivery	14–21 Gy as single doses (radiosurgery) or 4–12 Gy in schedules of 3–10 fractions as therapeutic irradiation	Same	Not expected as normal tissue is completely avoided with small target volumes	Increased cell kill (complete tumour ablation)

Tumours also have been shown to be heterogeneous with regard to cell survival parameters and growth kinetics with areas of resting cells as well as areas of high cell turnover and even necrotic areas. Thus any one schedule will not be ideal for treatment of all tumours, and with advances in physiological and biological imaging, it is now advised to consider faction schedules based on differential dose prescription to different target volumes in the same treatment field (like SIB) which would be based on the individual kinetics and radiobiology for each tumour. This individualized scheduling based on biological assay is already taking place though in settings of clinical trials and is likely to be a routine in the future.

11.6 Treatment Schedules

As explained in Chap. 7, the damage caused radiobiologically by ionizing radiation has a late and an early component which are, respectively, dependent on the fraction size (and its variations) and the total dose (+ treatment duration) as well as its variations. To explain this if the dose variation across the target volume as determined on a plan is 5%, this means that the target volume receives a range of doses from 95 to 105%. This means that 70 Gy in 35 fractions will be received by the target volume in a range from 66.5 to 73.5 Gy but in total 35 fractions with a fraction size range from 1.9 to 2.1 Gy. This means that some tissues would get not only a higher dose but a higher dose per fraction. As a result, there is now a *double* effect which affects most severely the late-responding tissues especially when large volumes are being treated or in curative hypofractionated treatment schedules.

The use of techniques such as IMRT allows for specific doses to specifically delineate volumes within the treated volume, thus allowing for a planned inhomogeneity within the target volume. This allows for dose escalation to the gross tumour volume or areas of metabolically active disease and limiting the dose even to those areas of the PTV which are near a critical organ. Also computerized planning allows for insertion of different fraction sizes in same plan and thereby using principles of biologically equivalent doses to different volumes instead of mathematically equivalent dose plans (in conventional planning from isodose charts). Computerized TPS will help compare the late effects of these equivalent doses by using either the LQ model or using LQ transformed DVHs (creating DVH bands instead of lines to check the effect of variation in fraction size within the volume as well as compare the hot and cold spots). Other methods include the use of alternate fractionation schedules taking into account the type of tumour being treated and the likely variation of acute and late-reacting tissues expected in the target volume. Table 11.1 describes the various altered fractionation schedules being followed across the world today.

The reason for the propagation of various hyperfractionation schedules is because small dose fractions result in higher total dose within tolerance of late-responding normal tissue with a higher biologically effective dose to tumour if α/β ratio for tumour is greater than that for dose-limiting normal tissue. Also a larger number of fractions result in greater chances of cells in radioresistant phase to be caught in more sensitive phase at the time of subsequent fraction, and with proportional decrease in hypoxic cells, there is increased cell kill in subsequent fractions. This results in lesser dependence on oxygen effect since OER is lower at low doses due to domination of single hit events.

11.7 Effect of Overall Treatment Time

Most conventional irradiation schedules last between 5 and 8 weeks, and in this time there is considerable cell re-proliferation, both in the tumour and in the critical normal tissues.

Early reactions: The early-responding normal tissues are those which have a relatively high rate of cell proliferation as well as turnover, and while these tissues are more easily damaged by irradiation, in between doses they swiftly undergo repair, this being the rationale for fractionation in radiotherapy. The ability of these tissues to withstand irradiation is due to the accelerated phase of repopulation they undergo over a period of weeks after the start of irradiation. If the overall treatment time is shortened to within 4–5 weeks with no breaks in between, then there will be less time for repopulation to occur, and the early reactions will be more severe.

Late reactions: Late-reacting tissues are usually well-differentiated function-specific tissues which usually proliferate slowly. Changes in overall time have less effect on these tissues, and a more deciding factor for these tissues is the dose per fraction. If the total dose as well as the fractional dose remains unchanged, small changes in overall treatment time may not significantly alter tissue dynamics.

Tumours: Tissue doubling times and repopulation rates as well as α/β values in tumours vary over wide ranges. Tumour doubling times conventionally have been estimated at been 5–7 weeks with most studies recommending completion of therapy within 8 weeks for best results. Withers et al. [7] demonstrated that a tumour during irradiation exhibits considerable increase in repopulation rate after about the third or fourth week of treatment with doubling times estimated to be less than 7 days. Therefore the overall treatment time is a very important predictor of tumour response with extensions adversely affecting response and survival. On the other hand, even a modest shortening of overall time, without lowering the total dose or even slightly increasing it, could result in improved local control. According to the study by Withers, it was estimated that the dose needed to achieve the same antitumour response increased by 0.6 Gy per day with increase in overall time. *This implies that for every day of treatment extension, every 2 Gy daily fractional dose is countered by a loss of 0.6 Gy due to repopulation, leaving an effective dose of only 1.4 Gy. Therefore when overall treatment time increases theoretically, additional dose of more than 0.6 Gy per day needs to be given* [7].

11.8 Taking into Account Treatment Disruptions and Calculating for Dose for These Treatment Gaps

Many cancer patients undergoing irradiation have been seen to suffer interruptions in their prescribed course of treatment. This can adversely affect their response to therapy as well as their survival. Most common reasons for patients missing out on treatment days can be divided broadly into patient-related causes such as severe acute reactions or co-morbidities requiring urgent intervention, machine-related causes such as machine breakdown, or even social or unrelated issues such as transport difficulties or public holidays. There are a number of options for adjusting these gaps into the treatment schedule:

1. Ignoring the treatment fractions missed by the patient: This would mean that effectively the patient would have received a dose less than that planned and that too irregularly, resulting in extremely poor response rates and by extension survival.
2. Ensure remaining course carried out with gap and adding the missed day's doses at the end of the course. This method is the one that is commonly followed but may not be the optimal corrective step. This method suffers from a vital disadvantage of an increase in the overall treatment time with resultant greater tumour cell repopulation without allowing for any correction for this accelerated repopulation.

   In most centres, a dose correction is taken into account (**Gap Correction**) for this repopulation by way of standard radiobiological formulae (which is usually 0.6 Gy per day for conventional fractions as given by Withers et al. [7] and explained in the previous section). This usually works out to one or two extra doses of the same fraction size when the gap is less than 2 weeks. Increasing the size of the dose per day to cover the extra gap dose is another option, but neither is ideal.
3. Many centres also practice increasing the fractional dose for the remnant of the course so that the radiotherapy treatment is finished within the planned time period (overall treatment time remains the same). This method can thus account for tumour cell repopulation but again only in situations in which the gap is less than 2–3 weeks. This method however has the disadvantage of an increased dose

per fraction with increased rates of late complications in cases where patient survival is expected to be better.

4. Another method of correcting for treatment gaps less than 1–2 weeks while remaining within the planned treatment time is to add extra fractions either during the weekends or as additional smaller fractions during a part of the schedule (as concomitant boosts). Extra doses during the weekends for more than 2 weeks has however the risk of higher acute toxicities (similar to accelerated radiotherapy). Radiobiologically, this technique appears most sound but may not be always logistically correct. If the gap occurs towards the end of the treatment course, it may be simpler to add gap correction.

11.9 Dose Prescription

The prescription in a radiation therapy treatment plan is a statement of intent which bears information pertaining to the site, intent, field, dose and duration along with any special interventions. Therefore a complete prescription of radiation therapy should include first the patient diagnosis with stage followed by site of irradiation, volumes of interest, patient treatment position, immobilization device used and any other specific protocol regarding immobilization or simulation (such as bladder protocol for pelvic treatments). This is followed by the total dose prescribed, dose per fraction, dose-volume requirements for the PTV and normal tissue constraints. Each prescription depending on type of technique is explained subsequently.

In general, cancers can be divided broadly into sarcomas, carcinomas, haematological cancers, germ cell tumours or even stromal cell tumours. Radiotherapy for cancers whether given radically or as adjuvant therapy should be optimally completed within 8 weeks after which there is increased chance of recurrence. If this is not possible, then it should be completed at the most within 8–11 weeks, but definitely any treatment extension beyond 11 weeks results in very poor outcomes.

Generally doses prescribed in conventional fractionation for radiotherapy range from 66–70 Gy over 6–8 weeks for radical radiotherapy in carcinomas or sarcomas to 45–55 Gy over 4.5–5.5 weeks as adjuvant radiotherapy in breast cancers, GI cancers, sarcomas and head and neck cancers 25–35 Gy for pure germinomas and Hodgkin's lymphomas and 35–45 Gy for non-seminomatous germ cell tumours and NHLs depending also on their radiosensitivities (Fig. 11.2). EBRT 2Gy equivalent doses for a few common cancers are:

1. **Head and neck cancers**:

   66 Gy in 33 fractions for T1/small T2 lesions

   66–70 Gy at 2 Gy per fraction for bulky T2/T3/T4 lesions or N+ lesions with concurrent chemo if indicated

   50–56 Gy in conventional fractions as adjuvant radiotherapy if all margins free

   56–60 Gy in conventional fractions as adjuvant radiotherapy if positive or close margins

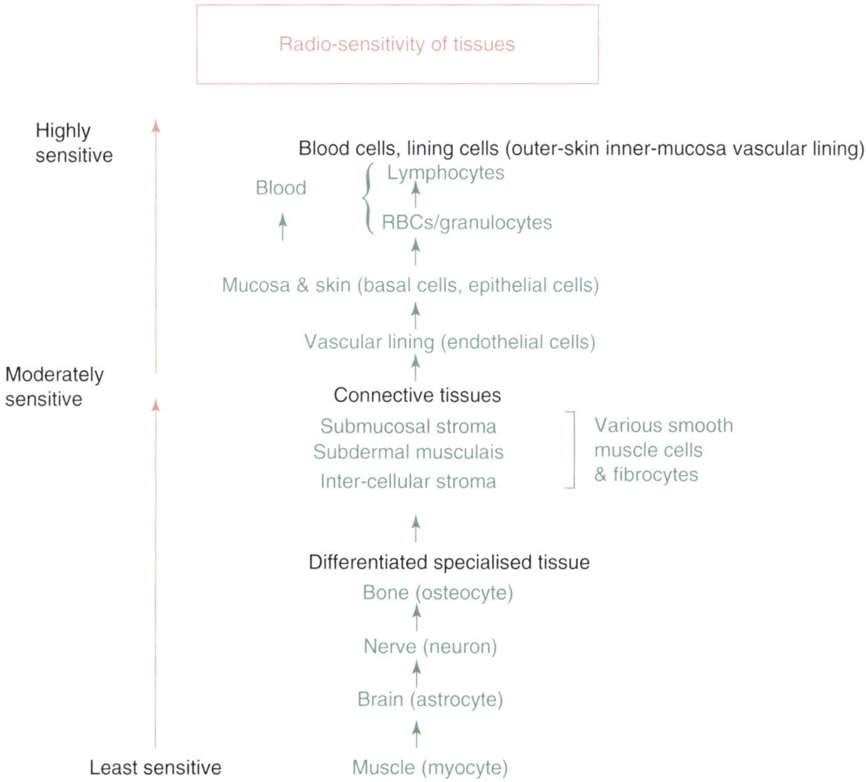

Fig. 11.2 Tumour tissue radiosensitivities

64–66 Gy in conventional fractions as adjuvant radiotherapy if post-operative residual disease present

45–50 Gy in conventional fractions if given as preoperative radiotherapy

30 Gy/10 fractions or 20 Gy/5 fractions or 8 Gy single fraction as palliative radiotherapy

2. **GI cancers**: This group includes oesophagus, stomach, pancreatic, rectal and anal canal cancers. It is preferable to treat with fraction sizes of 180 cGy rather than 200 cGy to limit normal tissue toxicity.

   45–50 Gy in conventional fractions if given as preoperative radiotherapy or adjuvant therapy with further 5–9 Gy boost depending on site. Low-dose regimes in the oesophagus and rectum have been described but are not universally used.

   In case of anal cancers, up to 66 Gy can be given with concurrent chemo with conventional fractionation.

3. **Gynaecological cancers**: Brachytherapy forms a major part of treatment protocols in many cancers like the cervix and corpus uteri. The aim in cervical cancers is to deliver at least 85 Gy to the paracervical region (Point A or area

bounded by 60% isodose line) and in the uterus usually treatment as adjuvant to a dose 45–50 Gy to the pelvis in locally advanced or just vault brachytherapy in early adjuvant cases, if pelvic lymphadenectomy has been done.

4. **Breast cancers**: 45–50 Gy by external beam RT as adjuvant dose followed by 6–10 Gy local boost with electrons, interstitial radiotherapy, IMRT or MammoSite. Hypofractionated RT has also been advocated in adjuvant setting with fraction sizes ranging from 2.3 to 3 Gy per fraction for 13–16 fractions.
5. **Lung cancers**: 60–66 Gy in conventional fractions with 3D-CRT or IMRT with concurrent chemo if required as radical radiotherapy. Also SBRT can be considered if facilities are available with fraction sizes ranging from 5 to 20 Gy.
6. **Genito-urinary cancers**: Doses for bladder and other urothelial cancers are:

   66 Gy in 33 fractions for T1/ T2 lesions

   66–70 Gy at 2 Gy per fraction for T3/T4 lesions or N+ lesions with concurrent chemo if indicated

   50–56 Gy in conventional fractions as adjuvant radiotherapy if all margins free

   56–60 Gy in conventional fractions as adjuvant radiotherapy if positive or close margins

   66–68 Gy in conventional fractions as adjuvant radiotherapy if post-operative residual disease present

   For prostate cancers, dose is 76–80 Gy in conventional fractions for radical radiotherapy. It is more advisable to consider hypofractionated radiotherapy in prostate with daily fractions ranging from 2.5 to 4 Gy for fractionated RT and up to even 20 Gy for SBRT.
7. **Bone and soft tissue sarcomas**:

   50–56 Gy in conventional fractions as adjuvant radiotherapy if all margins free

   56–60 Gy in conventional fractions as adjuvant radiotherapy if positive or close margins

   66–70 Gy in conventional fractions as adjuvant radiotherapy if post-operative residual disease present
8. **Germ cell tumours and lymphomas**: 25–35 Gy for pure germinomas and Hodgkin's lymphomas and 35–45 Gy for non-seminomatous germ cell tumours and NHLs
9. **Brain tumours:** Doses range from 50–60 Gy in conventional fractions for astrocytomas to 23–30 Gy for cranio-spinal axis irradiation.
10. **Skin cancers and melanomas**: Usually hypofractionated schedules are followed for skin cancers like squamous cell cancers like 50 Gy in 20 fractions or electron beam therapy for T-cell lymphomas of skin. Melanomas require hypofractionated adjuvant radiotherapy for nodal irradiation; usual doses given are 32 Gy in 4 fractions weekly therapy or 30 Gy in 5 fractions twice weekly over two and half weeks.

For dose prescriptions for 2DRT, the following details are entered into the treatment chart:

- Intent of radiotherapy, total dose, fraction size, no. of fractions per day, duration of treatment and any added concurrent chemotherapy/biomolecule or radioprotector
- Whether treatment plans are in single phase or multiple phase
- Treatment position, set-up indices, location of isocentre, SSD or SAD technique, simulation technique used and immobilization device (neck rest type, thermoplastic mask, vacloc, etc.) as well as any added instruments (like mouth gag, bolus, knee rest, etc.)
- **For PTV coverage**: prescription isodose, field size, treatment depth, prescription isodose and field weightage
- Machine used and beam energy used
- No. of beams used, beam angles, any beam-modifying device used, no. of MUs, beam-on time and schedule of portal verification

For dose prescriptions for 3D-CRT/IMRT, the following details are entered into the treatment chart:

- Intent of radiotherapy, technique used (3D-CRT/IMRT/VMAT), total dose, fraction size, no. of fractions per day, duration of treatment and any added concurrent chemotherapy/biomolecule or radioprotector
- Whether treatment plans are in single phase or multiple phase and whether repeat imaging are to be done and when
- Treatment position, set-up indices, location of isocentre, simulation technique used and immobilization device (neck rest type, thermoplastic mask, vacloc, etc.) as well as any added instruments (like mouth gag, bolus, knee rest, etc.) and any specific simulation protocol followed such as bladder protocol for pelvic treatments or respiratory gating in lung SBRT
- **For PTV coverage**: D98 (also called $D_{minimum}$), D95 (usually the prescription isodose), D50 or median dose, D_{mean} (is the area under curve in differential DVH divided by 2), D2% (or D_{max}) and D1% (i.e. dose received by less than 1% PTV volume)
- **For organs at risk**: D_{max} or D2%, D_{mean}, V20/30 (in case of lung), D33 and D66 in case of kidneys and the heart
- Machine used, photon or electron beam, beam energy used
- No. of beams used, beam angles, any beam-modifying device used, no. of MUs, beam-on time, schedule of portal and image verification

References

1. International Commission on Radiation Units and Measurements, (ICRU). Prescribing, recording, and reporting photon beam therapy. International Commission on Radiation Units and Measurements, ICRU Report 50, ICRU, Bethesda; 1993.
2. International Commission on Radiation Units and Measurements, (ICRU). Prescribing, recording, and reporting photon-beam intensity-modulated radiation therapy (IMRT). ICRU Report 83, ICRU, Bethesda; 2010.

3. Hall E, Giaccia A. Radiobiology for the radiologist. Philadelphia: Lippincott Williams & Wilkins; 2006.
4. Emami B, Lyman J, Brown A, et al. Tolerance of normal tissue to irradiation. Int J Radiat Oncol Biol Phys. 1991;21:109–22.
5. Bentzen SM, Constine LS, Deasy JO, Eisbruch A, Jackson A, Marks LB, Ten Haken RK, Yorke ED. Quantitative analyses of normal tissue effects in the clinic (QUANTEC): an introduction to the scientific issues. Int J Radiat Oncol Biol Phys. 2010;76:S3–9.
6. Wilson G. Cell kinetics. Clin Oncol. 2007;19:370–84.
7. Chao KSC, Majhail N, Huang C-J, et al. Intensity-modulated radiation therapy reduces late salivary toxicity without compromising tumor control in patients with oropharyngeal carcinoma: a comparison with conventional techniques. Radiother Oncol. 2001;61:275–80.
8. Emami B. Tolerance of normal tissue to therapeutic radiation. Rep Radiother Oncol. 2013;1(1):123–7. Updated version in 2017.
9. Withers HR, Taylor JMG, Maciejewski B. The hazard of accelerated tumor clonogen repopulation during radiotherapy. Acta Oncol. 1988;27:131–46.

12 Evaluating a Treatment Plan

This chapter constitutes an essential step in radiotherapy planning and treatment. Planning a radiotherapy schedule not only involves simulation and contouring but also setting up of the treatment fields, validating these fields, calculating the dose distribution and then evaluating these distributions to generate the optimum plan. Thus calculation of doses includes obtaining an optimum dose distribution with respect to a sequence or grid of points in the target volume or the contoured image or in conformal radiotherapy in a three-dimensional array covering the required anatomical region.

12.1 Plan Evaluation

Once dose calculation (called treatment planning) is over, the physician has to ensure that this dose distribution matches his initial treatment requirements (or dose constraints). This step is called plan evaluation and includes verification of the treatment fields (through simulation radiographs or DRRs), isodose distributions, point of maximal and minimal dose coverage and coverage of target volumes and sparing of normal structures. Evaluation also includes checking for the path of the beams as well as their exit routes as these areas will also get scattered doses. The following tools are used in the evaluation of the planned dose distribution [1, 2]:

- Isodose curves
- Orthogonal planes and isodose surfaces
- Dose distribution statistics
- Differential dose-volume histogram
- Cumulative dose-volume histogram

A. Mukherji, *Basics of Planning and Management of Patients during Radiation Therapy*, https://doi.org/10.1007/978-981-10-6659-7_12

12.1.1 Isodose Curves

Isodose curves are a series of lines connecting points receiving the same dose on a chart showing a dose distribution and are basically a two-dimensional representation of the resultant dose pattern caused by the combination of beam/s incident on a surface. Thus the interaction of one beam with another in the treated area as well as with other beam modifying devices such as shielding, wedges, bolus, etc. can be depicted by isodose charts. Standard isodose charts are derived from beam data that has been measured in water phantoms, and from these, using PDD and beam profile data, actual treatment distributions can be prepared. Thus since these isodose curves represent very specific beam interactions which can be affected by the beam energy, field size and the PDD, each set of isodose curves is valid only for a specific machine and field size. Also it is important to *normalize* or prescribe the dose to a specific point in the field which is usually at the target midpoint in the central axis of the beam. Two common point normalizations are:

- Normalization to 100% at the D_{max} on the central axis
- Normalization at the isocentre

Isodose curves can help evaluate treatment plans by matching the isodose covering the maximal part of the target volume with that at the isocentre. Usually, the difference between the two should not be more than 10–15% (e.g., target volume is covered by 90% isodose seen at the periphery, while D_{max} isodose is 100–105% – then this plan is acceptable). The isodoses are also checked for OAR tolerance doses and if these have been exceeded or not. This process can involve checking the isodose for a single central plane in case of a low-volume field or for multiple representative planes.

12.1.2 Orthogonal Planes and Isodose Surfaces

It is usual to treat a larger and more irregular target volume in which case a single axial section may not be representative of the volume (like in CT-based planning). These cases are then evaluated by generating a representative volume by using multiple orthogonal CT planes on which the isodoses are represented and an approximate dose distribution may be obtained (Fig. 12.1). Isodoses can also be used to obtain three-dimensional distributions by mapping the dose distributions in all three axes (*x*-, *y*-, and *z*-) and then overlaying this distribution on a 3D display featuring surface renderings of the target and/or other organs. These representations however can only show the dose coverage of the target volume and are not able to calculate the depth doses or provide any quantitative volume information.

12.1.3 Dose Statistics

Dose statistics provide quantitative information on the volume of the target or critical structure, and on the dose received by that volume. Since there may be varying distributions in different parts of irradiated area, dose distribution can be evaluated by the following measures:

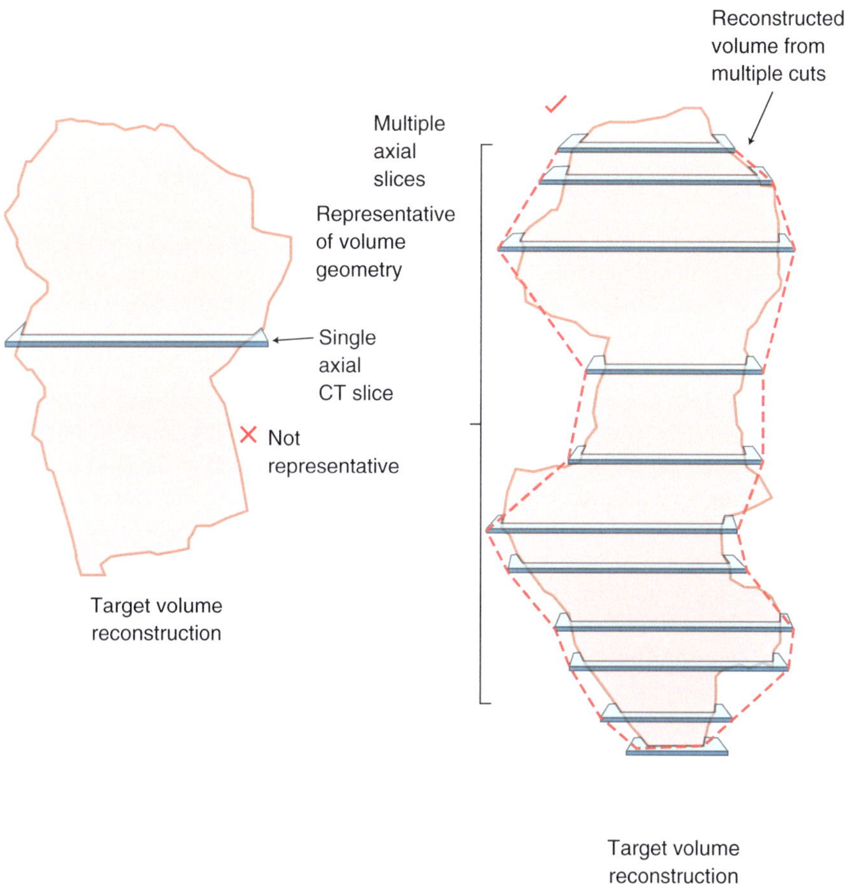

Fig. 12.1 Representative volume from multiple CT planes

- Minimum dose to the volume
- Maximum dose to the volume
- Mean dose to the volume
- Dose received by at least 90–95% of the volume
- Volume irradiated to at least 90–95% of the prescribed dose

The last two statistics are only relevant for a target volume. Organ dose statistics such as these are especially useful in dose reporting, since they are simpler to include in a patient chart than the dose-volume histograms. ***These tools have to be evaluated in conjunction with anatomical coverage evaluation tools such as dose colour washes or isodose lines as they do not convey any information regarding spatial distribution of dose***. For example, merely checking coverage of PTV by mean dose to volume or minimum dose coverage may show a plan meeting laid-out criteria; however, a hot or cold spot may be present over a vital critical structure or the GTV itself, which can only be checked by reviewing both dose statistics and anatomical coverage tools. The main advantage of dose statistical analysis is the ability to infer on the limiting doses and corresponding coverage of both target volumes and critical organs which are otherwise not possible from spatial distributions.

12.1.4 Evaluating Isodose Lines and CT-Based 2D Plans

As seen in Figs. 12.2 and 12.3, evaluating a 2D radiotherapy plan can mean analysing an isodose distribution based on field sizes, weightages, normalizations, effect of blocks, etc. In CT-based 2D planning, the process is slightly simpler with the use of computer; but here also the planner has to base his/her calculations on a single axial cut or at most a few more axial cuts and extrapolate for the whole field size.

In Fig. 12.2, an isodose distribution resulting from a parallel opposed field placement is shown. The plan evaluation here is based on estimating and then superimposing the likely dose distribution on to the patient anatomy. First the field sizes are checked along with the prescription for total dose, fraction size, number of fractions per day and duration of treatment. Also checked are treatment position, location of isocentre, SSD or SAD technique, simulation technique used, number of beams used, beam angles and any beam modifying device used. An equivalent square field size (EFS) of each field is calculated. Any blocks used are deducted from this area by calculating the EFS of the blocked area also. The percent depth dose of each

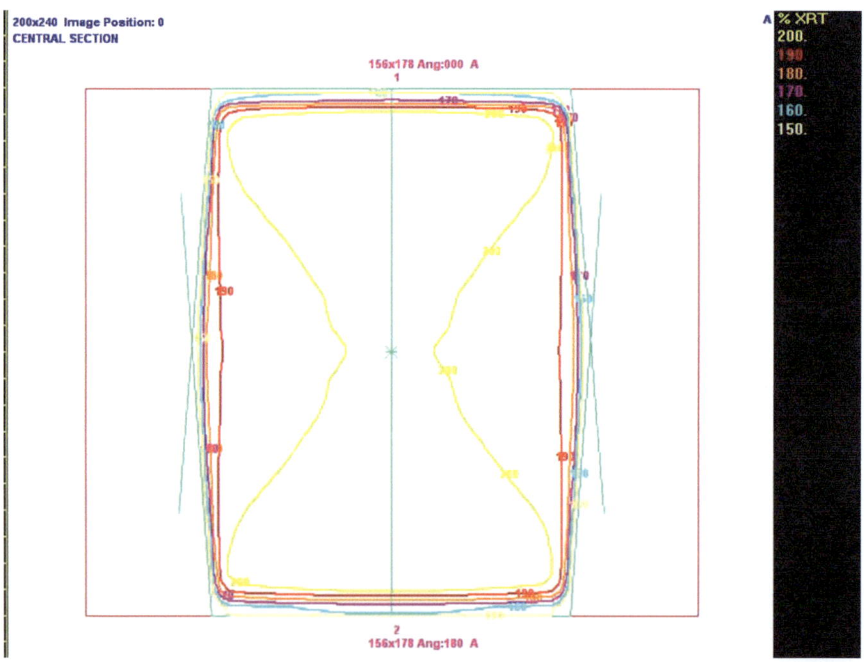

Fig. 12.2 2D planning by isodose lines

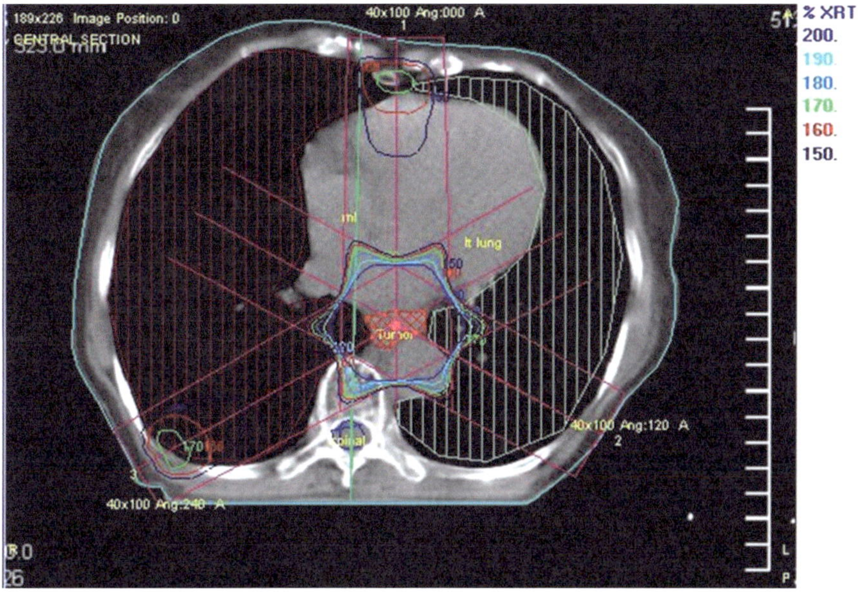

Fig. 12.3 CT based 2D planning

beam (PDD) is calculated using the EFS and prescription depth from standard tables. Once the net EFS and PDD are calculated, using standard formulae and percentage depth dose tables, the treatment time or number of MUs for each beam is obtained. This is further multiplied with field weightage and then with wedge factors or tray factors (for blocks, etc.) to correct it for beam weightage as well as for attenuation with the use of modifying devices.

The obtained isodose lines are then checked to see if they include the entire area under the field size as well as the extent of the 90 and 100% isodose line. Usually the 100% isodose line is shifted more towards the field surfaces with a narrow waist at the isocentre, and it is usually reasonable to prescribe the dose to 90% isodose line (Fig. 12.2). Based on the isodose distributions, the dose is prescribed to the isodose which best covers the full target volume and treatment times calculated as will be described subsequently in this chapter.

In 2D CT-based planning as seen in Fig. 12.3, contouring of target volume and critical structures as well as beam placement, use of any beam accessories and finally dose calculation are generally done on a single axial CT slice. In cases where there might be appreciable change in anatomical positions of target volume with body contour, a few representative axial slices are taken and sequenced according to portal length with proportional difference maintained between slices as in real patient. Beams are then placed, beam central axis point on skin identified and appropriate weightages used, and beam modifying devices introduced where required. The field doses are then calculated. In Fig. 12.3, the esophageal target volume has been contoured; a three-field beam placement has been utilized with one anterior and two posterior beams to avoid the spinal cord. After this, the dose is calculated for the given section and the isodose lines over the target volume reviewed. The isodose covering the target volume best with least dose variation in the centre (higher isodose lines) is chosen. The dose received by the spinal cord is also checked to see if it is within tolerance limits. In this figure, the 200% isodose line is chosen and dose prescribed to this level, while the spinal cord is well protected. The disadvantage with this method is that the entire field size is assumed to match this one CT slice which is usually not the case. This can be partially offset by choosing a few more slices representative of change in body contour and sequencing them as per their order in actual patient field length. In such cases, treatment planning can then partially take into account body contours and more accurate critical organ dosage. But for complete accuracy, full 3D CT-based treatment planning would need to be done with full body and contoured volume reconstruction and BEV-based beam placement.

12.1.5 Dose-Volume Histograms

These dose calculation and evaluation tools are typically used in CT-based planning and mainly in conformal radiotherapy plans, though rudimentary forms of differential dose-volume histograms (DVH) are available in some CT-based 2D planning systems also. These convey dose information over the entire three-dimensional array of the treated anatomical region and represent various frequencies of dose distributions in defined or contoured volumes which may represent the PTV or OAR [2]. But instead of displaying the dose distributions as frequency distributions, DVHs are usually displayed in the form of *percent volume of total volume* on the ordinate against the dose on the abscissa. Two types of DVHs are in use:

- Direct (or differential) DVH
- Cumulative (or integral) DVH

The main drawback of DVHs is that this distribution condenses the anatomical dose distribution into numbers and percentages and may not fully convey the spatial dose distribution for good plan evaluation. Here again, complete evaluation is done by analysing the DVHs and the dose colour washes/isodoses.

12.1.6 Direct Dose-Volume Histogram

DVHs are generated by computerized planning systems which create voxels over the entire range of dose distribution and then sum up the number of voxels for a given dose range (dose priorities) and plot the resulting volume (or more frequently the percentage of the total organ volume) as a function of dose. An ideal DVH for a target volume would be a single column indicating that 100% of the volume receives the prescribed dose but this is seldom the case with a part of the PTV getting various dose ranges near the prescribed dose from which the isodose which is nearest the prescribed dose and covers the most area is selected for evaluation. If this is an acceptable dose level, then this distribution is selected. In case of normal structures, a DVH may either be shown to have several peaks (differential DVH) indicating that different parts of the organ receive different doses or as a descending log curve with the area under curve denoting dose-to-volume distributions.

12.1.7 Cumulative Dose-Volume Histogram

In 3D treatment planning, an estimate of how much volume is covered by a dose under evaluation cannot be obtained directly from the direct DVH as the area under the curve for all dose levels above 95% of the prescription dose would need to be calculated. This can only be done on a cumulative DVH. In the cumulative DVH, the planning system calculates different volumes receiving different dose levels and presents it in the form of a log curve with the volume on the *y*-axis and absolute/percent dose on the *x*-axis and each point on the curve denoting a volume of the tissue receiving a certain dose.

A plan evaluation then can be based by checking the percent dose received by the volume of the tissue. However, it may not always be beneficial to check the percent dose; and evaluation should include checking both the percent dose and the absolute dose. This is because sometimes the CT simulation may not include an entire tissue volume and the percent dose then would be a false representation. Also many serial type organs have specified absolute tolerances with volumes in cu.cm, and in these, it is better to check for absolute figures in dose and volume.

12.1.8 How to Use a DVH

The use of computerized planning and incorporation of CT images into a treatment planning system now allows for prescription of doses and dose constraints to specific volumes rather than points. This can give a better estimate of expected effects both acute and late. A graphical representation of the dose distribution in the various delineated volumes in the form of a 2D graph wherein the dose is represented on the *x*-axis and the volume on the *y*-axis is called a Dose Volume Histogram or DVH (Refer also Chap. 11). The shape of the DVH curve for each organ or tissue whether cumulative or differential DVH gives an idea of the relative dose distribution in that tissue or organ and determines the fidelity of the dose distribution to decide on dose constraints and tissue tolerances. From this graphical representation, the percentage of the volume of an organ receiving a given dose (*d*) can be read as *Vd* (volume of tissue receiving dose "*d*") or as *Dv* (dose received by volume "*v*" of tissue). From the *x*-axis, various dose parameters such as the mean, median doses, and minimum or maximal target volume doses can be calculated. DVHs by themselves do not have a predictive function or provide spatial dose representation but they may give an idea of likely cause of sequelae whether acute or late by comparing doses received by the tissue volumes with the clinical effects seen. Taking an example, the likelihood of xerostomia in a patient who has received IMRT would be much less when the mean doses to the parotids and the minor salivary glands are below 25–26 Gy. Similarly, the probability of lung fibrosis is decreased in patients with a V20 of less than 30%, V30 less than 20%, and V5 less than 60%. These DVH limits try and compress a full distribution to a single assessment point; but even then it is important to still check the full spatial distribution rather than one essential point. This can be particularly useful when comparing two plans for the same patient.

Figure 12.4 shows a typical cumulative DVH. If we have to analyse this DVH, how would we go about it? Taking the DVH (Fig. 12.4), the main questions asked would be whether PTV coverage is adequate and whether the OARs are being adequately spared. At a first glance, this DVH looks like that representing a good plan with the target volumes bunched together at the right top and the OARs bunched together at the left lower part of x-axis. Basically, the area under curve is the volume of tissue getting a dose, and the smaller this area, the better for an OAR. Also the tail of the curve should not ideally taper too much to the right as this will mean a smaller volume getting a higher dose. This is true even for the target volumes, i.e. the more the dose line tails towards the right bottom (x-axis), the more is the maximum point dose to the target volume. This can be clinically significant if this maximal dose to OAR is in a serial organ like the spinal cord where even a small volume getting a very high dose can have catastrophic results.

Once this first look is done, next to be noted is the target volume maximal dose. Ideally, it should not be more than 5–7% of the prescribed dose. Similarly, the minimum dose to the target volume should be noted. If properly contoured, it should not be less than 5–8% of the prescribed dose depending on the treatment technique. In Fig. 12.4, both the PTV and GTV coverage is adequate. The PTV can be described as 95% of the volume receiving 94–96% dose which is usually in line with planning

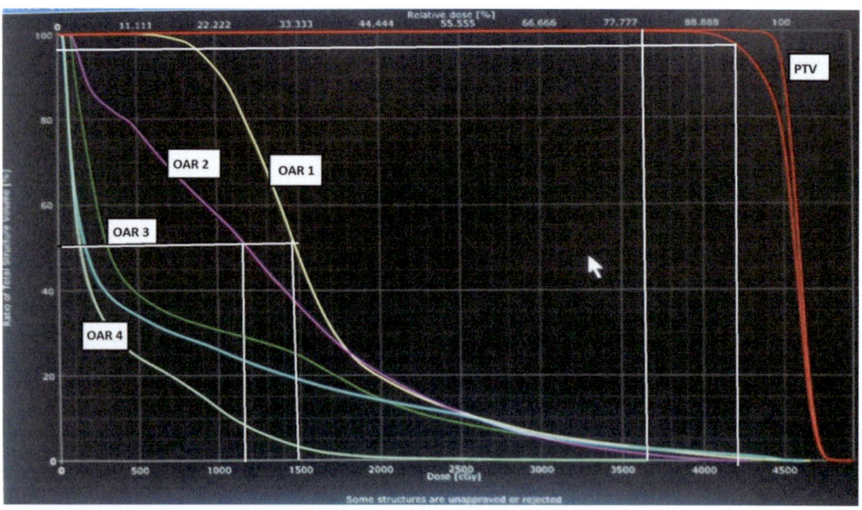

Fig. 12.4 A typical DVH showing target volume and OARs

criteria. The D_{max} of the PTV is seen to be not more than 4800 cGy for a prescribed dose of 4500 cGy which is about 106% and thus within acceptable parameters. Further, the quantum of the D_{max} is also important. From the DVH, we can deduce that the volume of PTV receiving a dose more than 4650 cGy (i.e. 103%) is less than 1% (most likely to be point doses). This is also checked in the dose colour wash to see the location of the hot spot – whether it is inside the PTV or overlying some critical structure where even if only a point dose has a risk of causing significant sequelae. Ideally, it should be inside the GTV.

After having evaluated the target volume, we now evaluate each organ at risk (OAR). First are the serial OARs. For serial OARs, the $D_{nearmax}$ is the limiting dose as the loss of function of even one FSU will cascade for the entire structure. In this DVH (Fig. 12.4), OAR4 is the serial DVH and its $D_{nearmax}$ is well within limits. For OARs with parallel FSUs, D50% is an acceptable estimate of probability of acute or late effects. In some OARs like the brainstem, optic chiasma or kidney, it may be necessary to check both median and near-maximum dose as these structures have both a mean tolerance limit and also develop significantly if point maximum doses exceed tolerance limits. The DVH in case of the OARs can give information regarding their D98%, D2%, D50% as well as their integral doses (calculated from differential DVH as area under curve).

12.2 Algorithm for Plan Evaluation

12.2.1 Target Volume

- As explained in Chap. 10, Section B, correct depiction of target volumes and organs at risk is necessary for good planning and evaluation. GTV is drawn based on imaging modalities, and from this basic target volume, the CTV and PTV are drawn. Other volumes such as ITV, RVR and OARs are then identified as per the case requirements.
- Organs at risk usually are contoured with a 3 mm margin to form the planning risk volume (PORV), and in case there is immediate proximity to a PTV such that dose to the OAR cannot be constrained within protocol limits, a second PTV may be defined as the overlap between the PTV1 and PORV. Dose to this overlap part of the PTV must reach as far as possible microscopic disease dose but not cross the OAR tolerance dose limit.

12.2.2 Planning Evaluation Guidelines

- First to be noted is the target volume maximal dose. Ideally, it should not be more than 5–7% of the prescribed dose. Similarly, the minimum dose to the target volume should be noted. If properly contoured, it should not be less than 5% of the prescribed dose. The inhomogeneity within the target volume should be kept to ±10% of the prescribed dose. According to ICRU 62, the absorbed dose in the

PTV should be confined within from 95 to 107% of the prescribed absorbed dose for 3DCRT [1].

- ICRU 83 report is used for reporting IMRT and requires description of D98%, D50% and D2% [2].
- Next the D98 and D95 of the target volumes are noted as also is the D2% and D1%. These are the minimum and maximum point and volume doses to target volume and are checked if they are within prescribed parameters.
- Also the above said D_{max} are checked in the dose colour wash in each slice to note its location; whether it is within the PTV and also whether it is overlying any critical structure which can later cause severe complications irrespective of plan generally meeting prescribed parameters. It should ideally lie within the PTV and not within the organ at risk. Ideally, the hot spots should be located inside the GTV.
- After this, the conformity and homogeneity indices should be checked. (This is explained in the next section.)
- After this, each OAR is checked for their mean and maximal doses, and depending on whether they are serial or parallel organs, their tolerance to the radiotherapy course can be predicted. In case of serial OARs, their D_{max} is checked as to whether it is limited to within tolerance doses; while for parallel OARS, D_{mean} is seen for analysis. D_{max} is also noted to check for any undue hot spots.
- Next the dose colour washes are used to see the volume of the body getting a dose 50% of the prescription dose and whether this is in line with previously stated treatment objectives. Also the dose is increased on the sliding scale of the dose colour wash to note the position and size of the areas receiving more than 105% of the prescribed dose. If it is significant, then these are converted to a contour, reiteration done with fresh objectives to decrease this dose so as to obtain a plan free of excess hot spots.
- Once the hot spots have been accounted for, target volume and OAR sparing checked and DVHs analysed, create a plan sum of all phases of the treatment plan to ensure once more that all dose parameters are within prescribed limits.
- Next one should then check all the field parameters like beam angles and number of MUs and corrections may be applied where necessary and recalculation done. The method of prescription dose normalization is checked; in 3DCRT, it can be normalized as either 95% dose to 95% volume or as 100% at target mean. In IMRT or VMAT, usually no plan normalization is done as the computer makes its own iterations.
- Finally, view all treatment fields through beam's eye view (BEV) to ensure adequate coverage and critical organ sparing. Generate DRRs for set-up comparison, add set-up fields and sequence the fields to be used.

12.3 Conformity and Homogeneity Indices (CI and HI)

Plan evaluation is basically a subjective issue with each radiation oncologist interpreting plans differently. While the DVHs may provide some objective means of comparison, they do not provide information on the plan quality. The quality of a plan depends on what is the dose gradient in the target and the irradiated volumes as

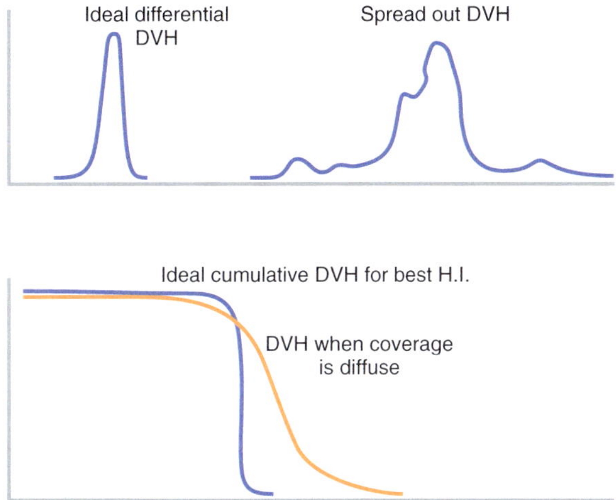

Fig. 12.5 Homogeneity index from the DVH

well as how well the prescribed dose has conformed to the target volume. This information can be assessed by two measures which are the dose homogeneity and dose conformity [2]. Dose homogeneity basically shows the uniformity of dose distribution within the target volume, and while it is usually good to have uniform doses in a 3DCRT plan, in modern IMRT/VMAT especially with simultaneous boost techniques and in SBRT, dose homogeneity is really not an aim of planning. On the other hand, dose conformity is a reflection of the success of conformal radiotherapy planning process, and it denotes how much of the high-dose volumes and the prescribed dose volumes have been restricted to the PTV and even better if to the GTV.

These two measures can also be identified from a DVH. A typical differential DVH for a PTV or an OAR is a near Gaussian shape in which the values should ideally be tightly distributed around the mean absorbed dose. If this curve is more spread out or has subsidiary peaks, then this means that there are areas of dose inhomogeneity. Therefore, a perfect homogeneity index (HI) would mean a steep narrow differential DVH with a small base around the mean value; and in a cumulative DVH, this ideal HI will be seen as a vertical drop in the curve from the 98 to 100% value to nearly the zero value within a dose gradient of 1–3 Gy (Fig. 12.5). Calculation of the standard deviation of the mean can give an idea on the extent of dose inhomogeneity along with the HI, and therefore, both the mean dose to PTV and the standard deviation of this mean should be reported.

Thilmann et al. [3] *defined the homogeneity index, $HI_{95\%/107\%}$, as the fraction of the CTV with an absorbed dose higher than 95% and lower than 107% of the ICRU-prescribed absorbed dose*. This definition however does not indicate the magnitude of under- or overdosage. Because the use of the minimum, the maximum and the ICRU reference point doses is no longer recommended, presently as per ICRU 83 [2], the *following definition for homogeneity index is suggested:*

$$\mathrm{HI} = (\mathrm{D2\%} - \mathrm{D98\%}) / \mathrm{D50\%} \quad [2]$$

An HI of zero indicates that the absorbed-dose distribution is almost homogeneous. D50% is suggested as the normalization value because reporting of D50% is strongly recommended in Level 2 reporting.

As explained before, dose conformity reflects the quality of the conformal plan to restrict high doses to the PTV and is one of main advantages of IMRT/3DCRT, and even between them, IMRT scores over 3DCRT in its ability to conform doses inside concave areas. *As per present ICRU definitions, conformity of the prescription dose to the PTV is expressed by the conformity index (CI), which represents the volume of the body receiving more than 95% of the prescribed dose, divided by the volume of the PTV* [1, 2]. A value of 1 reflects an ideal plan, and good plans have values approaching 1. CI is calculated by the following formula as per ICRU 62:

$$\mathrm{CI} = V_{95\%} / V_{\mathrm{PTV}} \quad [1]$$

12.4 Set-Up Evaluation

The aim of this step is to check for the physical feasibility of the planned beam arrangement, account for any change in position between the simulation set-up and the treatment set-up and also quantify the change in positioning of the patient on the couch from the simulation position to moving to the isocentre. These can be achieved through verifying the portal images at the couch with the simulation radiographs or DRRs as well as quality assurance for the physical dose distribution and matching with planned dose distribution using in vivo dosimetry.

Set-up verification methods can range from the use of port films for localization and verification as in 2DRT to online and even real-time verification and correction in conformal and image-guided RT using diodes, X-rays, CBCT and MVCT. This section will now explain each of these techniques.

Port Films: These are an emulsion-type film kept inside envelopes (as they don't have to be developed unlike radiography) and are placed in the treatment beam with the patient placed between the beam and the film. These films can be used for both localization of beam and field verification:

- **Localization**: This type of use of a port film is done to check if the patient positioning is correct for a particular beam and uses a fast and small exposure for films placed before and after irradiation exposure in each beam. These films have a thin layer of metal (copper/aluminium) facing the beam (for electron build-up) and an emulsion backing layer to provide backscatter.
- **Verification**: In this use, the film is placed in each beam for the duration of exposure to irradiation to check for fidelity of plan delivery and account for patient movement during therapy. Both fast and slow films are used: fast films for small or multiple fields and give a sharper image, while slow films are used for larger fields with longer exposure.

Port films can be taken either in single- or double-exposure techniques. In a **single-exposure technique**, the film is exposed to the treatment field only and is helpful in localization of beam for regions where the anatomy has prominent bony landmarks and can be covered in a single field. Usually all beam verification films are also single exposure. On the other hand, in a **double-exposure technique**, the beam position for a region with less bony landmarks and more soft tissue is verified by first exposing the film to the treatment field and then opening the collimators (and removing all shields) to expose the film to an area 5–10 cm beyond each field to show the surrounding anatomy.

Online Portal Imaging: With the advent of conformal radiotherapy, tighter margins have become common to allow for more normal tissue sparing, and this has necessitated the development of stricter protocols for patient set-up verification and treatment delivery. The computerization of the planning and treatment console system has allowed for online and real-/near-real-time portal imaging which can allow the correction of any positional change just before and even during treatment. These systems are composed of radiation detectors (fluoroscopic, diodes, MV- or CBCT) which are attached to the LINAC by robotic arms. They can be remotely brought into position at the time of treatment delivery to verify patient position and allow treatment delivery [4]. Currently these systems include:

1. **Fluoroscopic portal imaging detectors**: This system is made up of a combined metal plate and a fluorescent phosphor screen along with a 45° mirror and a television camera. The metal plate creates the build-up for electrons which are converted to photons by the phosphor screen with emission of light. This light is deflected by the mirror to the camera which can create an image after capturing only a fraction (<0.1%) of these photons. Good anatomical image resolution depends on phosphor thickness.
2. **Matrix ionization chamber detectors**: These are basically ion chamber-type electrodes which are arranged in a grid pattern and are composed of two metal electrodes separated by a distance of 1 mm of isobutene. Each of these plates has 256 electrodes, and the electrodes in these plates are placed perpendicular to each other. This arrangement measures the ionization at each point, and from this, a 2D ionization map is created and converted to a greyscale image.
3. **Amorphous silicon detectors**: This system uses an arrangement of solid detectors made of amorphous silicon which are connected to field effect transistors in a rectangular pattern. Light photons produce electron hole pairs in the photodiodes proportional to the intensity allowing an image to be obtained. This system produces an image with a greater resolution and contrast than the other systems.

12.5 Treatment Time and Monitor Unit Calculations

Calculating the treatment time or monitor units (MU) determines the length of patient exposure to irradiation. This factor is however affected by variables such as treatment technique used, PDD, the use of beam modifying devices, depth of prescription, beam energy, weightage of each beam and field size. In a fixed SSD technique, the dose distribution is affected by the PDD at the prescribed isocentre for each of the beams in the treatment plan and also by the weightage (W) accorded to each beam (which means how much of a daily fraction size will be contributed by each beam). **For example,** in a pelvic box field plan prescribed for daily 200 cGy, if no weightage is specified, then each of the four fields will contribute 50 cGy per day. While this looks ideal, it may or may not be an optimum distribution as the isocentre will not be at an equal distance in all four fields and hence PDD will vary. So to get a better dose distribution, the beam weightages may have to be altered like 1.1:1.2:0.8:0.9 which means the four fields will now give 55, 60, 40 and 45 cGy per day. This change will result in change in the treatment times/MUs calculated.

The isocentric technique calculates the dose to a fixed isocentre that is equidistant for all beams, so here, PDD does not depend on the SSD. The dose at depth is dependent on the tissue-maximum ratios, and each beam delivers a fixed fraction of the total MUs required at the isocentre for the prescribed dose. It is also important to note that for both the fixed SSD and isocentric techniques, calculation of treatment time or monitor units will depend on the machine output calibration which, for example, in megavoltage photon machines, is commonly expressed as cGy/MU for LINACs and in cGy/min (dose rate) for cobalt units. The conditions under which these output measurements were taken however have to be mentioned such as (1) measured in a water phantom, (2) measured on the central axis of the radiation beam, (3) measured at the prescribed point at depth of maximum dose, (4) measured for a specific field size such as 10×10 cm^2 and (5) measured at a nominal SSD (most commonly 100 cm). The output may be designated by and is used directly in metre-set calculations involving fixed SSD techniques.

12.5.1 Calculating the Treatment Time or MUs for Fixed SSD Set-Up

An equivalent square field size (EFS) of each field is calculated based on the formula $[2ab/(a + b)]$ if the field is rectangular. In case of a non-rectangular field, the field can be divided into two or more triangles by representative lines and area calculated accordingly or by using the Clarkson's method. Any blocks used are deducted from this area by calculating the EFS of the blocked area also. The percent depth dose of each beam (PDD) is calculated using the EFS and prescription depth from standard tables. Once the net EFS and PDD are calculated, using standard formulae and percentage depth dose tables, the treatment time or number of MUs for each beam is obtained. This is further multiplied with field weightage and then with wedge factors or tray factors (for blocks, etc.) to correct it for beam weightage as well as attenuation with use of modifying devices.

If calculating the PDD from the isodose charts, the isodose line (IL) through the ICRU reference point, the maximum dose and that isodose curve which completely covers the PTV are noted. This PDD is used then to calculate the treatment time as explained above and also to obtain the D_{max} doses (+2% and −2% of the $D(Q)$ dose). In order to calculate the MUs for a LINAC-based fixed SSD treatment, it is first necessary to calculate the dose rates for each of the fields. These can be obtained by multiplying the basic LINAC output with the relative dose factor RDF(A) where A refers to the approximate field size and any other applicable transmission factors (such as the wedge factor or the tray factor).

12.5.2 Calculating the Treatment Time or MUs for Isocentric Set-Ups

This can be explained by an example like in the previous section. To calculate doses for LINAC in MU, the doses from each beam at the isocentre at a depth of maximum dose $D(Q_{\max})$ have to be calculated so that SSD = SAD − $D_{\max}$. Once the dose at $D(Q_{\max})$ is known for each beam, it is possible to calculate the MU from the basic LINAC output $D(d_{\max},10,f,h\nu)$ multiplied by the RDF(A_Q), the ISF and other transmission factors as applicable.

For example, if a dose (DQ) of 200 cGy is prescribed for a three-field technique at the ICRU reference point Q located at the treatment isocentre. If the isodose line at this point is 240% (sum of the weights in %), with a maximum dose in the distribution being 242%, and the 235% isodose completely covers the PTV, then each of the beams (weighted 1:0.7:0.7) would need to deliver 100, 70 and 70 cGy at the isocentre for a total of 240 cGy. Then by the unitary method of calculation, to obtain the prescribed dose of 200 cGy at a point Q, doses of 83.4, 58.3 and 58.3 cGy should be delivered by the respective beams at the isocentre.

Normalization of Dose Distributions: As explained previously, normalization of a dose distribution means basically the resetting of individual beam prescription dose, weightages and points in such a way so as to obtain a total of the required prescription dose. For example, if each beam is calculated as 100%, then the isodose selected at the isocentre could be a near sum total of each such as 280 or 290%. This will create confusion for the beam while converting these isodose percentages to absolute doses. After normalization, this isocentre dose may become 85–90%, a value most planners are more comfortable with. The ICRU recommends normalization of the dose distribution to 100% at the prescription point Q. With this in mind, it is important to remember that in isocentric techniques, the isodose value at the isocentre is simply the sum of the absolute weights of each beam. Also after normalizing the dose to 100% at the isocentre, the relative dose distributions from each beam at the isocentre have to be readjusted with the fresh normalization.

12.5.3 Inclusion of Output Parameters in Dose Distribution

The final beam output has to be corrected before calculating the treatment time or MU as this will otherwise affect the dose distribution. This correction has to be done to take into account PDD for extended field SSDs, wedge and tray factors, effects of the use of shielding blocks, compensators or boluses as well as correction for shutter error in case of cobalt machines. While previously these had to be done manually or on isodose charts, modern planning systems incorporate each of these factors as drop-down menu inclusions to a basic planning algorithm, and the computerized software calculates the effect of these on the MUs required. These can then be rechecked in a good quality assurance programme using either gamma or electron scatter analyses or by measurement in a water or tissue equivalent phantom.

References

1. International Commission on Radiation Units and Measurements, (ICRU). Prescribing, recording, and reporting photon beam therapy (Supplement to ICRU Report 50). ICRU Report 62, ICRU, Bethesda; 1999.
2. International Commission on Radiation Units and Measurements, (ICRU). Prescribing, recording, and reporting photon-beam intensity-modulated radiation therapy (IMRT). ICRU Report 83, ICRU, Bethesda; 2007.
3. Thilmann C, Zabel A, Milker-Zabel S, Schlegel W, Wannenmacher M, Debus J. Number and orientation of beams in inversely planned intensity-modulated radiotherapy of the female breast and the parasternal lymph nodes. Am J Clin Oncol. 2003;26(5):136–43.
4. Marks JE, Haus AG, Sutton HG, et al. The value of frequent treatment verification films in reducing localization error in the irradiation of complex fields. Cancer. 1976;37(6):2755–61.

13 An Introduction to Brachytherapy

13.1 Brachytherapy

Brachytherapy can deliver a high dose to the tumour while limiting irradiation dose to the surrounding normal tissues and is based on the principle of rapid dose fall-off with increasing distance based on the "inverse square law". Brachytherapy techniques in general require that the source is placed in close apposition or within the tumour-bearing tissue in the form of seeds, wires or pellets. Such implants may be of temporary or permanent duration depending on the tumour tissue and hence the implanted device. In brachytherapy, very high doses are always obtained close to the sources, and there are actually no large volumes for which the dose is nearly homogeneous as in external beam therapy, while on the other hand, in external beam therapy with photons or electrons, the differences between the maximum and the minimum doses in the target volume are usually between 10 and 15% or even 20%. However in brachytherapy, because of the inverse square law, a 1 cm difference in coverage can result in dose falling by even half.

The objectives of brachytherapy are to achieve disease control and cure, enable a high tumour-to-normal tissue dose ratio (reducing radiation morbidities), preserve organ function and cosmesis and be occasionally used in re-irradiation for recurrent tumours. The basic differences between brachytherapy and teletherapy are summed up in Table 13.1.

Table 13.1 Differences between brachytherapy and teletherapy

Brachytherapy	Teletherapy
Concentrates tumour dose and spares normal tissues	Irradiates significant volume of normal tissues
Shorter treatment course (1–2 weeks)	Prolonged course (5–8 weeks)
Continuous cell killing due to dose rate effect	Fractionated cell killing guided by 4Rs of radiobiology

A. Mukherji, *Basics of Planning and Management of Patients during Radiation Therapy*, https://doi.org/10.1007/978-981-10-6659-7_13

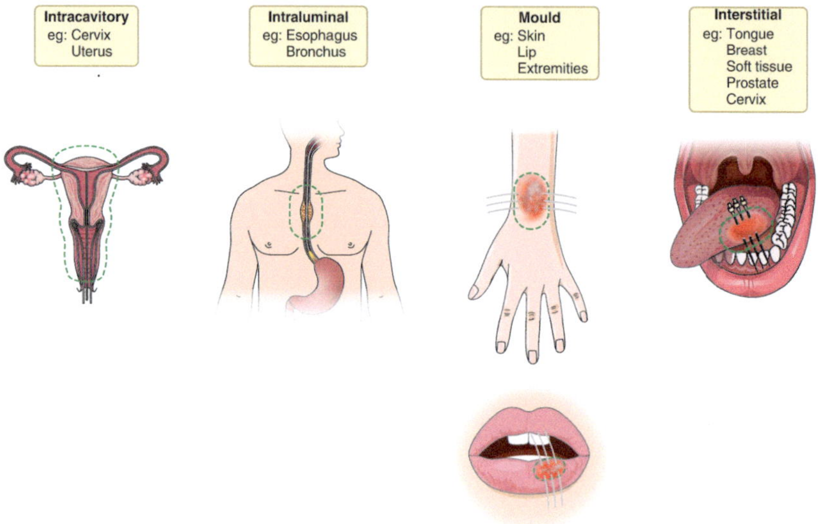

Fig. 13.1 Brachytherapy: methods of delivery

However brachytherapy cannot be successfully used in all situations and has its limits. Brachytherapy can be successfully applied for tumours which are accessible and well-demarcated. In addition, brachytherapy cannot be the single modality of therapy in tumours with high risk of regional lymph node spread and has to be combined with external beam radiation therapy as a form of local disease dose boost.

The practice of brachytherapy can involve the placement of radioactive sources through the tumour volume via needles (interstitial), in a body cavity (intracavitary), inside a lumen in cylindrical organs (intraluminal) or approximated to the tumour surface in case of superficial cancers (mould) (Fig. 13.1).

13.2 Indications of Brachytherapy

1. Mould brachytherapy can be used in small and superficial tumours like in T1 lip cancers or in oral cavity, basal cell cancers of the skin and superficial skin cancers in accessible areas like limb or scalp. In most of these cases, the requirement for mould brachytherapy is that these lesions are less than 1 cm thick and/or less than 4–5 cm in horizontal dimension. The reason these tumours are treated by mould and not by surgery can be due to their location where surgery can cause unacceptable cosmetic derangement or where there is not enough subcutaneous tissue plane to achieve desired surgical margins or when the patient is unable to tolerate surgery (advanced age, extreme co-morbidities). It is also used in deep-seated tissues like the nasopharynx, palate or vagina as a boost therapy following definitive treatment.

2. Plaque therapy is another type of surface mould therapy characteristically used in treating choroidal or retinal lesions with plaques containing radioactive sources.
3. Intraluminal brachytherapy is characteristically used in hollow cylindrical organs like the rectum, oesophagus, bronchus or biliary structures. Here an intraluminal catheter is introduced through which radioactive sources are approximated close to tumour surface. This technique is used as radical therapy in early stages where the entire tumour depth can be included in the prescription isodose or as a boost therapy after external beam irradiation where it is an excellent form of conformal radiation therapy.
4. Intracavitary brachytherapy is classically used in organs with hollow cul-de-sac where an applicator can be inserted and the surrounding tissues treated. It is usually used in gynaecological cancers like the cervix or uterine body. Again in early stages, it can be used as radical therapy or as adjunct to external beam radiation therapy in more advanced stages.
5. Interstitial brachytherapy implies placement of hollow catheters through a trocar and needle set through the substance of the tumour. This method is used in early-stage head and neck cancers as either radical or boost treatment, in soft tissue sarcomas as boost therapy pre- or post-surgery, in breast cancers as local boost or accelerated partial breast irradiation (APBI) and in prostate cancers or in gynaecological cancers as perineal implant.
6. Permanent implants are used in the prostate and consist of low-energy short-half-life radioactive sources implanted as seeds into the tumour tissue.

Thus brachytherapy is used in both superficial and deep-seated lesions where the tumour is well localized and can be accessed by either a mould or applicator, where there is a benefit vis-à-vis sparing of surrounding tissue and dose escalation which cannot be obtained through even IMRT. Situations where brachytherapy is not suitable include diffuse and extensive growth, node-positive or metastatic disease, tumour very close to bone or other critical structures and patient not fit for anaesthesia.

13.3 Brachytherapy Sources

Source specification or strength in brachytherapy is expressed by various quantities like equivalent mass of radium (mg-hour), activity (in Ci), apparent activity for sealed source (i.e. activity equivalent to an unsealed source in terms of exposure rate) or exposure rate constant. *In modern dosimetry, the AAPM recommends the use of air-kerma strength, Sk, to characterize the source strength.* The SI unit for exposure (exposure rate) is C Kg^{-1} (C Kg^{-1} s^{-1}). The exposure rate and air-kerma rate are used to describe the energy imparted by a radioactive source used keeping in mind the decay in activity with time. The air-kerma rate varies as a function of distance to the source because of the inverse square law and attenuation in air, which however is negligible, leaving the inverse square factor as the dominant one. The product of the

Table 13.2 Characteristics of radioactive sources used in modern brachytherapy practice

Radionuclide	Atomic mass (A)	Atomic number (Z)	Half-life	Decay product	Energy range (MeV)	Mean photon energy (MeV)
Radium (Ra)	226	88	1522 years	α	0.047–2.45	0.83
Gold (Au)	198	79	2.7 days	β	0.069–1.088	0.41
Caesium (Cs)	137	55	30 years	β	0.032–0.662	0.662
Cobalt (Co)	60	27	5.3 years	β	0.347–2.56	1.25
Iridium (Ir)	192	77	74 days	β, EC	0.062–1.38	0.38
Ytterbium (Yb)	169	70	32 days	EC	0.021–0.78	0.093
Thulium (Tm)	170	69	129 days	β, EC	0.07–0.084	0.066
Palladium (Pd)	103	46	17 days	EC	0.02–0.5	0.21
Iodine (I)	125	53	59.4 days	EC	0.027–0.035	0.028
Caesium (Cs)	131	55	9.7 days	EC	0.029–0.034	0.03

air-kerma rate with the square of the distance is roughly constant over a range of distances that are useful in clinical practice. The air-kerma strength, Sk, is defined as the product air-kerma rate in free space at the distance of measurement and the square of that distance along the perpendicular bisector and has been adopted as a reference quantity for low-energy sources used in permanent seed implants (PSIs).

In 1998, the AAPM (American Association of Physicists in Medicine) published recommendations on the conditions required for clinical use of new low-energy photon sources. These recommendations include definition of responsibility for source calibration and standardization to the manufacturer including periodic validation by independent laboratory, calibration and publishing dosimetric parameters of a new source as well as its Monte Carlo experiments as per TG43 protocol and maintenance of registry of sources [1]. Table 13.2 lists characteristics of commonly used brachytherapy sources.

13.4 Radiobiology of Brachytherapy

Brachytherapy has been traditionally divided according to the ICRU-38 [2] report into *low-dose-rate or LDR brachytherapy (rates of 0.3–1.0 Gy* h^{-1}*), medium-dose-rate or MDR brachytherapy (2–12 Gy* h^{-1}*) and high-dose-rate or HDR brachytherapy (greater than 12 Gy* h^{-1}*)* [2]. In addition there is also PDR or pulsed dose rate brachytherapy which has been explained in the following section and very-low-dose-rate (vLDR) brachytherapy in which the dose rates are less than 0.4 Gy h^{-1}. These can be used for permanent implants.

In brachytherapy dose rate is one of the main factors determining response. As the dose rates decrease, there is a corresponding decrease in the effects of irradiation which is because of the action of repair of tissue irradiated. It has been assumed that the dose required to achieve optimum tumour cell kill can double when the dose rate decreases by a factor of 10 and for the late-reacting tissues, the required dose to produce similar effects at low and high dose rates is 2.5–3 times. Thus there is always a differential between the tumour and acutely reacting tissues and the late-reacting tissues at low dose rates wherein the advantage of LDR brachytherapy lies. Thus in LDR brachytherapy, the principal determinants are the dose rate and the treatment time. Fractionation is usually not required in LDR as it may have any significant bearing on local control and normal tissue reactions are avoided by delivering brachytherapy at a dose rate which would allow normal tissue sublethal damage repair to proceed even during irradiation.

Radiobiology of High-Dose-Rate Brachytherapy: *LDR and HDR brachytherapies differ in their radiobiological response mainly because of the effect of the dose rate on repair of sublethal damage*. As discussed before there is dose differential between tumour or early-reacting tissue and late-reacting normal tissue which can be graphically seen in the survival curves of most tumour tissue being more linear than those for late-reacting normal tissue cells which at low doses show large shoulders displaying higher ability for repair of sublethal damage [3]. In a fractionated course of radiation therapy, there is greater scope for repair of the normal tissue compared to tumour tissue which may take time and for which therefore the fractions in HDR brachytherapy are separated by at least 6 h [4–6]. Thus the radiobiological advantage of sublethal damage repair in HDR brachytherapy is achieved by dividing the total dose into many smaller fractions which are separated by a time interval sufficient to ensure normal tissue damage repair.

This results in the creation of a *window of opportunity* in which treatment at a dose per fraction below the crossover point of the two survival curves causes more killing of tumour than normal tissue cells. To achieve this same effect by using HDR brachytherapy instead of LDR, one has to replace the effect of the continuous cell kill and sublethal damage repair at low dose rates with the effect of fractionation of total dose into smaller doses at determined intervals to allow tissue repair in HDR [7]. This effect is known as the **dose rate effect** [8]. Thus equivalency between HDR and LDR regimes can be achieved if the HDR fractional dose is low enough to allow cell repair making the survival curve shallower, while a high dose per fraction increases cell kill and causes the survival curve to become steeper.

13.4.1 Practical Uses of Radiobiology in Brachytherapy

The radiobiological principles involved in the effect of brachytherapy are used often in day-to-day practice either in deciding the dose and fractionation of brachytherapy regimes while using a combination of external beam radiation therapy and brachytherapy or in conversion of dose or obtaining isoeffective or conventional dose equivalents from a delivered brachytherapy regime whether HDR or LDR.

In case of LDR brachytherapy, the dose by LDR can be simply added to external beam radiation therapy doses (at conventional doses) to obtain equivalent total doses. Conversion or obtaining isoeffective doses in HDR from an LDR regime in the past used to be done by either using a dose reduction factor or time dose factor or the nominal standard dose (NSD). A simplified computer program developed by

Nag and Gupta [9] can obtain the isoeffective doses for HDR in which the clinician needs only to enter the EBRT total dose and dose/fraction, the HDR dose and the number of HDR fractions, and the program then calculates the EQD2 (2 Gy equivalent dose) for tumour and normal tissue.

The LQ model which takes into calculation the repair of sublethal damage can also be used to obtain the EQD2 doses. However there are many unaccounted variables in this method such as the effect of reoxygenation, redistribution or repopulation, which while for conventional dose may not cause significant contribution to the dose effect but may assume importance if the dose per fraction is large enough to negate reoxygenation or redistribution leading to an overestimation of the tumour effect of a single large dose per fraction. Also the accuracy of the LQ model in estimating EQD2 may vary because of the large variation in the α/β values for early reactions (6–13), late reactions (1–7) and tumour tissues (0.4–13).

Another problem of using the LQ model is that it assumes complete repair between fractions which is however dependent on the time interval between the fractions and will be accurate only if sufficient interval is provided between fractions. It is also important to note that during prescription, it is a common practice to prescribe the fractional dose to the isodose covering the target volume adequately. This means that the dose prescribed is the minimum dose the entire volume receives, while regions which are closer to the applicator may receive much higher doses. Therefore the radiation oncologist has to be careful when prescribing dose and volume bearing in mind the tissue tolerances and location of critical OARs. This point will be further explained in the next chapter. Thus the LQ model should be used judiciously as a guide correlated with clinical judgement and outcome results with special caution whenever large fraction sizes are used [10].

13.4.2 Pulsed Dose Rate (PDR) Treatment

What Is PDR: The commonly used brachytherapy equipment has been traditionally based either on low dose rate (LDR) or high dose rate (HDR). LDR brachytherapy has the advantage of almost following the tissue repair mechanisms with resultant decreased toxicities, while HDR brachytherapy is advantageous in terms of optimization of dose distribution and radiation safety in spite of high dose rate because of less treatment and thus exposure time. Pulsed dose rate brachytherapy is a recent brachytherapy modality that tries to combine physical advantages of high-dose-rate (HDR) technology with radiobiological advantages of low-dose-rate (LDR) brachytherapy. In PDR, the machine uses a single-stepping iridium source (Ir-192) of strength 15–37 GBq (0.5–1 Ci) which sequentially moves through all the implanted catheters for fixed dwelling time periods at each position specified by the treatment plan. The irradiation dose is delivered by dose rates of up to about 3 Gy h^{-1}, in the form of short durations of timed exposures of 10 min to up to 30 min of duration as hourly or two hourly pulses.

Mechanism of PDR: In PDR brachytherapy, while the source used has higher strength, the treatment is delivered as short pulses (10–30 min) of exposure hourly over the same total duration as LDR brachytherapy with the net result being the same hourly dose as LDR brachytherapy. In PDR the sequence and duration of pulses through the implanted catheters can be programmed by a dedicated computer. This computerization provides the advantages of precise calculation of the pulse sequences, optimizing the dwell positions and durations to achieve required target volume coverage, and allows remote control of dose delivery, thereby enhancing radiation safety of treating personnel. In this respect, PDR resembles HDR brachytherapy.

13.4.2.1 Advantage Over HDR

- In PDR, the source strength is 10–20 times lesser than in HDR, and thus the requirements for shielding become less stringent. An ordinary brachytherapy room would require less than two extra-half, value thickness of protection, and an accelerator-type bunker is not necessary.
- Computerization and remote afterloading and treatment delivery in PDR are similar to that in HDR with resultant improved radiation safety due to its weaker source strength.
- PDR brachytherapy has a theoretical radiobiological advantage over HDR as this technique allows some amount of tissue repair in late-reacting normal tissue during the intervals between pulses of dose exposure.

13.4.2.2 Advantage Over LDR

- In PDR brachytherapy due to availability of optimization, dose distribution is better controlled and tailored, with better target volume coverage by prescribed dose, better reproducibility of treatment plans and greater flexibility to change the dose distribution during treatment if necessary.
- The iridium source in PDR needs to be replaced at the most two to three times a year allowing to provide improved radiation safety for clinical and physics staff.
- A single machine like in HDR can perform all brachytherapy procedures such as intracavitary, interstitial and intraluminal.
- Nursing care compared with LDR brachytherapy is improved for PDR brachytherapy as the implanted patient can be monitored and attended to in between the pulses of dose exposure.

13.4.2.3 Advantage of HDR Brachytherapy

- The HDR remote afterloader treatments are performed in a fully shielded room comparable with those required for a cobalt teletherapy unit. 192Ir is the most commonly used radioisotope, while 137Cs or 60Co sources also are used in some units.
- Remote-controlled insertion of sources inside hollow applicators or catheters which are operatively placed into the target tissue has significantly contributed to the increase in radiation safety for medical personnel. The applicators are connected by transfer tubes to the radioactive material, which is stored in a shielded safe. The radiation source is driven through the transfer tubes and into the tumour by remote control from outside the room.

- By programming dwell position (the sequence of stops the source makes during its passage through the implanted catheter in the tumour tissue) and dwell time (amount of time a source in the implanted stops at a planned position within the target volume) of the source, desired isodose distributions can be obtained. The determination of the individual dwell position and optimization of the dwell time are part of the planning process. The use of a single-stepping source allows optimization of dose distribution by varying the dwell time at each dwell position which is consistent and reproducible.
- In HDR brachytherapy, the source sizes are very small. This translates to an advantage over LDR brachytherapy in that the cross section required for applicators in HDR brachytherapy would be less than LDR brachytherapy and hence while insertion into tissues will cause less damage and thus faster recovery.
- The treatments usually take only a few minutes, which can be given on an outpatient basis with minimal risk of applicator movement and minimal patient discomfort. Better packing or retraction of normal tissues is thus possible with HDR, because of the short treatment duration.
- However all these benefits of HDR come at the cost of increased expense in infrastructure and working costs, with no significant improvements in outcome over state-of-the-art conventional LDR brachytherapy and with significantly greater quality assurance requirements.

13.5 Use of 3D Planning in Brachytherapy

Brachytherapy has often been called as the *poor man's IMRT* because of the ability of this technique of radiation therapy to achieve a very high degree of dose conformity around the target volume with rapid dose fall-off beyond. This is because of its properties of inverse square law working in tandem with generally low mean energies of the sources used and can be optimized by interplay between source distribution and dwell times. This can be best achieved by 3D guided planning and dose optimization by direct visualization of the dose colour wash/isodoses on the CT images rather than estimating location of normal tissues and their volume dose effects based on the dose cloud obtained otherwise in 2D planning systems. Using CT images for viewing the position of implanted catheters or applicators especially with respect to the target volume as well as defining the tumour volume and the surrounding anatomy can be better achieved by 3D imaging using either CT or MR images. These will also provide for better visualization of the location and distance of the organs at risk and their relation to the target volume or dose distribution.

In 2D planning the radiation oncologist uses orthogonal check X-rays to assess catheter or applicator placement with respect to bony landmarks, and in this respect; 3D planning by the use of CT or MR images allows better appreciation of patient anatomy as well as assesses the degree of dose optimization and studies the dose distributions in surrounding tissues by way of dose-volume histograms (DVHs). Also when many different imaging techniques have been used (like CT, MRI or PET/CT), an accurate transfer of information from these different techniques as well as better target volume delineation onto the planning system can be achieved only through image registration and fusion [11] for which availability of 3D planning is a must. Other advantages of CT-based planning include a degree of automation in the anatomy delineation and catheter definition [12], as well as reduction in the time taken for the catheter reconstruction process using an auto reconstruction method compared to manual CT or film-based reconstruction.

Furthermore, 3D planning has brought into practice the concept of dose escalation. Several studies have shown that the traditional method of estimating the dose distribution by calculating the dose delivered to specific single points has not correlated with the observed pattern of post-therapy sequelae. In this respect, therefore, recent advances in dose-volume concepts have been applied to brachytherapy as well, and it has been noted that volume-based estimation of received doses to target and critical organs correlates better with observed effects [13]. Good quality assurance requires full volumetric data on dose distribution which can be only provided by reviewing the entire 3D volume. Thus in 3D planning, the objective of the treatment plan is to achieve a specific dose distribution to a defined volume and not to a fixed source configuration which would mainly depend on the dose delivered without reference to dwell time pattern or source distribution.

13.5.1 CT-Based Brachytherapy

The proper dose delivery of fractionated HDR brachytherapy relies on the stability of the implant and on reproducible catheter positions for each fraction. This is particularly critical with the current trend to reduce the number of fractions and increase the dose per fraction. *The tumour volume may change because of the insertion of catheters or the delivery of radiation.* The dosimetric errors resulting from these volume changes can be minimized by the anatomic information provided by 3D imaging.

Another factor is the uncertainty in the localization of the longitudinal catheter tip positions due to the discrete slice thickness for which fine-thickness CT scans are done to minimize the dose error induced by uncertainty of CT reconstructions. But in this situation, the treatment planning needs additional time and effort from the oncologists for contouring the target volume in the additional slices and from the medical physicist to define the catheter positions in the increased number of CT scan slices. In a study [14], different scenarios were considered to mimic the longitudinal imprecision of the catheter tips and dwell positions, with catheters randomly distributed within the space defined by one CT slice thickness, for thicknesses from 2 to 5 mm. It was found that the dose uncertainties caused by the finite slice thickness increase with the slice spacing, from 3 to 8% for slice thickness values from 2 to 5 mm, respectively, and limiting the slice thickness to below 3 mm without compromising much on the total slice numbers brought down this dose uncertainty to less than 1%.

Use of needles to insert permanent implants into the prostatic tissue can itself induce local tissue trauma and cause rapid volume changes in the tissue over the next few hours or days [15–17] and taking often several weeks to resolve. The effect of this oedema on dose coverage has been investigated [14–18], but with differing results and significance as usually the irradiation is completed in a few fractions within the first 2–3 days after catheter insertion and may actually have less effect than estimated. *What is important to the clinician is whether this oedema and the resultant change in volume will be significant between each fraction, necessitating a replanning for each fraction.* Another study on the effect of change in the prostatic volume following temporary interstitial HDR brachytherapy [14] reported either an expansion or a contraction of up to 17% of the tissue between the fractions delivered, which amounted to less than 5% variation from the prescription dose.

In addition to the dose uncertainty attributable to the intrinsic characteristics of the finite CT slice thickness and the dosimetric effect of volume change resulting from the trauma caused by the insertion of catheters and from resolution of oedema between fractions [19], cranio-caudal catheter displacement attributable to patient and organ motion between fractions can also affect the dose distribution. A study performed by Kim et al. [20] showed an average catheter displacement of 4.1 mm between the first and second fractions. Using fluoroscopy in another study, Martinez et al. [21] measured a mean displacement of 20 mm between the first and second fractions, which decreased between the subsequent fractions to an average of 4 mm. Using measurements of catheter tips by plain films taken before treatment, Damore [22] reported a mean displacement of 7.6 mm and a maximum displacement measurement by the bony marker method of 28.5 mm between the first and second fractions and a reduction in needle movement after the first day. Mullokandov and Gejerman [23] using template-based brachytherapy in prostate cancers reported that no displacement of catheters relative to template occurred and that the mean consecutive catheter displacement was 2, 8 and 10 mm before the second, third and fourth fractions.

13.5.2 Robotic Brachytherapy

Robotic mechanisms can achieve precise positioning and registration using precision mechanisms and mathematic coordinate transformations and have the potential to guide seeds to many more locations in the body because they do not rely on rigid mechanical grids or real-time imaging for human guidance and are increasingly being introduced into clinical practice. Such recent advances in medical robotics have been studied and commented upon by Taylor and Stoianovici [24] and Cleary [25]. Image-guided needle insertion procedures in particular can benefit from the more precise control over the needle insertion and pathway by using robotic hand-guided instrumentation; and custom robotic devices can address the clinical challenges of space constraints, safety requirements and imaging modality compatibility such as in CT- or MR-guided intervention techniques [26–31]. Using robotic assistants inside MR scanners is even more challenging not only due to space constraints but also because of the presence of magnetic fields which necessitates use of non-metallic body parts for the robotic assistant. The use of these robotic assistants allows for faster, more accurate and more representative biopsies in tissues which were otherwise difficult to access especially under CT or MR guidance. Also, the delivery of seeds or catheters using robots offers the unique advantage of performing real-time or quasi real-time imaging during the procedure. This allows the validations of the correct location of the needle relative to the anatomy before seeds are dropped, potentially eliminating a lot of errors. A series of experiments performed at UCSF showed that the several imaging systems (MRI or CT), the planning system and the robot control could be registered to guide the delivery of a seed to within 1 mm of a target. Similarly, even MRS information could be used to guide the robot to certain cancer-validated areas.

Recently dosimetric planning studies have shown that inverse planning [32] could be used to optimize new seed distributions [33] or new catheter patterns for HDR in the limited space inside a closed MRI. These can potentially deliver equivalent dose distribution to the target and reduce physical trauma to organs. Thus robotic hardware can offer the ability to drive a needle along any desired path three dimensionally to reach an imaged point. This will allow high precision of dose delivery resulting in increased treatment effectiveness, reduced side effects and expanded treatment availability.

References

1. Rivard MJ, Coursey BM, DeWerd LA, et al. Update of AAPM Task Group No. 43 Report: a revised AAPM protocol for brachytherapy dose calculations. Med Phys. 2004;31:633.
2. Report No. 38. Dose and volume specification for reporting intracavitary brachytherapy for gynecology. Bethesda, MD: International Commission on Radiation Units and Measurements; 1985.
3. Hall EJ. Radiobiology for the radiologist. 5th ed. Philadelphia: Lippinott Williams & Wilkins; 2000. p. 401.
4. Dale RG. The application of the linear-quadratic dose-effect equation to fractionated and protracted radiotherapy. Br J Radiol. 1985;58:515.
5. Fowler JF. Why shorter half-times for repair lead to greater damage in pulsed brachytherapy. Int J Radiat Oncol Biol Phys. 1993;26:353.
6. Thames HD. Effect-independent measurements of tissue responses to fractionated irradiation. Int J Radiat Biol Relat Stud Phys Chem Med. 1984;45(1):1–10.
7. Orton CG. High and low dose rate remote afterloading: a critical comparison. In: Sauer R, editor. International radiation therapy techniques—brachytherapy. Berlin: Springer; 1991. p. 53.
8. Hall EJ. Radiobiology for the radiologist. 5th ed. Philadelphia: Lippincott Williams & Wilkins; 2000. p. 74.
9. Nag S, Gupta N. A simple method of obtaining equivalent doses for use in HDR brachytherapy. Int J Radiat Oncol Biol Phys. 2000;46:507–13.
10. Dale RG. The use of small fraction numbers in high dose-rate gynecological afterloading: some radiobiological considerations. Br J Radiol. 1990;63:290.
11. Krempien RC, Dacuber S, Hensley FW, et al. Image fusion of CT and MRI data enables improved target volume definition in 3D-brachytherapy treatment planning. Brachytherapy. 2003;2(3):164.
12. Milicokovic N, Giannouli S, Baltas D, et al. Catheter auto reconstruction in computed tomography based brachytherapy treatment planning. Med Phys. 2000;27(5):1047.
13. Milickovic N, Lahanas M, Papagiannopoulou M, et al. Multiobjective anatomy-based dose optimization for HDR-brachytherapy with constraint free deterministic algorithms. Phys Med Biol. 2002;47:2263.

14. Kim Y, Hsu I-C, Lessard E, et al. Dose uncertainty due to computed tomography CT slice thickness in CT-based high dose rate brachytherapy of the prostate cancer. Med Phys. 2004;31(9):2543.
15. Yue N, Dicker AP, Nath R, et al. The impact of edema on planning 125I and 103Pd prostate implants. Med Phys. 1999;26:763.
16. Yue N, Dicker AP, Corn BW, et al. A dynamic model for the estimation of optimum timing of computed tomography scan for dose evaluation of 125I or 103Pd seed implant of prostate. Int J Radiat Oncol Biol Phys. 1999;43:447.
17. Waterman FM, Yue N, Corn BW, et al. Edema associated with I-125 or Pd-103 prostate brachytherapy and its impact on post-implant dosimetry: an analysis based on serial CT acquisition. Int J Radiat Oncol Biol Phys. 1998;41:1069.
18. Prestidge BR, Bice WS, Kiefer EJ, et al. Timing of computed tomography-based postimplant assessment following permanent transperineal prostate brachytherapy. Int J Radiat Oncol Biol Phys. 1998;40:1111.
19. Kim YB, Hsu I-C, Lessard E, et al. Prostate volume change and dosimetric impact of edema between HDR brachytherapy fractions. Int J Radiat Oncol Biol Phys. 2004;59(4):1208.
20. Kim Y, Hsu I, Pouliot J. Cranio-caudal catheter displacement between fractions in CT-based HDR brachytherapy of prostate cancer. J Appl Clin Med Phys. 2007;8(4):1.
21. Martinez AA, Pataki I, Edmundson G, et al. Phase II prospective study of the use of conformal high-dose-rate brachytherapy as monotherapy for the treatment of favorable stage prostate cancer: a feasibility report. Int J Radiat Oncol Biol Phys. 2001;49(1):61.
22. Damore SJ, Syed AM, Puthawala AA, et al. Needle displacement during HDR brachytherapy in the treatment of prostate cancer. Int J Radiat Oncol Biol Phys. 2000;46(5):1205.
23. Mullokandov E, Gejerman G. Analysis of serial CT scans to assess template and catheter movement in prostate HDR brachytherapy. Int J Radiat Oncol Biol Phys. 2004;58(4):1063.
24. Taylor RH, Stoianovici D. Medical robotics in computer-integrated surgery. IEEE Trans Rob Autom. 2003;19(5):765–81.
25. Cleary K, Melzer A, Watson V, et al. Interventional robotic systems: applications and technology state-of-the-art. Minim Invasiv Ther Allied Technol. 2006;15(2):101–13.
26. Kwoh YS, Hou J, Jonckheere EA, et al. A robot with improved absolute positioning accuracy for CT guided stereotactic brain surgery. IEEE Trans Biomed Eng. 1988;35(2):153.
27. Masamune K, Ji LH, Suzuki M, et al. A newly developed stereotactic robot with detachable drive for neurosurgery. In: Medical image computing and computer assisted intervention (MICCAI); 1998. p. 215.
28. Fichtinger G, Burdette EC, Tanacs A, et al. Robotically assisted prostate brachytherapy with transrectal ultrasound guidance phantom experiments. Brachytherapy. 2006;5(1):14.
29. Maurin B, Doignon C, Ganglo J, et al. CT-Bot: a stereotactic-guided robotic assistant for percutaneous procedures of the abdomen. Proc SPIE Med Imag. 2005;2005:241.
30. Chinzei K, Hata N, Jolesz FA, et al. MR compatible surgical assist robot: system integration and preliminary feasibility study. In: Medical image computing and computer assisted intervention (MICCAI). New York: Springer; 2000. p. 921.
31. DiMaio SP, Pieper S, Chinzei K, et al. Robot-assisted needle placement in open-MRI: system architecture, integration and validation. In: Westwood JD, et al., editors. Medicine meets virtual reality, vol. 14. Washington: IOS; 2006. p. 126.
32. Lessard E, Kwa SLS, Pickett B, et al. Class solution for inversely planned permanent prostate implants to mimic an experienced dosimetrist for pre and real-time treatment planning. Med Phys. 2006;33(8):2773.
33. Marion PR, Van Gellekom MP, Marinus A, et al. MRI-guided prostate brachytherapy with single needle method—a planning study. Radiother Oncol. 2004;71:327.

14 Brachytherapy Planning and Evaluation

14.1 Definition of Treatment Volumes in Brachytherapy

In general in brachytherapy, target and OAR volumes are similar to that in external beam radiotherapy, while prescriptions are based on ICRU Reports 38 and 58 [1, 2]. The gross tumour volume (GTV) in brachytherapy as in external beam irradiation is basically the visible tumour which can be identified either clinically or by imaging and consists of the primary cancer with any involved lymph nodes. Thus the GTV is always the part of the growth with highest tumour density. The GTV can be different in its shape and contour depending on the examination and localization technique used (such as use of only palpation or combined with mammography or ultrasound for breast tumours, whether CT or an MRI has been used in soft tissue solid tumours), and this should be indicated on the treatment planning chart by the radiation oncologist. A GTV can be part of an organ (e.g. an early-stage breast cancer or part of the tongue or lip), or even a whole organ like a large sarcoma of the extremity or locally advanced breast cancer. Also this contoured GTV could extend outside or even be limited within the normal anatomical borders of the organ tissue involved. In brachytherapy, this GTV is mainly defined as the primary tumour or GTV-T. With advent of MRI in brachytherapy, new concepts in volumes have been postulated and studied. GTV can be divided into GTV_D which is the GTV at time of diagnosis and GTV_B which is the GTV at time of brachytherapy.

In brachytherapy planning, one of the most important steps is the correct identification and delineation of the gross tumour volume. This is necessary to allow for firstly a proper staging and therefore correct decision making in treatment intent and technique. Correct and complete identification of the GTV allows accurate recording of tumour response and therefore computation of various prognostic factors. Finally in view of the "inverse square law" being applicable in brachytherapy, it is of utmost importance in correctly identifying the volume to be treated to ensure adequate dose coverage. There is however no big change in the definitions for various target or avoidance volumes in brachytherapy compared to external beam radiotherapy as per ICRU Report 50 and ICRU Report 62 (supplement to Report 50) [3, 4].

A. Mukherji, *Basics of Planning and Management of Patients during Radiation Therapy*, https://doi.org/10.1007/978-981-10-6659-7_14

Similarly the CTV (according to GEC-ESTRO) is also divided based on clinical examination and MRI study into a **high-risk CTV (HR-CTV)** and an **intermediate-risk CTV (IR-CTV)** [5]. The area designated as the HR-CTV is one which has a high risk of disease relapse as it may contain either the tumour itself (for radical brachytherapy in early-stage disease) or residual gross tumour (post-surgery or external beam irradiation), while the area designated as IR-CTV may have had initial macroscopic disease but, at the time of brachytherapy, is thought to have microscopic subclinical disease [5]. The treatment aim is to deliver a total dose as high as possible to eradicate all residual macroscopic and microscopic disease [5].

For PTV in brachytherapy, width of margin should, ideally, be based on systematic evaluation of the uncertainties. It may differ according to the organ being treated, the clinical target volume and also the type of applicator and technical devices used. With some techniques, there are uncertainties about consistency of source position (moving sources, fractionated techniques) or alteration of source or applicator position (intracavitary applications, permanent implants) during the application. In general, in brachytherapy, PTV is considered the same as CTV with some exceptions such as in intraluminal brachytherapy where longitudinal movements may have to be taken into consideration.

14.2 Application Techniques

14.2.1 Surface Mould

It is used in superficial tumours. Contour of the lesion is simulated, and tissue equivalent material as a mould is placed over the skin surface. These customized devices are designed to hold the catheters in position as closely as possible to tumour surface to provide adequate dose coverage of tumour volume and increase distance to other normal surrounding structures. Local control of disease exceeds 90% in early-stage (T1/T2N0) tumours treated with brachytherapy alone [6]. Mould therapy is excellent in treatment of superficial oral cancers as it provides a high localized dose of radiation, with rapid fall-off and short treatment course duration, [6] and enables highly reproducible irradiation [7, 8]. Superficial lesions, compared to more deep infiltrating lesions even in the same stage, usually have a higher cure rate with mould irradiation [9]. Source is in form of tube, needle and seeds. Distance between the source and skin depends upon the depth below the surface to be irradiated and is generally 0.5 or 1 cm but not beyond 1.5 cm depth, for example, the ear, lip, floor of the mouth, penis and limbs. Material used for mould includes plastic compounds (Perspex, Bexoid), self-adhesive Elastoplasts, plaster of Paris and even wax.

The moulds are prepared from a variety of frameworks such as thermoplastic sheet/wax/Perspex/plaster of Paris. These are approximated to the area planned to be treated in such a way that the frame exactly or as far as possible matches the patient's anatomy. The frame is then converted into the actual mould by either layering wax over the frame or using the wax frame as a negative to create the actual Perspex or acrylic mould (Figs. 14.1, 14.2, 14.3, and 14.4). This mould which has

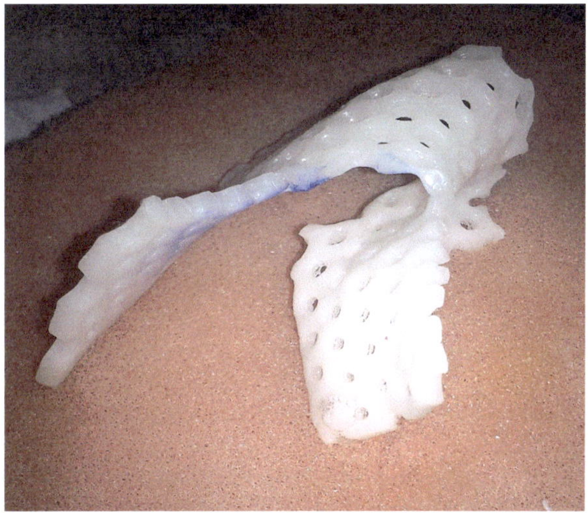

Fig. 14.1 Creating a frame for a surface mould

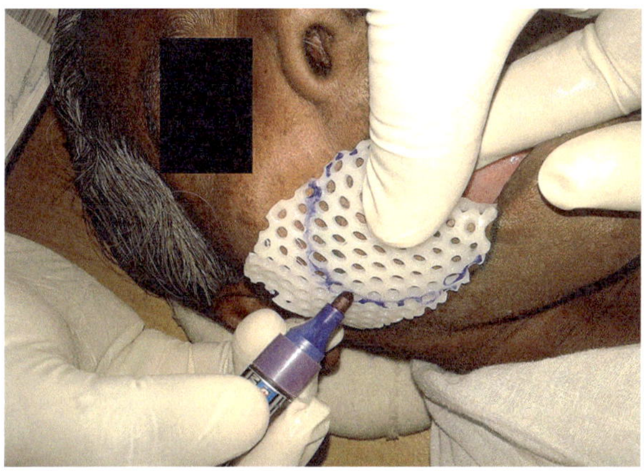

Fig. 14.2 Marking the lesion on the frame of the surface mould

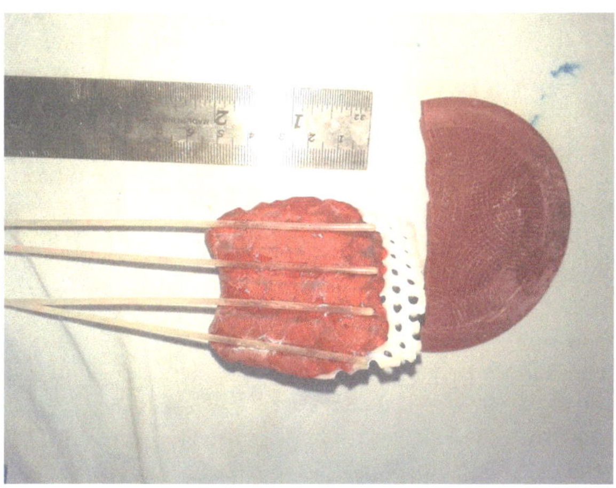

Fig. 14.3 Dental wax layered on the frame for a surface mould and catheters fixed

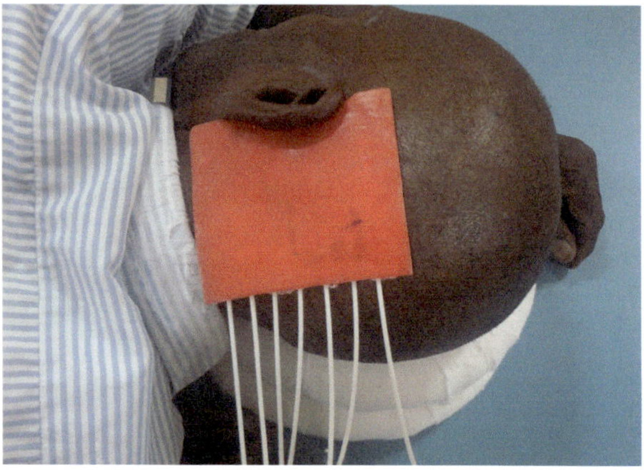

Fig. 14.4 Planar surface mould with catheters fixed

been prepared and marked is again matched with the surface of the lesion, the area to be treated is marked on to the mould, catheters are then fixed and checked for position and fidelity, and then the patient is imaged with the mould in place. On the CT images, the CTV is drawn, dwell positions marked and dosimetry done.

Mould types include planar, linear and cylindrical. In planar moulds, the plane or its curvature is less than that of hemisphere or semi-cylinder. Source arrangements in moulds can be as circle, square or rectangle. Selection of treatment distance "*h*" where "*h*" is the distance between the source plane and treatment surface depends on the depth dose required and also dose to other tissues surrounding the implant.

In planar circular mould, area to be treated is circular in shape. Source distribution depends on diameter of the circle d and the distance between the planes h. If a single circle is used, then $d/h = 3$ (ideal is $d/h = 2.83$). The inner circle is half the diameter of outer circle. Distribution rule for circular moulds: If d/h is <3, then outer circle gets 100% dose; if d/h is 3 to <6, then outer circle gets 95% dose and inner circle gets 5% dose; while if d/h is >6, then outer circle gets 80% dose, inner 17% dose and the centre 3% dose.

In square-/rectangular-shaped moulds, source distribution is on four sides and inside, parallel to longer side (Fig. 14.4). Separation between any two lines of sources is $\leq 2h$, and separation between active ends of any two sources in the same line is $\leq h$. The linear activity of added line, inside the area, should be one-half of the peripheral (single added line) and two-thirds for more than one added line. For rectangular areas, the dose should be increased by a factor to correct for the elongation.

14.2.2 Sandwich Mould

A block of tissue can be sandwiched between the parallel planes of sources kept in the moulds. To achieve the dose homogeneity across the tissues block, two moulds are kept parallel to one another, enclosing between them tumour-bearing tissues (Fig. 14.5). The fall-off in intensity from one mould is balanced by the rise from the other. Examples include cancers of the lip, ear and floor of the mouth.

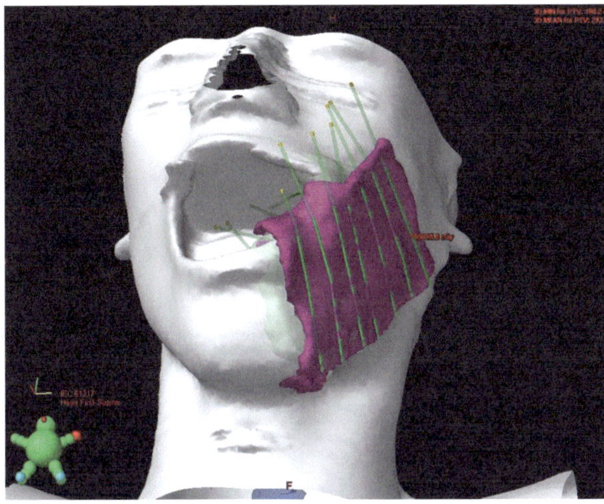

Fig. 14.5 Sandwich mould

In earlier times calculation of dose in mould brachytherapy was done according to Paterson-Parker rules. In present times, with the increasing use of CT-based planning and stepping source type machines, source dwell positions can be optimized by both automatically computer-aided software or even manually by applying specific source position patterns depending on the PTV and loading the catheters as well as altering dwell times accordingly.

14.2.3 Linear Moulds

Sources loaded end to end in appropriate applicator. Examples include the oesophagus, rectum, vagina, nose, etc. Space between the active ends of any two sources shouldn't be more than the radius of the applicator. If the tumour is too long compared to radius of the applicator, sources should be loaded well beyond the lesion of interest, or end activity may be increased. The dwell times required for delivering 1000 cGy on the surface of the applicator for different active lengths and treatment distances are standard.

14.2.4 Cylindrical Moulds

Examples include use in the neck, finger, penis, etc. Source distribution is in a single ring or over the surface of a cylinder. Uniform dose is obtained over cylindrical surfaces coaxial with and of smaller diameter than the source bearing cylinder. Sources are arranged in series of coaxial rings with series of equidistant lines parallel to the axis of cylinder (Fig. 14.6).

It is usual to prescribe the required dose to the 85–90% isodose which is adequate for brachytherapy. The aim is to cover the maximum tumour volume within this prescription dose and to prevent higher isodoses from entering the skin-mould

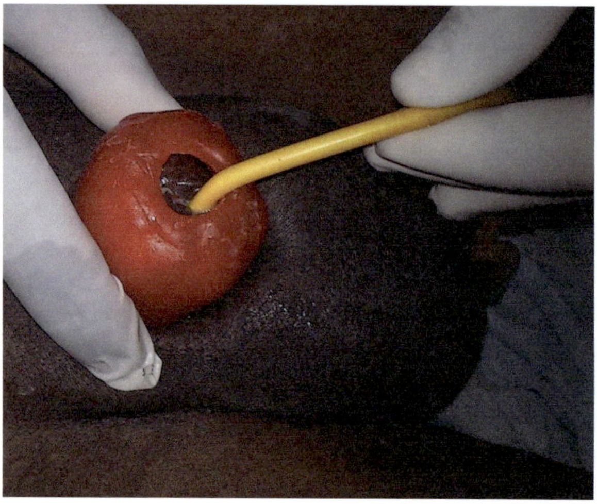

Fig. 14.6 Cylindrical mould

interface and remain within the mould. Ideally no part should receive more than 130–140% of prescribed dose, but usually planners aim to keep tissue receiving more than 150% to less than 5%.

14.3 Interstitial Implant

In this technique, the sources are directly implanted into the tissues in and around the malignant growth. This technique aims to deliver a uniform dose (ranging about ±10% from the prescribed dose) in the substance of the volume to be treated. This technique thus combines the advantage of obtaining very high tumour volume doses while restricting sharply doses to surrounding normal tissues. But the main drawback is that absolute dose homogeneity is not possible because of the intensely high zone of the radiation immediately surrounding the implanted needle and seed sources. Examples include use in the oral cavity, breast and extremity soft tissues (Figs. 14.7, 14.8, 14.9, 14.10, 14.11, and 14.12). Interstitial implants are divided into planar and volume implant. Planar implant is used when tumour spread is under the skin surface or when the lesion can be sandwiched between the parallel planes of implant. Volume implant is used when lesion to be treated is more than 2.5 cm thick and planar implant leads to low-dose region midway between the planes.

Rules for needle insertion in interstitial implant have been traditionally based on Paterson-Parker, Quimby or Paris system. But in modern-day brachytherapy, computerized planning system-based source strength and dwell-time optimizations have taken place of implantation rules. The classical **Paterson-Parker system** aims to obtain a uniform dose throughout the target volume, and in this system, the sources are distributed non-uniformly based on the size of the target volume. The pattern of implantation follows a set principle of rules and tries a distribution with more source strength in the periphery of the target volume. There is very less variation of dose within the implanted volume with difference between the prescribed dose and

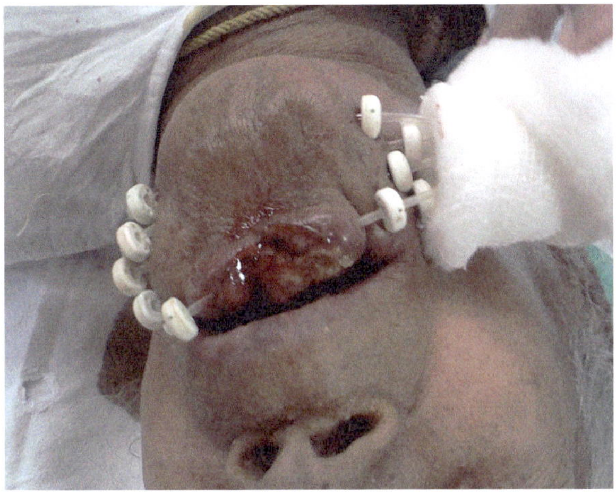

Fig. 14.7 Single plane lip implant

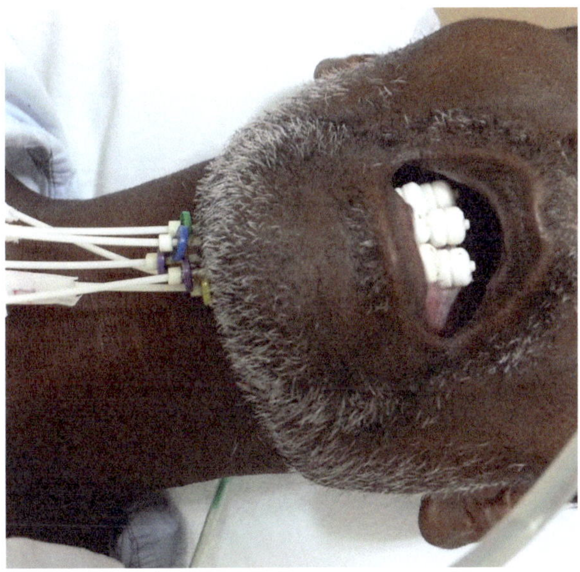

Fig. 14.8 Three-plane tongue implant

minimum target volume dose not being more than 10%. Needles spacing are not more than 1 cm from each other. For uncrossed ends, effective area is reduced by 10% for each uncrossed ends. In a multi-planar implant, planes should be parallel to each other, and if separation is more than 1.0 cm between the planes, then multiplication factors are used.

In single-plane implant, reference dose plane is 0.5 cm from source plane. The dose at 0.5 cm is the minimum dose throughout the 1-cm-thick slab. The high spots immediately surrounding each source are assumed to be tolerated by tissues, and its presence is ignored. Distribution laws of sources in planar implants: when area is <25 cm^2, two-thirds of strength of source is at periphery and one-third at centre.

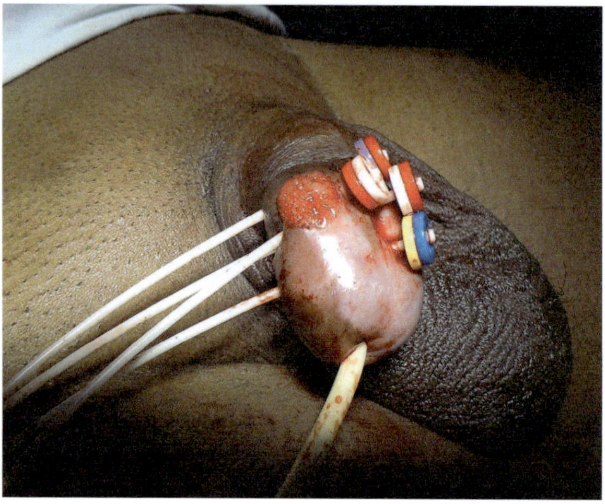

Fig. 14.9 Two plane flexible penile implant

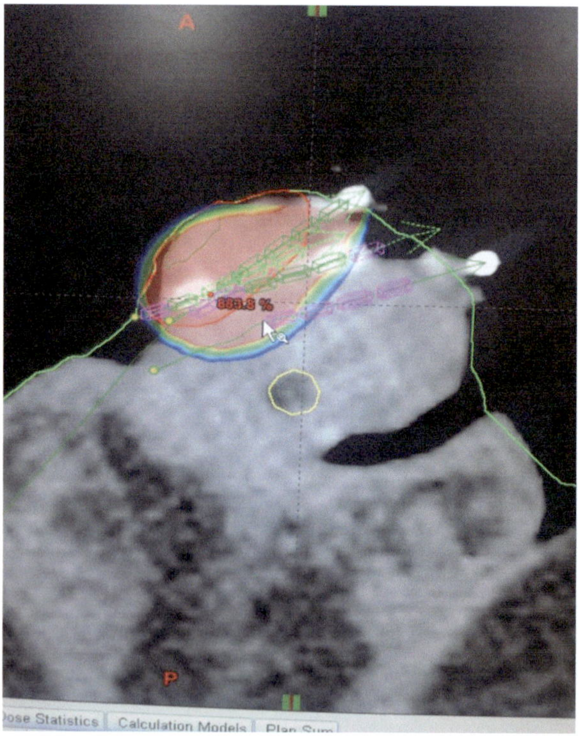

Fig. 14.10 Dose distribution in penile implant

When area is 25–100 cm^2, half is at periphery and half at centre, and when it is more than 100 cm^2, then it is one-third at periphery and two-thirds at centre.

Volume implants are used when the lesion is >2.5 cm thick. Two plane implants lead to low-dose region midway between the planes (Figs. 14.8 and 14.9). Tumour

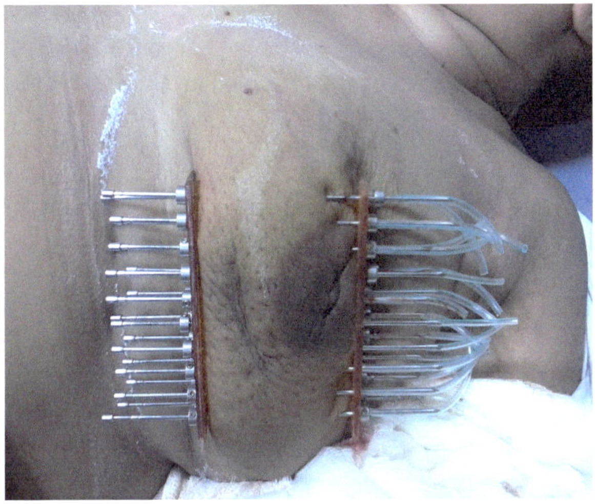

Fig. 14.11 rigid template breast interstitial implant

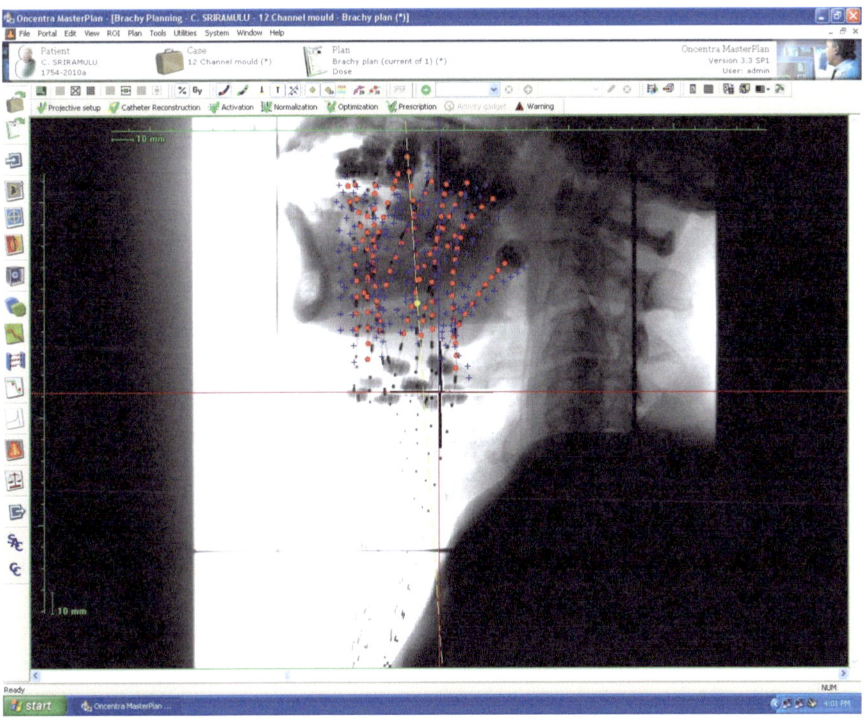

Fig. 14.12 Source positions in a tongue implant case

shape is sphere, cube and cylinder. Elongation factor is applied when length, breadth and height are not equal. In the implant, the volume is divided into two parts: rind and core. For a spherical implant, rind → shell/surface; in a cube, rind → six faces;

and in a cylinder, rind → belt and two ends. Rules for calculating volume implant are the following: Sources should be spaced evenly possibly. Separation between the two needles should not be more than 1.0 or 1.5 cm. In a cylindrical implant, belt should not be more than eight needles and the core not less than four. In certain cylindrical cases, it is impossible to close either one end or both ends. In such cases, the volume as determined by the active length of the belt must be reduced by 7.5% for each open ends. Uniform linear activity sources are distributed uniformly over the area or volume to be treated. This will lead to non-uniform dose distribution, with higher dose in the central region.

The **Quimby system** differs from the Patterson-Parker system in that this system has a non-uniform dose distribution in the target volume, but the distribution of source strengths through the target volume is uniform. In this system, the dose in the central region of the implanted volume is higher than the dose near the periphery. The isodose chosen from the tables in the Quimby system is the minimum dose which covers the full implanted volume, while in surface applicators, the computed dose is the maximum dose in the treatment plane. The **Paris system** is used for both single- and double-plane implants, but it is not used for volume implants. In this system of interstitial implant, sources are linear and placed in a parallel pattern equidistant from each other with their centres located in the same plane (central plane). The source strength for each position is always uniform and identical for all sources. Spacing between sources could be increased when using long sources. In Paris system, *basal dose rate (BD) is defined as the arithmetic mean of the local minimum doses midway through an array of equally spaced ribbons for single-plane implants* [2]. For double-plane implants, the basal dose rate is the dose rate in the central cross-sectional plane at the intersection of perpendicular bisectors projected from the side of the triangle for triangular arrangement and at the geometric centre for square arrangements. The reference dose (RD) rate is equal to 85% basal dose rate and is the dose rate used for dose prescription.

The concept of mean central dose was introduced to bring some standardization in dose reporting in interstitial brachytherapy. Various parameters have been therefore defined in the ICRU Report 58 for reporting dose. **Mean central dose** *is defined as the arithmetic mean of the local minimum doses between sources in the central plane (or in the central planes if there is more than one)* [2]. Firstly in all cases, a central plane for dose calculation is selected. In source patterns in which the source lines are straight, parallel, of equal length and with their centres lying in a plane perpendicular to the direction of the source lines, this plane is defined as the central plane. In cases where such homogeneity is not possible, the central plane is chosen perpendicular to the main direction of catheter lines and in estimated centre of implant volume. In cases of complex volume implants, the entire volume is divided into more than one subvolume and central planes calculated for each of these subvolumes, from which the mean central doses are calculated.

In a single-plane implant, the mean central dose is, in the central plane, the arithmetic mean of the doses at mid-distance between each pair of adjacent source lines, taking into account the dose contribution, at that point, from all sources in the pattern. In the case of an implant with line sources in more than one plane, the mean central dose is the arithmetic mean of the local minimum doses between each set of three (triangles) or four (squares) adjacent source lines within the source pattern. This point is equidistant from all three source lines. For squares, the minimum is at the intersection of the diagonals. The mean central dose can broadly be calculated by many methods. In one method, the implant volume is divided into equilateral triangles, and the intersection points of the perpendicular bisectors of each triangle are determined, and the local minimum doses are calculated for each of these points. The mean of these local minimum doses is the mean central dose. In another method, the dose profiles are calculated for one or more axes through the centre of the implant passing through as many local minima as possible, and the mean of these local minima is the mean central dose.

It is now pertinent to introduce few definitions at this stage. A *low-dose region is defined as a region, within the CTV, where the dose is less than 90% of the prescribed dose, while a high-dose region should be defined as that encompassed by the isodose corresponding to 150% of the mean central dose (MCD) around the sources in any plane parallel to the central plane where a high-dose region is suspected* [2]. *The dose homogeneity index is defined as the ratio of minimum target dose to the mean central dose. Minimum target dose is the dose selected and specified by the radiation oncologist as adequate to treat the PTV. Treated volume is the tissue volume that, in the actual implant, receives at least a dose selected and specified by the radiation oncologist as appropriate to achieve the purpose of the treatment* [2].

As per ICRU 58, reporting for interstitial brachytherapy requires description of the clinical conditions, including GTV and CTV; description of the technique; source specification, including RAKR and TRAK; complete description of time-dose pattern; treatment prescription; mean central dose (MCD); minimum target dose; homogeneity index; and volumes and their dimensions, including PTV, treated volume, high-dose regions, low-dose regions, reference volume, irradiated volume and organs at risk [2].

14.4 Intracavitary Brachytherapy

It implies the insertion of radioactive sources through designed applicators into body cavities. Various lesions in sites such as the bladder, anus, rectum, antrum, oesophagus and nasopharynx and treatment of female gynaecological malignancies use this technique. Intracavitary treatment of cervical cancers has been the most common and most studied type of this technique (Figs. 14.13, 14.14, 14.15, and 14.16). Various schools of treatment have come up which have prescribed different dosages and times to the treatment volume. ICRU Report 38 [1] has since tried to standardize the prescription volume and prescribing as well as reporting parameters.

In the Paris technique, small quantity of radium is used and LDR brachytherapy is performed. It has a longer period of treatment at about 6–8 days, and total amount of radium for application was 8000 mg/h. A part of the radium was applied

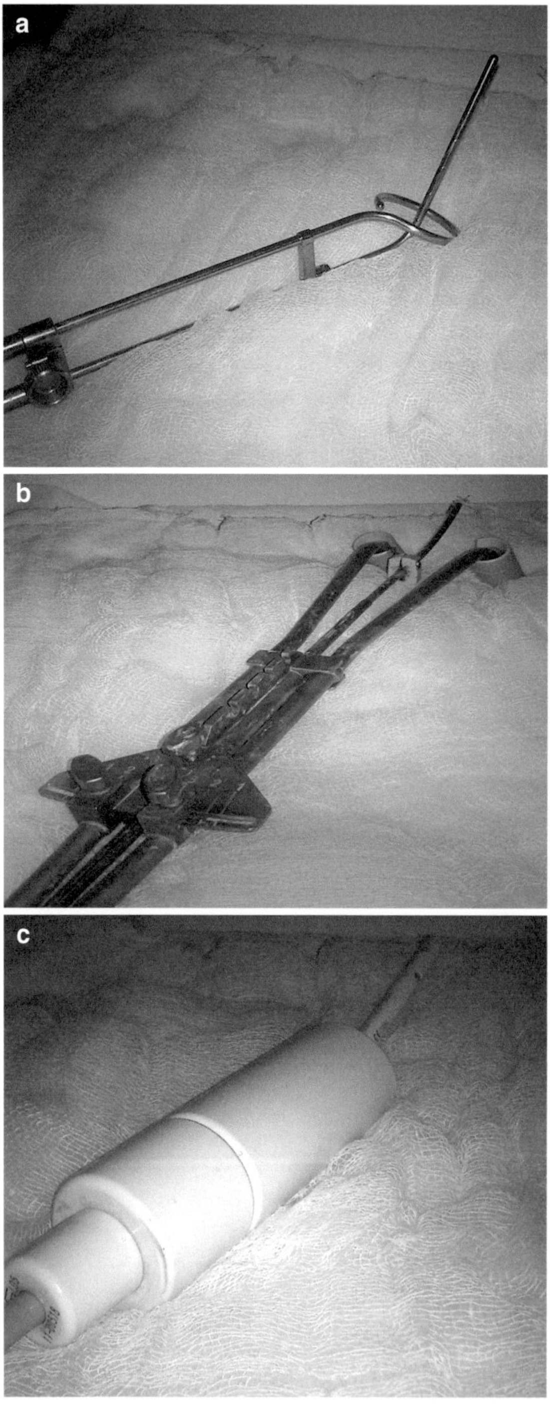

Fig. 14.13 (**a**) After loading applicators (Ring Applicator). (**b**) After loading applicators (Fletcher-Suit Applicator). (**c**) After loading applicators (Vaginal Linear applicator)

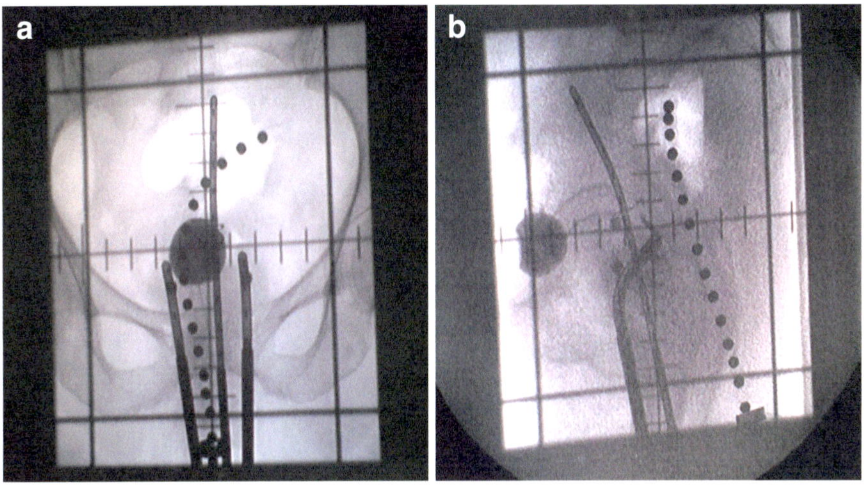

Fig. 14.14 Orthogonal films taken with fletcher-suit applicator and bladder-rectal markers in place

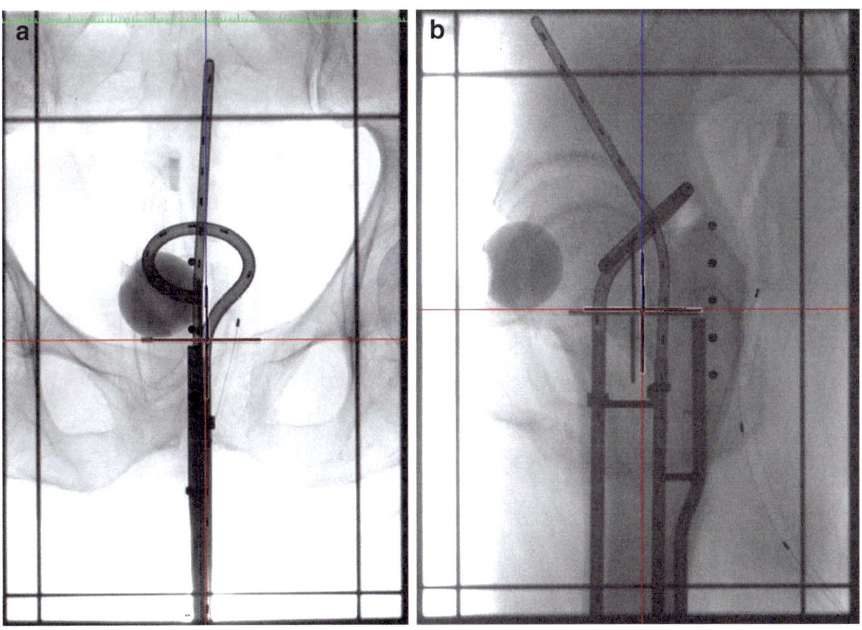

Fig. 14.15 Orthogonal films taken with ring applicator and bladder-rectal markers in place

in the uterine canal and the rest divided into two halves and placed in two colpostats (cylindrical applicators made of cork or "sorbo rubber") applied high up in the vaginal vault. Colpostats were separated laterally by a spring. This system was modified by the Manchester group and known as Manchester system.

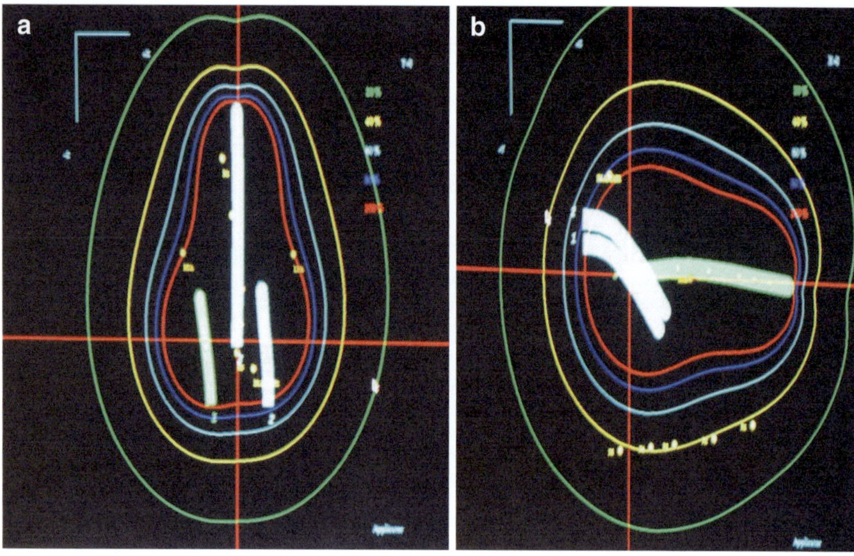

Fig. 14.16 HD-ICRT for Ca cervix. Dosimetry profiles-ant and lateral

In the **Stockholm technique** developed by Forsell and Heyman, large amount of radium was used with a shorter treatment time. The applicators were of stainless steel with bigger cross-sectional lengths to avoid very high doses to the uterine wall. These were permanently loaded, i.e. tandem with 53–88 mg of radium, and designed to provide 75 R/h (of the order) dose rate at 2 cm from the centre of the applicator, while the ovoids varied in shape and size with 60–80 mg radium. Treatment time was generally about 27 h × two sitting at 3 weeks interval.

The main feature of the **Manchester system** was the selection of a reference point in the pelvic cavity for dose specifications and dose specification in terms of R. The advantage of this was that this system was anatomically comparable from patient to patient, not highly sensitive to small and clinically insignificant alterations in applicator position and allowed for correlation of dosage and clinical effects. Source loading was with 20 and 35 mg of radium in intrauterine applicators and 15 and 25 mg of radium in vaginal ovoids. The ovoids are tissue equivalent materials of stainless steel or plastic or rubber and are placed in such a manner that the rectum (posterior) and the bladder (anterior) lie end on to the radium tubes. In order to reduce rectum dose, gauze packing is used behind the ovoids. The packing also avoids movement of the ovoids during treatment.

The dose was prescribed to a **point A** which was described as follows:

Anatomical position: Chosen in the paracervical tissues, lying 2 cm lateral to the central canal of the uterus and 2 cm above the superior surface of the vaginal vault. **Anatomically point A lies in the region where the uterine artery crosses the ureter** and lies on the apex of a triangle formed by the uterine canal, uterine artery and ureter (called the "paracervical triangle") (Figs. 14.16 and 14.17).

Point A can also be defined in relation to the applicator positioned in situ and as viewed on orthogonal planar films. *This position is defined as being located in the oblique frontal plane* (**ICRU Report 38**) [1] *containing the intrauterine source(s) and bisecting the vaginal sources. In that plane and from its intersection with the plane containing the vaginal sources, a point is taken, on the midline, cranially at a distance equal to the source to vaginal mucosal distance (cranial contour of the vaginal sources) + 2 cm. The left and right points' "A" are located in the oblique frontal plane, perpendicularly to the intrauterine source(s), at 2 cm laterally from the midline* [1].

Significance: This region is important in respect of tissue tolerance and is often the site of early infiltration and hence not to be underdosed. Also being the point where the uterine vessels cross the ureters, this point represents the critical site of onset of late reactions.

The other important dose prescribing parameter is the **point B**:

Anatomical position: 3 cm lateral to point A in the same distance vertically from the vaginal vault. In an average patient, point B lies close to or on the pelvic wall.

Significance: Give an indication of the fall-off of dose in the pelvic region. The dose rate at point B is very useful for supplementary external beam irradiation.

The main feature of Manchester system is the constancy of dose rate at point "A", irrespective of the size of the applicators used. In the original Manchester system, it was considered that half the tolerance dose to point A could be safely delivered through the vaginal sources. In the revised Manchester system (1953) [10], on the basis of clinical experience, the ratio of intrauterine to vaginal contribution at point A was changed to 1.84:1.00. Total dose to point was also raised from 7000R in 140 h to 8000R in 150 h delivered in two sessions with a 4–7-day interval between them. Thus the total dose rate at point A is calculated to be about 53 cGy/h irrespective of the length of the uterine tube or the size of the vaginal ovoid. The dose rate at point B is approximately 30% of point A. According to ICRU 38 [1], the reference volume has since been changed to the volume encompassed by reference isodose surface which is 60 Gy of adsorbed dose for low-dose rate therapy. When the BT is combined with EBRT, then reference isodose will be 60 Gy minus the dose delivered by EBRT. For MDR and HDR, the therapist has to decide the dose level, which would be equivalent to 60 Gy of LDR.

Recommendations put forward by the American Brachytherapy Society for LDR brachytherapy of cervical cancer make use of the original Manchester system point A referring to it as point Ao while adding a modified point A (Af) [11]. When tandem and ovoids are used in a patient, *point A is defined and located in radiographs by drawing a line connecting the middle of the sources in the vaginal ovoids on the AP radiograph and moving 2 cm (plus radius of the ovoid) superiorly along the tandem from the intersection of this line with the intrauterine source line and then 2 cm lateral on either side of the tandem* [11]. In case a tandem and vaginal cylinder is used where there is involvement of the lower vagina, the ABS recommendations then define point A *by moving from the flange of the tandem 2 cm superiorly along the tandem and then laterally 2 cm perpendicular to the tandem on both sides of the AP radiograph* (Fig. 14.17) [11]. Also for reporting dose delivered or prescription dose according to ABS recommendations in PDR and HDR brachytherapy, it is necessary to include type of applicator used; dose fractionation and prescription point/volume (point A or HR-CTV); dose to point A; total reference air kerma of the isotope used; loading pattern (dwell pattern and times) for target volumes D90, D100 and V100 and for OARs $D_{0.1cc}$, D_{2cc} and D_{5cc} (organ wall); and isodose lines in (a) sagittal plane including tandem, (b) oblique frontal coronal through point A and middle of vaginal sources and (c) axial through vaginal sources and dose to the lateral vaginal mucosa and 0.5 cm depth in vaginal surface [11].

ICRU [1] has in its report number 38 steered away from using point A or B as dose prescription reference points because of the observed ambiguities in the location or even interpretation of these points in view of various anatomic variations or personal or institutional practice. This resultant variation even in definitions of commonly accepted treatment guidelines or principles could potentially cause promulgation of different values for the calculated dose rate to point A and would only provide differing values adding to confusion. Therefore aiming to standardize practice and avoid ambiguity, the ICRU 38 report has suggested the use of a target volume enclosed by a specific dose for dose prescription and reporting. The **reference volume** [1] as recommended by ICRU 38 is the volume enclosed by isodose level 60 Gy (for definitive treatment for very early disease or combination treatment with surgery for limited disease) and 75/85 Gy (for definitive treatment for limited and extensive disease) and is only to be used as a base for comparison of treatments performed in different centres using different techniques in ICRU Report 38 and is not as a therapeutic dose recommendation. This "volume" approach is defined by three dimensions, (a) height (d*h*), (b) width (d*w*) and (c) thickness (d*t*), which are measured from the oblique frontal and oblique sagittal planes. These orthogonal dimensions of the volumes are reported individually and not their product; because of the "pear shape", the actual computed volumes may be much smaller (about 50%) compared with the product of their dimensions. Also the lateral and AP-PA dimensions are clinically meaningful for tumour control with regard to parametrial extension and complications, respectively.

The **bladder and rectal points** (Figs. 14.14 and 14.18) [1, 12] are used as a surrogate markers for bladder and rectum dose limitation where image-based planning is not done. The bladder can be localized with the help of a Foley catheter and filling the balloon of the catheter with contrast. This contrast-filled balloon which is lying on the urethral orifice of the trigone is then visualized on AP and lateral X-rays or on CT images, and the **bladder point** *is then marked at the centre of the balloon in the AP view and on a line joining this centre of the balloon to the posterior surface in the lateral view*. The **rectal point** (Figs. 14.14 and 14.18) [1, 12] is *defined on the frontal radiograph and CT image at the midpoint of the ovoid sources (or at the lower end of the intrauterine source), and on the lateral view, the rectal point is located on a line drawn from the middle of the ovoid sources, 5 mm behind the posterior vaginal wall. The posterior vaginal wall may be visualized by using radiopaque gauze for the*

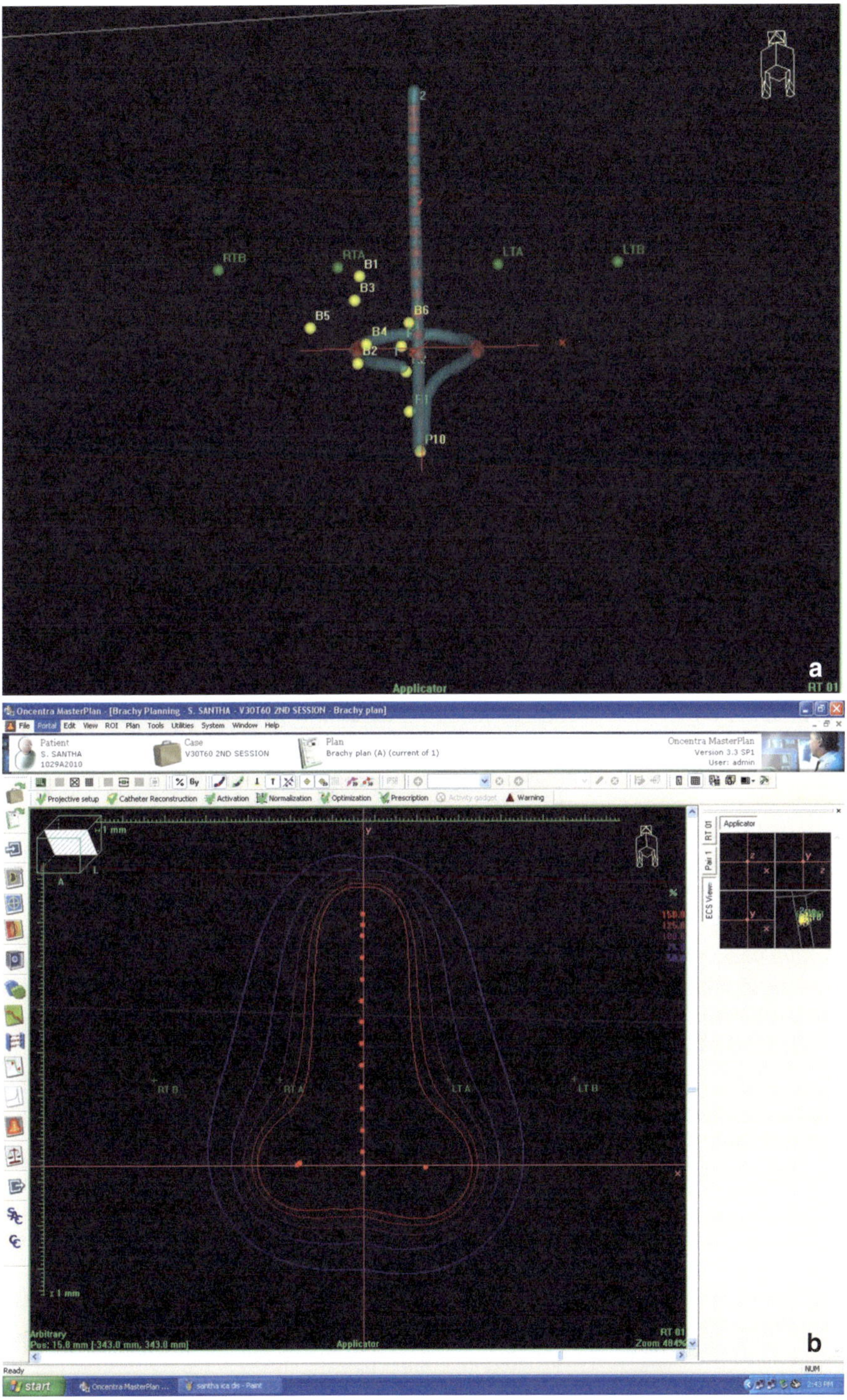

Fig. 14.17 (**a**) Positions of point A and B. (**b**) Pear shaped dose distribution at point A and B

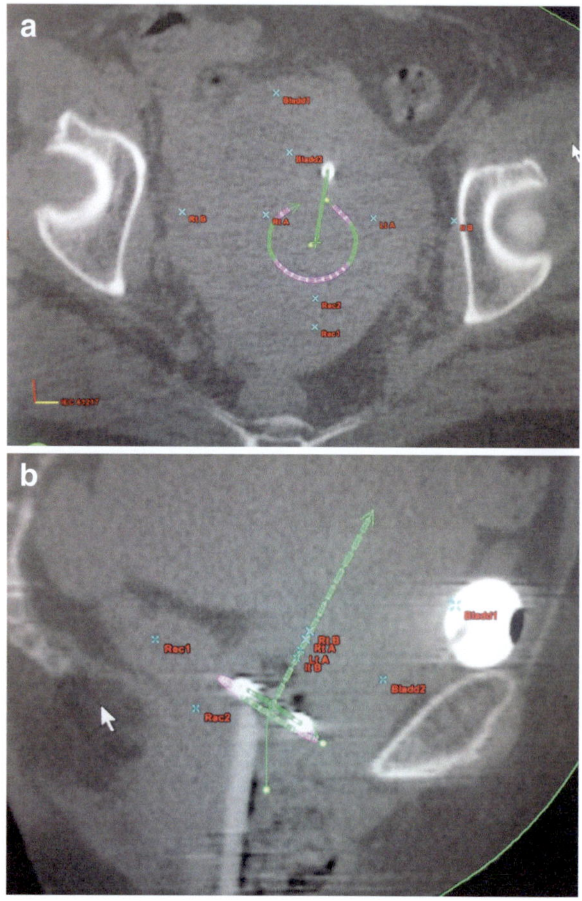

Fig. 14.18 (**a**) ICRU Bladder and rectal point as seen in CT images (axial view). (**b**) ICRU Bladder and rectal point as seen in CT images (lateral view)

vaginal packing [11]. On anteroposterior X-rays, the pelvic wall points are located at the intersection of a horizontal tangent to superior aspect of the acetabulum and a vertical line touching the medial aspect of the acetabulum. On the lateral view, these points are marked as the highest mid-distance points of the right and left acetabulums [1, 12]. Even then the doses at point A must always be reported both from external beam radiotherapy and brachytherapy as point A is still used today for prescribing and reporting brachytherapy in a majority of centres worldwide, providing a large amount of clinical information, and literature reports have shown association of the dose at point A to tumour control and side effects [13, 14].

The lymphatic trapezoid of the pelvis represents the dose to the mid-external iliac, low common iliac and low para-aortic lymph nodes [15] and is obtained by a line drawn from the S1/S2 vertebral bodies' junction to the top of the symphysis pubis from the middle of which a line is drawn to the middle of the anterior aspect of L4 and a trapezoid is constructed in a plane passing through the transverse line in the pelvic brim plane and the midpoint of the anterior aspect of the body of L4. A point 6 cm lateral to the midline at the inferior end of this figure is used to give an estimate of the dose rate to mid-external right and left iliac lymph nodes (labelled, respectively, R. EXT and L. EXT); at the top of the trapezoid, points 2 cm lateral to the midline at the level of L4 are used to estimate the dose to the bilateral low para-aortic areas (labelled R. PARA and L. PARA); the midpoint of a line connecting these two points is used to estimate the dose to the bilateral common iliac lymph nodes (labelled R. COM and L. COM) [15].

The **treated volume** in intracavitary brachytherapy as per ICRU can be defined according to specific isodoses rather than a point dose and reported as prescribed dose either as an absolute value (in Gy) or as a percentage of the dose delivered at reference points selected for prescribing and reporting. Two additional volumes can also be defined related to the treated volume. These are the **high-dose volume**, *defined as the volume encompassed by the isodose corresponding to 150% (and 200%) of the dose defining the treated volume* [16] and may be useful for interpretation of tumour effects and side effects and for purpose of comparison, and the **irradiated volume** *which is defined as the volume encompassed by a lower isodose to be specified, e.g. 90–50% of the dose defining the treated volume* [16]. Reporting irradiated volumes has been considered to assist in the explanation or prediction of side effects outside the treated volume and for purpose of comparison. When MRI or CT scan is used for defining the target volume, the **HR-CTV** should include gross tumour volume, width of the cervix and any parametrial extension superior border of which should be extended at least 1 cm above uterine vessels. The **IR-CTV** should include HR-CTV along with any extension of disease at the time of brachytherapy [16].

Dosage guidelines according to ICRU 38 [1] **are**:

- The clinician should use the largest possible ovoid size for each particular patient with longest possible tandem, the length of which is estimated by sounding the uterus but should not be more than 6 cm. This will limit dose to the mucosal linings and enable better lateral dose distribution.
- Dose recommendations according to ICRU 38 [1] for specific prescription points are the following: Point A, 8000R; uterine wall, 30,000R; cervix, 20,000–25,000R; vaginal mucosa, 10,000R; and rectovaginal septum, 6750R.
- For the principal organs at risk, dose limitations include:
  - Bladder <80 Gy
  - Rectum <75 Gy

In definitive treatment the total dose at point A and/or in the PTV2 (tumour extension at the time of brachytherapy) ranges between 75 and 90 Gy (as per current recommendations). This includes limited disease (e.g. stage IB1, stage IIB proximal) and extensive disease (stage IB2 to IIIB/IVA). Therefore, for selecting as reference volume, the volume encompassed by a higher-dose level like the 75 or 85 Gy isodose should be selected (Fig. 14.19). Selection of 60 Gy (definitive treatment for very early disease; combination treatment with surgery for limited disease) and 75/85 Gy (definitive treatment for limited and extensive disease) to define the

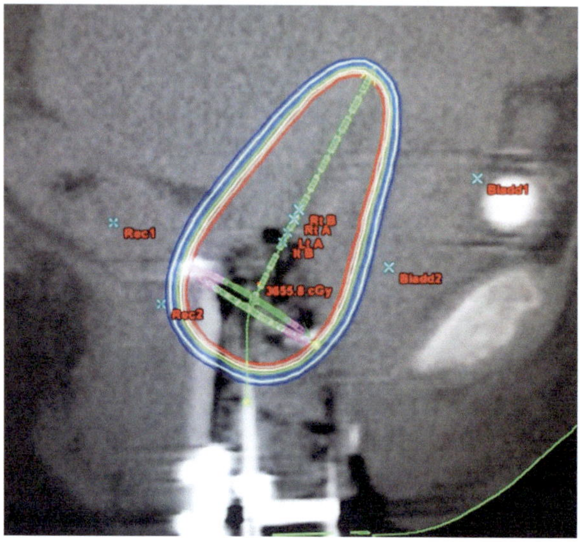

Fig. 14.19 ICRU Bladder and rectal point as seen in CT images with dose distribution in reference volume

reference volume is for purpose of comparison as per concept of reference volume, introduced in ICRU Report 38.

14.5 Intraluminal Brachytherapy

Intraluminal brachytherapy (ILBT) is another type of intracavitary brachytherapy characteristically used in hollow cylindrical organs like the rectum, oesophagus, bronchus or biliary structures. Here an intraluminal catheter is introduced through which radioactive sources are approximated close to tumour surface. In intraluminal brachytherapy, the length and depth of the target volumes such as the GTV, CTV or PTV are important for prescription, delivery and reporting purpose. During prescription, delivery or reporting, the lengths of the target volumes are defined in relation to the apposed mucosal surface, while the depths of these volumes are defined in relation to the luminal surface.

Dose prescription in ILBT: The principles of dose prescription usually involved are similar to other types of brachytherapy, namely, adequate coverage at depth and limiting excess surface dose. These include:

- Dose is usually prescribed 0.5 cm from applicator surface or 1–1.5 cm from source depending on the applicator circumference.
- In ILBT, all doses are calculated and reported with respect to the central plane of the applicator. *This central plane can be defined as the plane perpendicular to the axis of the organ lumen, halfway between the proximal and distal ends of the PTV* [17].

- For reporting irradiation of such target volumes, a set of three reference depths/points are defined which include the surface (mucosa) itself, the minimum target dose and a reference depth of 5 mm in the tissues, from the surface (mucosa).
- For prescribing dose depth, commonly accepted principles advocate covering a depth of 5 mm, from the surface of the organ luminal wall, in the central plane, in case of organs like the the oesophagus, bronchus and vagina. In endovascular brachytherapy, this reference depth is calculated from the endothelium (surface wall) in the artery and is taken as 1 mm for coronary arteries and 2 mm for peripheral arteries [17].

According to ICRU, the **reference volume, in intraluminal brachytherapy**, *is defined as the tissue volume encompassed by the isodose corresponding to 90% of the dose at the reference point, while length of the reference volume is defined parallel to the (main) lumen axis or source axis, at the reference depth, i.e. 5 mm from the mucosa (1 and 2 mm for intravascular brachytherapy)* [17]. These lengths are defined along the direction of the main axis of the source.

As we can see from the quantum of the reference depths, any small change in the dimension of luminal cross section of the catheters inserted can appreciably change the prescribed depth dose. Therefore for purposes of reporting, it is better to consider the distance from the central plane of the applicator to the mucosal or luminal surface rather than from the surface of the applicator. The isodose achieved is like a "banana", an elongated cylinder (Fig. 14.20). If, in a large irregular tumour, the mucosal dose in the central plane is not representative, reporting an average mucosal dose around the central plane may be more relevant. This technique is used as radical therapy in early stages where the entire tumour depth can be included in the prescription isodose or as a boost therapy after external beam irradiation. The dose at the mucosa represents the highest (maximum) dose in the PTV and is thus clinically relevant in relation to tumour effects and/or complications.

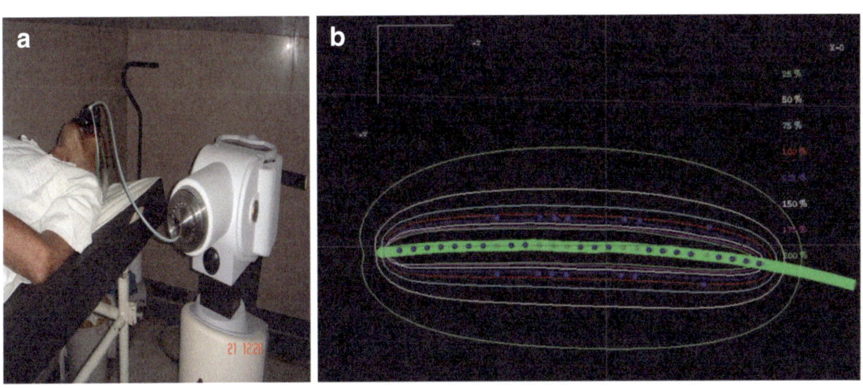

Fig. 14.20 Delivery and isodose distributions in Intra-luminal brachytherapy

14.6 Role of Dose Optimization and Inverse Planning in Brachytherapy

In modern brachytherapy, the development of both better anatomical imaging and physiological or functional imaging has enabled the radiation oncologist to have a clearer view of the anatomical extent of the tumour as well as tumour activity within the gross volume clearly demarcated both from surrounding tissues and within the same organ [18]. With the increasing use of CT-based planning techniques and the extensive use of remote afterloading HDR devices, brachytherapy calculations now use a variety of dose distributions for each given application to achieve the desired or as close to desired dose distribution. This can be either by adjusting the length of time (dwell time) that the source remains at a location (dwell position) or by differing active and inactive catheter positions or even various combinations of these methods. Dwell times or positions can be manually optimized based on user experience, or full volume-based optimization can be done by the computer.

The target for dose optimization as in external beam radiation therapy remains obtaining the desired dose distribution. This in brachytherapy is affected by the relative position and extension of the tumour volume and the surrounding organs at risk as well as positional variations in target and OAR volumes in between applicator insertion and dose delivery. This optimization process as mentioned earlier can either be manual or computer based. In the manual method, the constraints for tumour and OAR volumes are used to prepare sets of plans which are then selected by the oncologist according to his or her experience to select the solution that provides the best fit for the clinical goals [19]. This is done by varying dwell positions or times and by selectively activating or deactivating specific channels. The aim is to obtain the desired dose distribution. The other method is computer-based **inverse planning** [20, 21], in which the constraints required after having delineated all the target volumes and critical OARs on CT slices are determined. Weight factors or importance factors are then entered into the planning system just as in IMRT to prioritize the dose constraints [22–24]. Conflicting constraints are then presented as a weighted sum so that coverage, conformity and uniformity of dose distribution are uniformly balanced for all target and OAR volumes. Since this method is computer generated, the planning system draws up various dwell times and positions and aims to achieve an optimal arrangement using dose constraint potentials (DCPs). This process of optimization is done by awarding a system of penalty points to each dose distribution point being assessed and the penalty changes with change in the magnitude of deviation from the prescribed dose range to that point. Thus the range of penalties and points scored can be assessed by parameters such as minimum and maximum dose constraints (D_{min} and D_{max}) as well as their slopes (S_{min} and S_{max}).

Various inverse planning tools in treatment planning systems are available, and comparison studies of different optimization techniques in manual and computerized inverse planning systems have been done by several centres including geometrical optimization [20], graphical optimization [25, 26], and dose point optimization [26], All these studies have reported a significant dosimetric advantages of the computerized inverse planning system over other optimization techniques which include better dose coverage, conformity and homogeneity of the target and a significant reduction in normal tissue doses as well as planning time. Thus use of inverse planning systems in brachytherapy allows for complex computations of dose distributions taking into account many more organs at risk, with use of an irregular target volume, and helps in prescribing global dose values rather than point-based dose prescriptions.

Clinical application of inverse planning: Inverse planning has resulted in many advantages:

- As a result of this computer-generated dose distribution and optimization process, the clinician can now focus more on better delineation of target volumes as well as proper plan evaluation and delivery.
- CT- or MRI-based contouring of the CTV and OAR provides the clinician with more options and the freedom to shape the dose distribution as well as add new organs at risk such as the penile bulb in prostate cancers [27] or even neurovascular bundles seen with MRI , which could not be taken into account before.
- The inverse planning process can now identify many more dose distribution patterns that could achieve required distribution than was possible by manual optimization process.

14.7 Plan Evaluation from DVH

The shape and area under the DVH curve are used to ensure that the target volume is adequately covered with a homogeneous dose and that dose to critical structures is within acceptable limits. From this, the percentage of the volume of an organ receiving a given dose (*d*) can be read as V_d (volume of tissue receiving dose "d") or as D_v (dose received by volume "v" of tissue). From the *x*-axis, the mean, median doses, etc. can be calculated. If DVHs are obtained from a series of patients in whom acute or late effects are recorded, points on the DVH can be correlated with the probability of these effects occurring.

Figure 14.21 shows a typical cumulative DVH. In this DVH, the main questions asked would be whether PTV coverage is adequate and whether the OARs are being adequately spared. Basically the area under a curve is the volume of tissue getting a dose, and the smaller this area, the better for an OAR. Also the tail of the curve should not ideally taper too much to the right as this will mean a smaller volume getting a higher dose. This is true even for the target volumes, i.e. the more the dose line tails towards right bottom (*x*-axis), the more is the maximum point dose to the target volume. This can be clinically significant if this maximal dose to OAR is in a serial organ like the spinal cord where even a small volume getting a very high dose can have catastrophic results.

Once this first look is done, next to be noted is the target volume maximal dose. The Dmax in a brachytherapy treatment is generally not evaluated as it can go even up to 2000% right adjacent the source. What should be looked for is the V90%, V150% and V200%, i.e. the volumes of PTV receiving, respectively, 90%, 150%

and 200% of prescribed dose which is a clinically more relevant parameter. V200% in the target volume should ideally be located inside the applicator and V150% as far as possible at the tissue-applicator interface. The PTV should be covered by 85–90% isodose but not less than 80% isodose. It is difficult to aim for 100% isodose coverage as it would entail shifting of the higher isodoses to within the tissue resulting in late reactions like necrosis and strictures. The minimum dose to the target volume should be noted. If properly contoured, it should not be less than 5–8% of prescribed dose depending on the treatment technique. In Fig. 14.21, both the PTV and GTV coverage are adequate. The PTV can be described as 85% of volume receiving 94–96% dose which is usually in line with planning criteria. This is also checked in the dose colour wash to see the location of the hot spot—whether it is inside the PTV or overlying some critical structure where even if only a point dose has a risk of causing significant sequelae. Ideally it should be inside the GTV.

After having evaluated the target volume, we now evaluate each organ at risk (OAR). First are the serial OARs. For serial OARs, the Dnearmax is the limiting dose as the loss of function of even one FSU will cascade for the entire structure. For OARs with parallel FSUs, D2% is an acceptable estimate of probability of acute or late effects, and it should be preferably less than the prescription isodose. The DVH in case of the OARs can give information regarding their D98%, D2% and D50% as well as their integral doses (calculated from differential DVH as area under curve). Dose distribution should now be evaluated in different volumes such as the GTV, CTV, PTV, treated volume and organs at risk, such as the mandible, bladder, rectum, sigmoid and bowel. The maximum bladder and rectum dose is the dose received in a volume of at least 2 and 5 cm^3. The minimum dose in the most irradiated tissue volume adjacent to the applicator (0.1, 1, 2 and 5 cm^3) is recommended for recording and reporting.

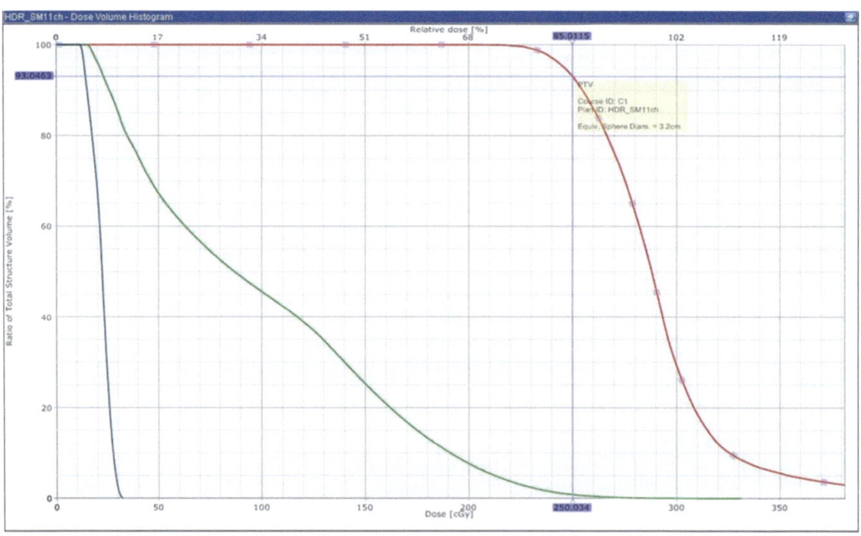

Fig. 14.21 DVH of a typical case of brachytherapy

Parameters for reporting dose in intracavitary brachytherapy in cervical cancer in the era of 3D planning and image guidance: Development of 3D image-based treatment planning in brachytherapy has significantly improved the 3D assessment of dose-volume relations. Dose distribution can now be evaluated in different volumes such as the GTV, CTV and PTV. The most relevant organs at risk (OARs) are the rectum, the sigmoid, the bladder, the bowel and the vagina. The maximum bladder and rectum doses to consider are the doses received in a volume of at least 2 and 5 cm^3 and volume of the OAR that receives a dose close to or higher than the dose considered to be significant in relation to tolerance. Because of lack of definitive data, volumes corresponding to dose levels of 60–90 Gy should be considered. The volumes should be reported in cm^3 (absolute values) and as a percentage of the organ volume. The dose to 2 cc and 5 cc (D_{2cc} and D_{5cc}) of the OAR is useful in evaluating toxicities, while $D_{0.1cc}$ is an indication of the maximum dose received [28] (e.g. in case of ICRT for cervical cancers, recommended D_{2cc} for bladder is 90 Gy EQD2 and 75 Gy EQD2 for sigmoid and rectum, and target coverage D90 should equal 100% of prescription). According to American Brachytherapy Society (ABS) recommendations for dose evaluation and reporting, evaluation should include doses to the ICRU rectal and bladder points and in case of MRI- or CT-based volumetric dosimetry then $D_{0.1cc}$, D_{2cc} of OAR (and D_{5cc} of OAR if organ wall is contoured) as well as D90, D100 and V100 for evaluating HR-CTV [11].

References

1. ICRU, International Commission on Radiation Units and Measurements. Dose and volume specification for reporting intracavitary therapy in gynecology. ICRU Report 38. Bethesda: ICRU; 1985.
2. ICRU, International Commission on Radiation Units and Measurements. Dose and volume specification for reporting interstitial therapy. ICRU Report 58. Bethesda: ICRU; 1997.
3. ICRU, International Commission on Radiation Units and Measurements. Prescribing, recording and reporting photon beam therapy. ICRU Report 50. Bethesda: ICRU; 1993.
4. ICRU, International Commission on Radiation Units and Measurements. Prescribing, recording and reporting photon beam therapy (Supplement to ICRU report 50) ICRU Report 62. Bethesda: ICRU; 1999.
5. Haie-Méder C, Potter R, Van Limbergen E, et al. Recommendations of gynecological (GYN) GEC-ESTRO Working Group (I): concepts and terms in 3D imaged based 3D planning in cervical cancer brachytherapy with emphasis on MRI assessment of GTV and CTV. Radiother Oncol. 2005;74(3):235–45.
6. Mazeron JJ, Ardiet JM, Haie-Méder C, et al. GEC-ESTRO recommendations for brachytherapy for head and neck squamous cell carcinomas. Radiother Oncol. 2009;91:150–6.
7. Rustgi SN, Cumberlin RL. An afterloading 192-Ir surface mould. Med Dosim. 1993;18:39–42.
8. Takeda M, Shibuya H, Inoue T. The efficacy of gold-198 grain mould therapy for mucosal carcinomas of the oral cavity. Acta Oncol. 1996;35:463–7.
9. Chalian VA, Drane JB, Standish SM. Maxillofacial prosthetics. Baltimore: The William and Wilkins; 1972. p. 181–3.
10. Tod M, Meredith WJ. Treatment of cancer of the cervix uteri: a revised Manchester method. Br J Radiol. 1953;26:252–7.
11. Vishwanathan AN, Thomadsen B. American Brachytherapy Society consensus guidelines for locally advanced carcinoma cervix. Part I: General principles. Brachytherapy. 2012;11:33–46.

12. Chassagne D, Horiot JC. Proposal for common definitions of reference points in gynecological brachytherapy [French]. J Radiol Electrol Med Nucl. 1977;58(5):371–3.
13. Potish RA, Gerbi BJ. Role of point A in the era of computed dosimetry. Radiology. 1986;158:827–31.
14. Pötter R, Van Limbergen E, Gerstner N, Wambersie A. Survey of the use of the ICRU 38 in recording and reporting cervical cancer brachytherapy. Radiother Oncol. 2001;58:1–4.
15. Fletcher GH. Squamous cell carcinoma of the uterine cervix. In: Textbook of radiotherapy. Philadelphia: Lea & Febiger; 1980. p. 720–89.
16. Vishwanathan AN, Dimopoulos J, Kirisits C, et al. Computed tomography versus magnetic resonance imaging-based contouring in cervical cancer brachytherapy: results of a prospective trial and preliminary guidelines for standardized contours. Int J Radiat Oncol Biol Phys. 2007;68:491–8.
17. Pötter R, Van Limbergen E, Dries W, et al. Recommendations of the EVA GEC ESTRO Working Group: prescribing, recording and reporting in endovascular brachytherapy. Quality assurance, equipment, personnel and education. Radiother Oncol. 2001;59:339–60.
18. Kurhanewicz J, Vigneron B, Nelson S. Three-dimensional magnetic resonance spectroscopic imaging of brain and prostate cancer. Neoplasia. 2000;2:166.
19. Lahanas M, Baltas D, Zambouglou N. Anatomy-based three-dimensional dose optimization in brachytherapy using multiple objective genetic algorithm. Med Phys. 1999;26:9.
20. Hsu I-C, Lessard E, Weinberg V, et al. Comparison of inverse planning and geometrical optimization for prostate high dose rate brachytherapy. Presented at the 23rd American Brachytherapy Society Meeting, Orlando, 24 May 2002.
21. Pouliot J, Charra-Brunaud C, Kim YB, et al. Inverse planning for HDR brachytherapy: Clinical implementation. Presented at the 23rd American Brachytherapy Society Meeting, Orlando, 24 May 2002.
22. Lessard E, Pouliot J. Anatomy-based dose optimization for HDR-brachytherapy of the prostate using fast simulated annealing algorithm. Med Phys. 2001;28:773.
23. Pouliot J, Tremblay D, Roy J, Filice S. Optimization of permanent 125I prostate implants using fast simulated annealing. Int J Radiat Oncol Biol Phys. 1996;36:711.
24. Kneschaurek P, Schiessl W, Wehrmann R. Volume-based dose optimization in brachytherapy. Int J Radiat Oncol Biol Phys. 1999;45:811.
25. Morton G, Sankreacha R, Halina P, et al. A comparison of anatomy-based inverse planning with simulated annealing and graphical optimization for high-dose-rate prostate brachytherapy. Brachytherapy. 2008;7:12–6.
26. Jacob D, Raben A, Sarkar A, et al. Anatomy-based inverse planning simulated annealing optimization in high-dose-rate prostate brachytherapy: significant dosimetric advantage over other optimization techniques. Int J Radiat Oncol Biol Phys. 2008;72(3):820–7.
27. Fisch BM, Pickett B, Weinberg V, et al. Dose of radiation received by the bulb of the penis correlates with risk of impotence after three-dimensional conformal radiotherapy for prostate cancer. J Urol. 2001;57:955–9.
28. Georg P, Lang S, Dimopoulos JC, et al. Dose-volume histogram parameters and late side effects in magnetic resonance image-guided adaptive cervical cancer brachytherapy. Int J Radiat Oncol Biol Phys. 2011;79:356–62.

15 Planning Electron Therapy and Evaluation of Plans

Electron beams are basically also charged particle beams and show many of the characteristics of charged particles. They are however covered separately as they have almost no mass unlike the heavy charged particles and proton beams. Electrons deliver a high surface dose along the central axis which falls rapidly with depth and tapers off beyond a defined depth. The surface dose of an electron beam is however not the point of maximal dose; in fact with increasing depth, this dose increases up to a certain point which is called the depth of dose maximum (D_{max}). Thus an electron beam can be summarized as:

High surface dose → point of maximal dose at D_{max} → dose falls rapidly and tapers off as bremsstrahlung.

From the above we can see that an electron beam therefore will have a definite depth or range at which it will give the required dose distribution. This is important in the treatment of superficial tumours wherein deeper structures are spared of irradiation. This range can be calculated from the beam energy as will be explained subsequently in this chapter. Most clinically useful beam energies range from 6 to 15 MeV (depth of 2–5 cm). Electron beams are used in the treatment of [1]:

(a) Superficial skin and lip cancers
(b) Chest wall irradiation for breast cancer in the adjuvant setting or as palliative treatment for local chest wall relapse
(c) Boost dose to nodes in head and neck cancers especially when these are overlying the spinal cord where photons cannot be used beyond 45–50 Gy
(d) Parotid gland tumours and other superficial head and neck cancers as mixed beams along with photons
(e) Scalp irradiation
(f) Whole skin irradiation
(g) Intraoperative radiotherapy for tumour bed irradiation immediately after surgery

A. Mukherji, *Basics of Planning and Management of Patients during Radiation Therapy*, https://doi.org/10.1007/978-981-10-6659-7_15

Many of these situations can also be treated by brachytherapy (electrons have the advantage of being less invasive with more dose uniformity), superficial X-rays (electrons have much less depth dose) or advanced conformal beams (electron therapy is a more simple technique with less body integral dose).

15.1 Properties of Electrons

In this section, we shall discuss the various physical properties of electron beams. Electron beams on production are monoenergetic, but as they pass through the collimator head, these electrons interact with the various filters and collimator edges and give rise to scatter electrons. These scatter electrons *contaminate the beam* and have variable energies, some of which may even be their characteristic beam energy or bremsstrahlung which is seen as a tail of the largely monoenergetic beam. In calculating treatment depths and use of electron beams, it is important to know the percentage depth dose of an electron beam which is usually calculated along the central axis (this is the point of least beam divergence and that gets the maximal scatter dose from surrounding irradiated tissue) and is calculated as the ratio of the dose at the required depth to that at the D_{max} calculated as a percentage. This depth dose is usually used to determine the treatment depth (or nominal treatment distance) and is dependent on electron beam energy (increased energy → increased forward scatter → increased depth dose) and field size (higher field size → more is the scatter component to central axis dose).

Interactions with tissue: Electrons have the following types of interactions with the tissue they pass through:

- Inelastic collisions with outer electrons of an atom. It is called inelastic as the energy transfer may not be equal (part of the energy is lost or transferred to the atomic electrons), and this results in ionization and excitation of atoms. This effect is termed collisional or ionizational loss. Inelastic collisions with atomic nuclei result in bremsstrahlung production.
- Elastic collisions with atomic electrons or with atomic nuclei. These do not result in any energy loss from the incident electron. There may however be a change in the direction of the electron, or the energy may be completely transferred to the new emerging particles from the irradiated nucleus.

The energy loss in an electron beam (called the mass stopping power) as it traverses through a medium usually depends on the number of electrons present per unit area (electron density) in that medium which in turn is dependent on the atomic number of the material making up the medium [1]. In this respect this stopping power is inversely proportional to the atomic number because materials with high atomic number though having a larger number of electrons have a larger mass; therefore the electron density in the outer shells is comparatively lesser than those with lower atomic numbers which have tightly bound electrons. As an electron beam passes through a medium, it interacts with the medium (tissue) electrons leading to scattering. The magnitude of this scattering depends on the speed of the incident electron beam, i.e. its beam energy. Higher energies as explained will get scattered forward. After such multiple interactions, the energy of the electron beam comes down, and its angle of spread increases (i.e. the beam becomes more divergent). This is clinically useful in the large-field superficial electron treatments as in total skin electron therapy in the production of scattering foils made up of high atomic number materials to induce divergence and decrease penetrance [1].

Bremsstrahlung is the characteristic radiation released as an excited electron goes back into its non-excited state, and this is proportional in effect to the atomic number (square of) and electron energy with higher beam energies and higher atomic number materials giving off more of bremsstrahlung [1].

Inverse square law (virtual source position): The inverse square law basically means that as the distance increases, the effect decreases. The electrons have a virtual source as there is no single point in the electron gun which can be termed as the definitive source. Hence in case of electrons, the effect of the inverse square law can be calculated by first marking out an effective SSD (SSD_{eff}) which would be from the virtual source to the treatment isocentre. This distance has then to be corrected by taking into account the air gaps between the applicator and the patient's surface as this may have a bearing on the dose distribution.

Range: Electrons being charged particles will have a definite range; as the electron beam travels deeper into the tissue, it keeps losing energy with increased angular scatter till it finally loses all energy by ionization [1]. Most interactions between the incident electron beam and the medium occur as individual transfer of small fractions of the incident particle's kinetic energy. Thus an electron beam can be thought to be losing its kinetic energy gradually and continuously in a process called continuous slowing down approximation (CSDA). The path of each single electron can be calculated as the total of the distance travelled between its entering the medium until the electron comes to a stop and the sum total of each of these paths when projected from the incident beam gives the projected path an electron beam.

Electron beam ranges are defined in terms of maximum range and practical range. *The maximum range R_{max} of an electron beam is defined as the depth at which extrapolation of the tail of the central axis depth dose curve meets the bremsstrahlung background* [1, 2]. Thus the range of an electron beam represents the deepest the beam has entered the medium, but because of the presence of the Bremsstrahlung tail, the range does not stop at a point but gradually tapers down to the baseline (Fig. 15.1). Therefore this range is not an actual physical range but a *practical range (Rp)* and can be described on a graph plot by extrapolating the downward vertical of the steepest part of the depth dose curve to where it intersects the baseline bremsstrahlung on the x-axis [1, 2].

Build-up region: The principle of dose build-up region in an electron beam is similar to that of photon beams though the magnitude is much less. The incident electrons in an ideal situation will enter perpendicular to the surface of the medium and interact with the electrons of the absorbing surface. These interactions may result in scattering in all directions with predominant directions being guided by the incident electron energy. There is also however significant back scatter which accounts for the higher surface dose in electron beams compared to photon beams. As the electrons are charged particles, their interactions with the irradiated medium are much more ionizing, and hence the depth penetration of these beams is less than

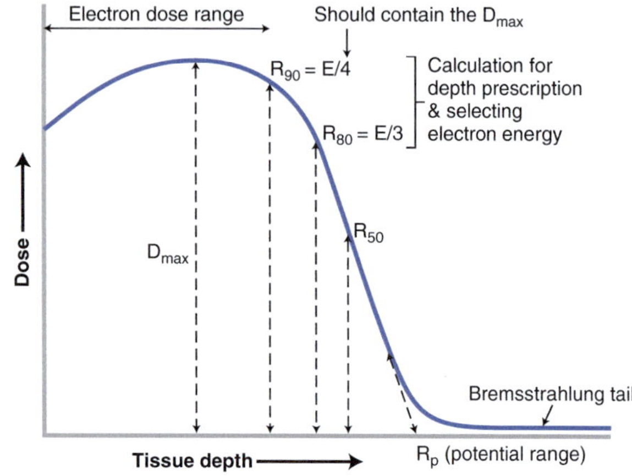

Fig. 15.1 Electron beam profile

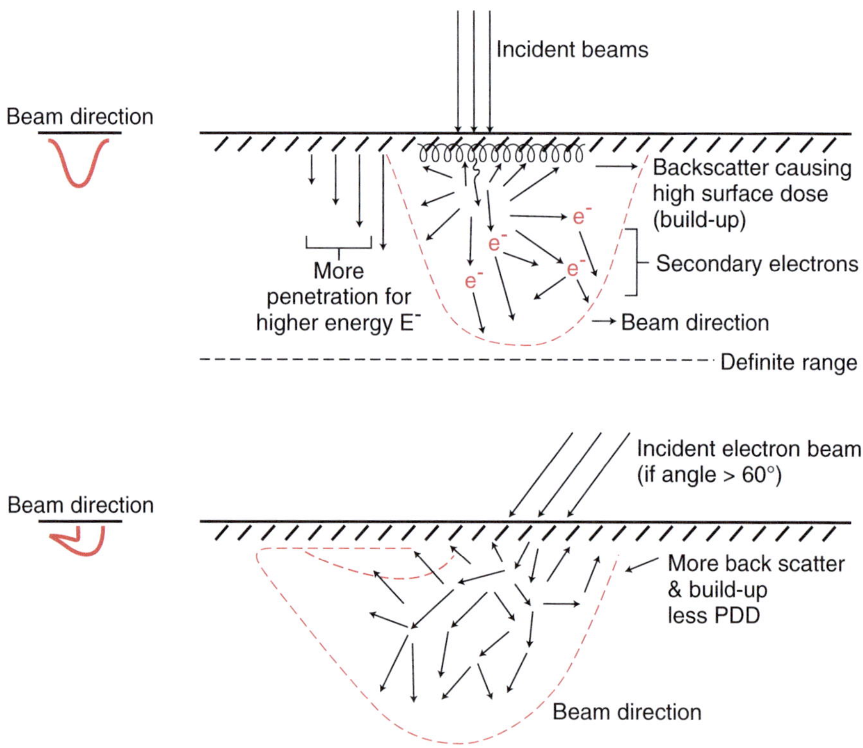

Fig. 15.2 Electron beam

photon beams. As with photon beams, the PDD of the electron beams also varies with beam energy and field size. Lower-energy beams undergo more angular scatter with lower resultant surface doses because of less build-up, and hence the ratio of surface dose to maximal dose is lower for lower-energy electrons than for higher-energy electrons (Fig. 15.2).

Dose distribution beyond D_{max}: Beyond the build-up region and point of maximal dose (D_{max}), there is a rapid dose fall-off followed by a bremsstrahlung tail. This is because of increased scattering of the lower-energy electrons; the low energy is caused by the continuous loss of energy due to interactions through the medium. The dose gradient for lower electron energies is more as previously explained because of the increased scattering of these low-energy electrons in all directions. Therefore the fall-off beyond the D_{max} is steeper for these low energies.

Percentage depth doses for small or large electron field sizes: As has been explained before, electron beams differ from photon beams in the magnitude of the effect of scatter. In electron beams, there is significant scatter in all directions, and therefore for a consistent dose to the field edges away from the central axis, the distance between the lateral edge and the central axis has to be more than the range of the scattered electrons. If the field size is decreased, the contribution of the lateral scatter to the central axis will come down, and the depth dose will decrease. Similarly the shape of an electron field also matters in deciding the depth dose. Square fields generally produce good scatter equilibrium; however if rectangular fields are used, care must be taken that each arm of the field border should have a value above the practical range (Rp); otherwise there will be a decrease in the depth dose.

Percentage depth doses for oblique beam incidence: Generally it is best to apply an electron beam on a flat surface or near flat surface with the central axis of the beam being perpendicular to the surface being irradiated. However this is not always possible. In case of an angulation of the beam, i.e. the beam is applied obliquely to the surface, the magnitude of this angle will determine the effect on the PDD. If the angle is less than 20°, there is hardly any change in either the range or the PDD, but if the angle of incidence exceeds 60°, there is significant change in D_{max} because of increased electron fluence via the central axis and even the characteristic shape of the dose distribution changes. The result might be a coma-shaped field (Fig. 15.2).

Therapeutic range R90: *The depth of the 90% dose level (R90 (cm)) beyond* D_{max} *is defined as the therapeutic range for electron beam therapy* [2]. This depth is important for treatment planners as this is the prescription depth and is generally calculated from the beam energy. Thus knowledge of this depth helps choose the correct beam energy for treatment. The R90 is the depth at which the target volume should be ideally covered, and the R80 (80% PDD beyond D_{max}) is the depth at which the target volume should be minimally covered in a good plan (Fig. 15.1). Any isodose beyond this is not acceptable as there is a steep fall in the beam energy beyond this isodose. The R90 is calculated as $E/4$ in which "E" is the selected electron beam energy, while R80 is calculated as $E/3$. For e**xample**, a skin tumour of size 2 cm × 2 cm × 2 cm is required to be treated. The beam energy required would be as follows: R90 is 2 cm in this case; hence $E/4$ = R90 or $E/4$ = 2 cm; hence $E = 2 \times 4 = 8$ MeV. In case this beam is not available, then this 2 cm can be considered as R80 in which case 6 MeV beam would be required. In general R80 is used to avoid further depth dose in very superficial tumours.

15.2 Treatment Planning with Electrons

Electron beam treatments are usually delivered using a treatment cone by a single enface field and ideally approximated to a flat tissue with homogeneous composition. But this is seldom the case, and many times the planner has to take into account a neurovascular bundle or underlying bone or other tissue inhomogeneities. Also the surface may not be flat but sloping, and these situations may present challenges in planning.

Choice of energy and field size: As explained before, the beam energy of an electron beam is decided by the depth required to be treated which in turn is influenced by target volume as well as the presence of any critical structure within this volume. This also determines the field size. While the R90 is the ideal depth required, selecting this value may result in a higher beam energy (R90 depth × 4) and result in a higher depth dose. In most cases, the isodose selected is the 80% isodose (R80) especially in postmastectomy chest irradiation or scalp irradiation [2]. Beyond the 80% depth dose, the dose fall-off is characteristically rapid at these beam energies, and the advantage of the R80 depth is the selection of lower beam energy (R80 × 3) (Fig. 15.3). This is especially seen at energies above 7 MeV [2]. Therefore in deciding the field size, the constriction in the isodose curves should be taken into account, and when compared to selecting photon fields for the same dimensions of target volume, electron beams use larger field sizes.

Corrections for air gaps and beam obliquity: In electron beam therapy, the treatment cone is placed directly on to the skin which collimates the beam to the required field size and shape and prevents beam divergence. This condition is best met when there is no gap between this collimator and the skin surface ideally over a flat surface. However sometimes because of surface curvature, there can be formation of small air gaps which results not only in increasing the SSD but also the beam divergence, thus causing a decrease in the absolute depth dose [3–5]. This effect has been explained by Ekstrand and Dixon [6] who have reported that any increase in beam obliquity within a maximum angle (as explained before) causes the following effects:

(a) Increased obliquity increases side scatter of the secondary electrons in the medium at D_{max}.
(b) D_{max} is shifted towards the surface.
(c) There is a decrease in the depth of penetration (R80 goes down).

Each of these points can be explained by considering an electron beam as a number of small pencil beams. Therefore when these beams are incident obliquely on a surface rather than perpendicular, each of these pencil beams travels through the medium at an angle. In such a case, at each point in the medium, these beams would have travelled a relatively greater distance and hence would have experienced greater side scatter. Thus at absolute greater depths, the beam energy remaining with the beam would be much less with much less scatter, and hence the depth dose will decrease, while surface side scatter will increase.

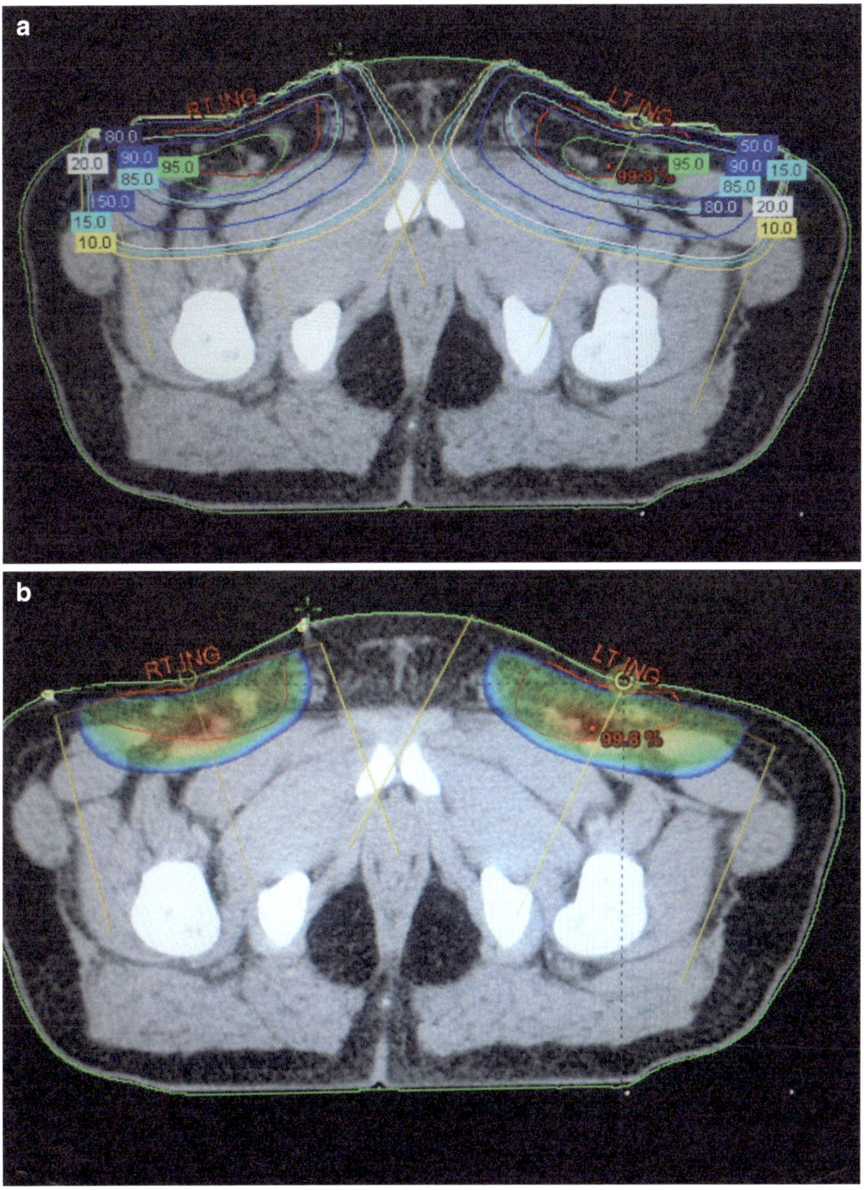

Fig. 15.3 (**a**) Electron beam isodose lines. (**b**) Electron beam percent depth dose and showing PTV coverage at 80% isodose

Effect of tissue inhomogeneity: In the previous sections, we have seen that the electron beams are mainly affected by two factors: the amount of scatter the beam has to undergo in a medium and the depth required to be covered by the effective range. These have been usually calculated in a water medium or equivalent medium which has a defined and homogeneous electron density. Therefore any presence of tissue inhomogeneity such as the bone, lung and air cavities having differing electron densities will result in different amounts of scattering at each of the tissue interfaces. This scattering will not just be one directional but will affect the scattering within each of the tissues themselves and will cause a net unpredictable scattering pattern making it difficult to calculate beam isodoses and depth doses. In general tissues with higher electron density will cause more scattering and allow less depth dose beyond, and this, if the dimension of this inhomogeneity is large enough, can be calculated from standard isodose distributions using a *coefficient of equivalent thickness (CET) method* [5, 7–10]. This CET is basically a ratio and is calculated by the electron density of the medium relative to the electron density of water and is essentially the mass density of the inhomogeneity.

There is also the phenomenon of *edge effects* in which the electron strikes at an angle the interface between two mediums of different electron densities. The net result on the isodose distribution will be an interplay between the scatter effects in the two mediums. The electron density affects the scattering of electrons and hence the depth or tissue dose at that point. Materials with higher electron density will have more scattering than materials with less density, and hence at the interface between the two materials, the higher scattering from the higher density will send more doses to the lower-density material. This effect assumes importance in the following situations:

- While calculating depth doses inside a patient where the tissue has two structures of different density
- In calculating surface doses for very irregular surface
- In calculating depth doses while taking into account either internal shielding or a shielding block placed very close to the patient's surface

Use of bolus and absorbers: As in photon beam therapy, bolus is used with electrons to basically increase the surface dose. In addition it can also be used to create a homogeneous flat surface over an irregular tissue surface (*acts as tissue compensator*). Bolus acts by drawing the dose to the surface and is used where penetration is not desirable for example in very superficial skin tumours where the R80 of the beam exceeds significantly the lesion thickness. In these cases, the bolus acts as "missing tissue" to smoothen out the surface and reduce the dose inhomogeneity. In electron beams, it is important for the bolus to conform as far as possible to the tissue surface as any large air gaps left between the bolus and the tissue will affect electron scattering and hence the depth dose. Commercially available materials used as bolus include paraffin wax, polystyrene, Lucite, Super Stuff and Superflab [11, 12]. The use of bolus and treatment planning can be made more accurate by the use of computed tomography (CT) which helps identify the tumour shape, depth and the patient contour. Sometimes low atomic number bolus materials such as Lucite and polystyrene are used to reduce the energy of an electron beam and are called *decelerators*, and these act when placed in close contact with the patient surface like a bolus.

15.2.1 Dose Specification and Reporting

By nature of their properties of scattering and range, electron beams are usually used in the treatment of superficial or subcutaneous disease, and the target volume is irradiated using a single enface field which is prescribed to a given depth. The beam is collimated by the use of cones and beam cut-outs to limit the electrons to around the target area. Thus beam specification and dose reporting are based on the dimensions and depth required to be treated. Treatments are usually prescribed at D_{max}, R90 or R80, so as to limit dose to deeper tissue and thus spare normal tissue as far as possible. In case of a treatment prescription given to either R90 or R80, the skin dose may be as much as 20% higher, and in such a situation, it would be better to assess the D_{max} also so that unwanted skin reactions are not encountered.

15.3 Field Shaping with Electrons

Electron applicators: Electron beam cones are applicators which are used to define the beam shape as well as the horizontal dimensions. These are placed on the skin surface and extend as an attachment from the treatment unit. These cones are of fixed sizes such as 5 × 5 cm or 8 × 8 cm or 10 × 10 cm. The smallest is usually 5 × 5 cm (Fig. 15.4).

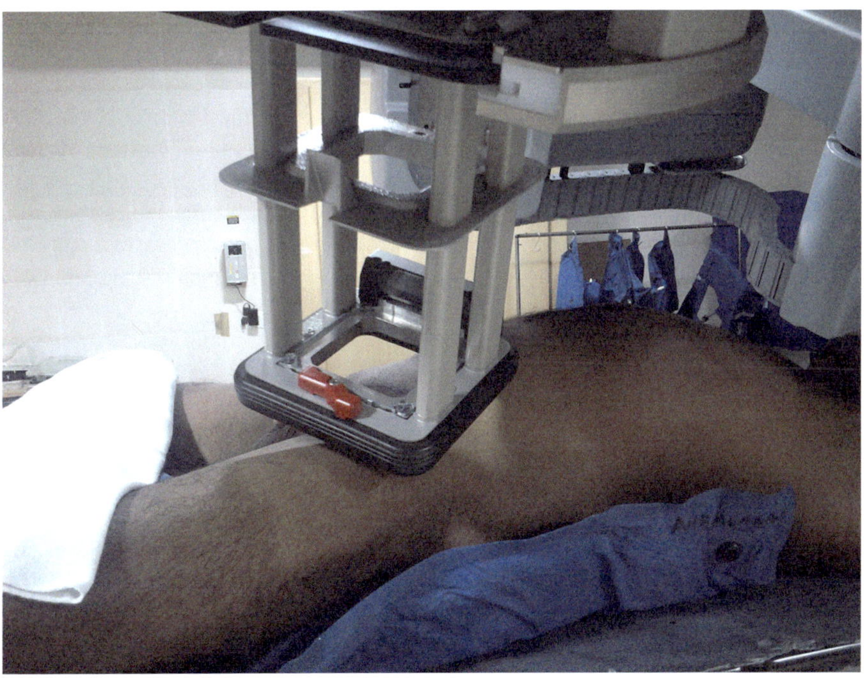

Fig. 15.4 Electron beam cone in use

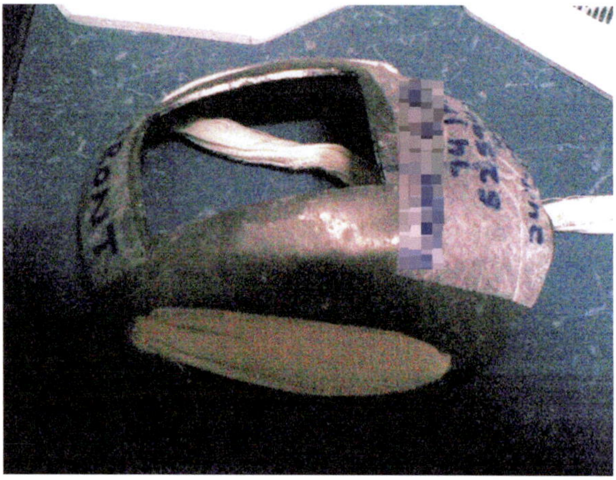

Fig. 15.5 Cut-out for use of electrons

Shielding and cut-outs: Sometimes there may be critical structures on the surface next to an irregular target volume, and the regular square fields achieved by the use of cones may not be desirable. In such situations, lead or metal alloy sheets are used in which the required field is cut-out and this cut-out is placed on or close to the surface being treated. These cut-outs are customized for the target volume based on imaging, and the thickness of metal used is based on the required level of transmission block such as 50, 10 and 5%, which is calculated by dividing the practical range Rp by 10 to obtain the approximate thickness of lead required for shielding (<5% transmission) (Fig. 15.5).

Internal shielding: In cases of superficial cancers of the lip, buccal mucosa, eyelids or ear lobes, where the target volume is related both to an external surface (skin) and an internal surface (mucosa), internal shield is used to protect the normal structures beyond the target volume. But these lead shields themselves may add dose to the normal structures due to backscatter and therefore need further addition of a layer of wax, aluminium or acrylic materials to absorb the backscattered electrons, which are usually low in energy.

Extended source to surface distance treatments: Sometimes it is necessary to treat from a greater distance, i.e. have a larger SSD, which may result in significantly different beam penumbra and output but little change in the PDD. The beam penumbra is usually corrected and restored by moving the collimator to the right over the skin so that the inside edge of the skin is now within the penumbra. This correction is required as the electrons are not produced from a single point source but from a "virtual point source" after the electrons hit the scattering foil in the treatment head, and hence this is an "effective" SSD that is used to correct for a non-standard SSD.

15.3.1 Electron Beam Combinations

There are many clinical situations in which two electron fields may lie next to (abut) each other or an electron and photon beam may abut each other. This is especially seen in the treatment of pelvic tumours (penile or vulvar cancers) in which the main pelvic photon field is bounded on its two sides by electron fields for the inguinal nodes or in head and neck cancers where a posterior neck is treated by an abutting electron field. This creates special interactions between the two fields and is explained below.

Matched (abutted) electron fields: Electron fields characteristically have lateral isodose bulges at depths, and when two fields abut, then these lateral isodose bulges can create differential hot or cold spots which may create dosimetric difficulties. It is better to have the two adjacent electron beams parallel to each other as otherwise any change in the angle of incidence will move the isodoses laterally and create wider bulges with higher surface doses, and while it would be better to avoid these adjacent beams at all, if it is required to do so, then film dosimetry at beam edges may identify hot or cold spots.

Matched photon and electron fields: This type of beam matching is more commonly seen and is an easier exercise with most treatment planning systems having dosimetric data for identifying and avoiding hot or cold spots from this type of beam matching at various prescription depths. However when the matching is done at the skin, then hot spots are usually seen to occur on the photon side of the matched beam pair.

References

1. Fletcher GH. Clinical applications of the electron beam. In: Textbook of Radiotherapy; Tapley N, ed. New York, Wiley, 1976; 1.
2. Khan FM, Doppke KP, Hogstrom KR, et al. Clinical electron-beam dosimetry: report of AAPM Radiation Therapy Committee Task Group No. 25. Med Phys. 1991;18:73–109.
3. Khan FM. The physics of radiation therapy. 2nd ed. Baltimore: Lippincott Williams & Wilkins; 1994.
4. Kirsner SM, Hogstrom KR, Kurup RG, et al. Dosimetric evaluation in heterogeneous tissue of anterior electron beam irradiation for treatment of retinoblastoma. Med Phys. 1987;14:772–9.
5. Klein EE, Li Z, Low DAA. Feasibility study of multileaf collimated electrons with a scattering foil based accelerator. Radiother Oncol. 1996;41:189–96.
6. Klein EE, Low DA, Purdy JA. Dosimetric changes with the new scattering foil applicator system on a C12100C. Int J Radiat Oncol Biol Phys. 1995;32:483–90.
7. Lee MC, Jiang SB, Ma CM. Monte Carlo and experimental investigations of multileaf collimated electron beams for modulated electron radiation therapy. Med Phys. 2000;27(12):2708–18.
8. Low DA, Starkschall G, Bujnowski SW, et al. Electron bolus design for radiation therapy treatment planning: bolus design algorithms. Med Phys. 1992;19:115–24.
9. Low DA, Starkschall G, Sherman NE, et al. Computer-aided design and fabrication of an electron bolus for treatment of the paraspinal muscles. Int J Radiat Oncol Biol Phys. 1995;33:1127–38.
10. Ma CM, Ding M, Li JS, et al. A comparative dosimetric study on tangential photon beams, intensity-modulated radiation therapy (IMRT) and modulated electron radiotherapy (MERT) for breast cancer treatment. Phys Med Biol. 2003;48(7):909–24.
11. Meyer JA, Palta JR, Hogstrom KR. Demonstration of relatively new electron dosimetry measurement techniques on the Mevatron 80. Med Phys. 1984;11:670–7.
12. Million RR, Parson JT, Bova FJ, et al. Electron beam: the management of head and neck cancer. In: Vaeth JM, Meyer JL, editors. Frontiers of radiation therapy and oncology, Vol. 25: The role of high energy electrons in the treatment of cancer. Basel: S. Karger AG; 1991. p. 107–27.

Planning Stereotactic and Adaptive Radiotherapy

16

16.1 Stereotactic Radiotherapy

Stereotactic radiosurgery (SRS) or radiotherapy (SRT) is a newer modality of delivering high doses of radiotherapy to a very precise volume with objective of achieving tumour ablation. This technique of radiotherapy uses multiple planar or non-planar beams which converge on a precisely defined target volume with very tight margins. This technique was initially started for cranial lesions, and when the target volume is treated by 1–3 fractions (usually 1), the dose per fraction is very high (10–20 Gy), and this procedure is called *radiosurgery* (*SRS*) as like in surgery the tumour is literally *removed or ablated*. When more fractions are used with lesser dose per fraction (3.5–9 Gy), then this technique is called *stereotactic radiotherapy* (*SRT*). In recent years this technique is being used for extracranial sites such as the lung, prostate, liver, pancreas, head and neck or even benign conditions and is called *stereotactic body radiotherapy* (*SBRT*). Stereotactic methods were first introduced by a neurosurgeon, Lars Leksell in 1951, using rigid frames on the skull which were used to pinpoint a small target volume (GammaKnife), while the first such stereotactic treatments for extracranial sites also originated in 1991 at the Karolinska Hospital in Stockholm by Ingmar Lax [1]. Hamilton et al. at the University of Arizona was one of the first to publish data on spinal radiosurgery using rigid skeletal fixation device [2].

The main features of this technique are the use of CT-guided treatment planning, use of tight margins (usual GTV to PTV conversion is 0.5–0.8 cm), highly localized target volumes (unlike conventional RT, extensive regional nodal or subclinical disease area irradiation is not done), considerable dose inhomogeneity within the target volume (usually dose is prescribed to the 70–80% isodose) so that the surrounding tissue gets less than 50% dose and image-guided dose delivery to prevent errors in dose delivery. These features result in high target dose and steep dose gradients beyond target. In a presentation, Timmermann has postulated the benefits of SBRT and the need for accurate imaging by advanced techniques and also the non-necessity of prophylactic fields [3]. This technique has been gaining ground over the past

A. Mukherji, *Basics of Planning and Management of Patients during Radiation Therapy*, https://doi.org/10.1007/978-981-10-6659-7_16

decade and half with increasing availability of machines which provide for real-time or near real-time image guidance as well as set-up verification and dose delivery in the same position as well as advances in medical imaging which allows precise tumour location and the availability of filter-free technology to allow for high-dose rates to a very small target and allow for treatment to be completed in less time.

16.1.1 Radiobiology

The general principle of cell kill by SRT/SBRT is hypofractionation or even extreme hypofractionation to ablate the tumour and preventing any or significant dose delivery to normal surrounding tissues to optimize the therapeutic ratio. Also because so few fractions are used, the questions of prolonged set-up reproduction and tumour regrowth do not come into play. The effect of radiotherapy has been traditionally defined by the linear quadratic model (LQM) [4], which usually explains radiotherapeutic cell kill in terms of double-strand DNA breaks (DSBs), sublethal damage to cells, reoxygenation, fractionation effects, redistribution, etc. According to studies by Brenner, the LQM has been validated for fractional doses of up to 10 Gy per fraction and can be reasonably used even for fraction sizes of 18 Gy [5]. However validity of the LQ model at very high doses has been questioned by Kirkpatrick et al. [6]. In this study, mice irradiated to doses of 8–13 Gy did not die of the gastrointestinal syndrome, but there was stem cell death by apoptosis thus resulting in gastrointestinal syndrome and death of the animals following single doses higher than 17–18 Gy [7]. This suggests that with doses greater than 17–18 Gy, a radiation threshold of either stem cell or vasculature cell killing is crossed which is not explained by the LQ model. But in the absence of any other suitable models, the LQ model remains widely used.

16.1.2 SRT/SBRT Technologies

Non-rigid stereotactic body frames with inbuilt markers for localization were first described by in 1994 by Lax et al. [8]. To reduce internal motion caused by breathing, slight constant pressure was applied to the abdomen, reducing the measured expansion of diaphragm from 1.5–2.5 to 0.5–1.0 cm [8]. Eight noncoplanar, isocentric beams, shaped to beam's eye view, were used to achieve a conformal dose distribution around the target. Similar to the initial SBRT treatments, the most widely used systems for SBRT use linear accelerators. The most widely used systems for SBRT fall into one of the following categories:

1. **Gantry-based linear accelerator system with CT-on-rails**: In this system the CT simulator and treatment unit are housed in the same complex. The patient does not leave the couch. After CT simulation, target localization and treatment planning is done; and the patient is positioned and immobilized on the couch.

The CT is brought into the treatment chamber for positional verification and then removed. Treatment is then delivered.

2. **Gantry-based linear accelerator system with on-board cone beam CT imaging**: Cone beam CT combines kV X-ray imaging and megavoltage radiation delivery for image-guided treatment delivery. The kV X-ray gantry rotates around the patient who is on the linear accelerator couch. This rotation generates tomographic images for three-dimensional (3D) reconstruction, used for position verification. Once position is verified, radiation is delivered by the linear accelerator (Fig. 16.1).
3. **Robotic linear accelerator system (Cyberknife®) with kV X-ray image guidance system**: The Cyberknife® system is an integrated image guidance and treatment delivery device with a computed controlled robotic linear accelerator with an X-ray camera device for near real-time image-guided radiation delivery. The Cyberknife® system tracks the tumour in real time during the treatment, and localization data are sent to a software program that readjusts the position of the robotic arm to deliver the treatment. Two tracking systems are available: Synchrony Respiratory Tracking System for tumours with respiratory motion, such as the lung, liver, kidney, or pancreas, or X-sight for spinal lesions. The Synchrony system couples motion tracking of implanted fiduciary markers placed in or around the tumour volume prior to treatment planning, with chest wall motion determined by an optical tracking system. The X-sight system uses a hierarchical mesh-tracking algorithm to track the bony anatomy for accurate treatment delivery. During the treatment delivery, the robot moves and retargets according to the tumour localization, and at each position (called nodes) radiation is delivered, and the process is repeated to each of the planned delivery positions.
4. **Helical tomotherapy**: This system uses a ring gantry to image the patient and for treatment delivery. A megavoltage CT detector array allows for image acquisition of megavoltage CT (MVCT) for image guidance. This integrated system

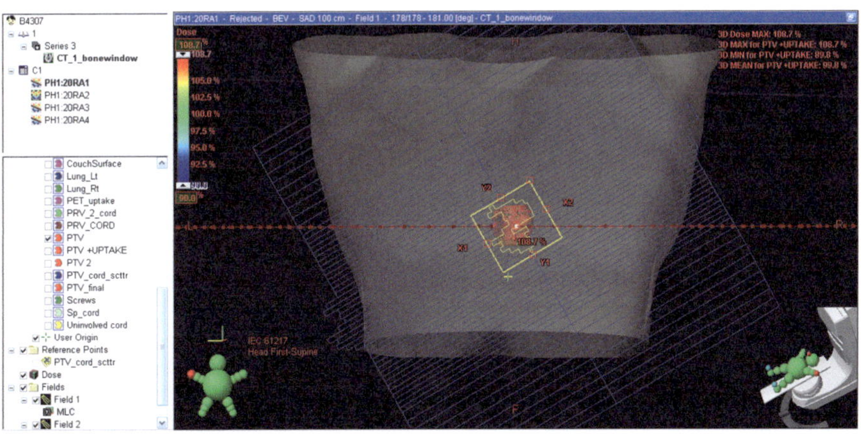

Fig. 16.1 SBRT with on-board imaging

uses a rotational beam delivery (continuous 360°) by a pneumatically driven beam modulator. The radiation is delivered as tens of thousands optimized, narrow beamlets in a continuous rotational manner with dynamic table movement creating a helical effect. Tomotherapy often uses immobilization coupled with four-dimensional target definition to achieve treatment accuracy.

5. **Use of filter-free beams**: In this technique (such as in Varian True Beam™), the flattening filters are removed and results in extreme dose rates along the central axis, less electron contamination and a sharp fall-off at the beam edge. The benefits of this method are in rapid treatment times with treatment over in seconds and significant reduction of dose at edge of beam or out of the field. However this method requires strict dosimetry, image guidance (to avoid errors) and quality assurance to prevent devastating late effects.

16.1.3 Patient Selection

Characteristics of Lesions Amenable to SRT/SBRT

- Small size of lesion (<3 for SRS and up to 5 cm for SRT)
- Low probability of multiple regional or distant spread at diagnosis
- Located in or near relatively radiation-tolerant organs
- Well-encapsulated lesions with well-defined margins

Current Indications

- Medically inoperable non-small cell lung cancer
- Early-stage prostate cancer
- Early-stage pancreatic cancer
- Oligometastases in the brain
- Shwanommas/acoustic neuromas
- Primary spinal tumours
- A-V malformations
- Uveal melanomas

Potential Indications Where Data Is Being Generated

- Medically operable non-small cell lung cancer
- Medically inoperable renal cell cancer
- Unresectable hepatoma
- Oligometastases in liver
- Vertebral oligometastases
- Recurrent head and neck cancers with well-localized recurrence

16.1.4 Simulation and Treatment in SRT/SBRT

Positioning and immobilization: Frame-based methods already have their stereotactic markers in place and therefore simply need pretreatment images for confirming proper tumour relocalization; on the other hand, in frameless methods there is always the risk of minimal patient-based or couch-based positional shift during planning and delivery, and hence these methods use fiducial markers in addition to more rigorous patient immobilization. These markers are typically radio-opaque and are applied on to the patient and registered before or during treatment set-up and delivery. These markers are placed in line with a stereotactic coordinate system in such a way so as to ensure that the target volume lies within the volume created by these markers. Scanning is done for a minimum distance of 15 cm beyond field borders to account for both coplanar and noncoplanar beams. For spine cases, the sacrum is included for lower spine as well as C1 spine for upper spine so that the vertebral levels can be easily identified.

Respiratory tracking control and simulation: Accounting for a patient's internal motion and its effect on the relative position of the target volume with respect to beam arrangements is an important part of stereotactic radiotherapy and especially SBRT (patient movements are minimal in intracranial SRT). Any significant change can have the double catastrophe of missing the target volume and ablating an important normal structure. Methods, like respiratory gating, tumour tracking, organ motion dampening or patient-directed methods are used so that the beam is delivered when the target volume is in that predetermined position for which the treatment has been planned. After patient's positioning and immobilization, bony landmarks are marked out to register the patient's position within a stereotactic coordinate system, and this is marked out on the CT contouring. Respiratory gating or active breath-hold techniques are used if the motion is more than 5 mm in the presence of regular, reproducible breathing which can be predicted by the software. If this is not there, then an inspiratory and an expiratory CT scan is taken with patient in treatment position from which an ITV is contoured (ITV, Chap. 9, Sect. 9.2).

Abdominal compression helps in limiting the movement of the diaphragm and also the target volume and is used to the degree of minimal patient comfortableness. After abdominal binder is placed, CT simulation is done and the range of target volume movement verified by tracked imaging as explained in previous paragraph. From this as explained in Chap. 9, the CTV to PTV expansion is determined. CBCT when used for set-up verification and delivery should have good alignment with the GTV with correction required being less than 1 cm. If this correction is more, then resimulation may have to be done.

16.1.5 Treatment Planning

Contouring for an SBRT involves precisely marking out the GTV based on anatomical imaging and if required biological imaging also. A margin 2–3 mm is usually added for PTV. It is usually difficult to get perfect fusions with MRI sequences unless the treating department has MR-based planning which may be more common in the future. Usually MR imaging angles do not match the simulation position, and hence the radiation oncologist is advised to incorporate the MR findings on to the contouring CT image. The use of coplanar or noncoplanar beams can be decided depending on patient's position, target volume location and treatment technique to be used. Noncoplanar beams are generally avoided with gating techniques, and similarly VMAT also may not be feasible with gating. Gating with fixed beam IMRT or dynamic wedge (EDW) is not advisable as it takes too much time, and therefore field-in-field (FIF) may be used. The aim of a good stereotactic plan is to absolutely conform to the target volume shape, providing high doses inside that volume while the normal tissues outside this volume get as less dose as possible (Fig. 16.2). Plan

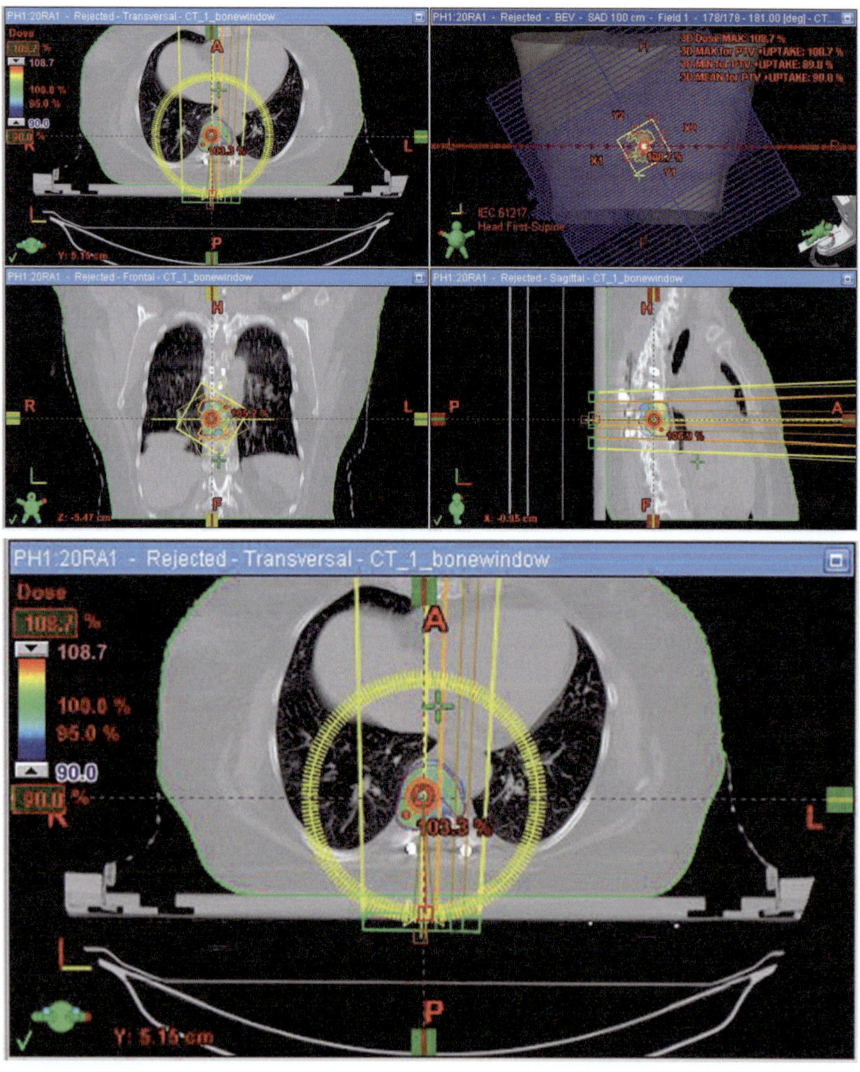

Fig. 16.2 High conformity of target volume with PTV covered by 90% of prescribed dose

evaluation is then done using dose/volume statistics for the target volume and normal surrounding tissues to avoid exceeding volume-based tolerances.

16.1.6 Planning Criteria (*Based on RTOG 0813* [9] *and RTOG 0915* [10])

The main prescribing constraints used for dose prescription are D_{max}, point D_{max}, target volume coverage by prescribed isodose, isodose prescribed to, high-dose spillage area and OAR constraints. The PTV and OAR constraints have been given in the Tables 16.1 and 16.2.

General rules for target volume dose prescription in stereotactic radiotherapy include: The target volume should be prescribed to an isodose between 60 and 90% so that the dose fall-off outside this volume remains very low (less than 40–50%). The D_{max} should be within the PTV as this area will undergo complete ablation, and the area of higher dose spillage should also be inside the PTV, getting not more than 105% of D_{max} and covering less than 15% of the total PTV volume. The prescribed isodose should cover more than on 95% of the target volume, and 100% of the target volume should not receive a dose less than 90% of the prescribed isodose.

16.1.7 Treatment Delivery and Verification

Accurate and reproducible treatment delivery is the hallmark of stereotactic radiation whether single or multi-fraction; and therefore dedicated quality assurance is an essential part of this technique. Set-up verification should account for not only internal organ motion (respiratory or peristalsis) but also daily positional errors with the error margin even tighter than for IMRT or VMAT. CBCT/4D CT or MVCT matching should be done before every fraction depending on the machine used and site being irradiated. The basic premise of stereotaxy is precise three-dimensional or

Table 16.1 Dose constraints for common OARs treated by SRT/SBRT

	One fraction SRS		Three-fraction SBRT	Five-fraction SBRT
Tissue	Volume threshold for D_{max}	Total point D_{max} dose (Gy)	Total point D_{max} dose (Gy)	Total point D_{max} dose (Gy)
Spinal cord	Less than 0.35 cc	14	21.9 @ 7.3 Gy/Fr	30 @ 6 Gy/Fr
Cauda equina	Less than 5 cc	16	24 @ 8 Gy/Fr	32 @ 6.4 Gy/Fr
Sacral Plexus	Less than 5 cc	16	24 @ 8 Gy/Fr	32 @ 6.4 Gy/Fr
Brachial plexus	Less than 3 cc	17.5	24 @ 8 Gy/Fr	30.5 @ 6.1 Gy/Fr
Oesophagus	Less than 5 cc	15.4	25.2 @ 8.4 Gy/Fr	35 @ 7 Gy/Fr

According to the AAPM task force 101 on normal tissue tolerance doses for SBRT; Benedict et al. [11]

Table 16.2 Dose constraints for common areas treated by SRT/SBRT

Site	Situation	Guideline and PTV dose	OAR D_{max} point dose in Gy (total dose)			
			One fraction	Three fractions [14]	Five fractions [9, 11]	Seven fractions [9, 11]
Lung PTV	Medically inoperable T1/2N0M0 NSCLC	CARO [12] Dose 60 Gy/8 Fr	–	–	–	–
	Metastases in the lung	CARO [12] Dose 50 Gy/5 Fr	–	–	–	–
	Primary size <5 cm	CARO [12] Dose 48–60 Gy/3–4 Fr	–	–	–	–
	Medically inoperable stage 1/2 peripheral NSCLC	RTOG 0236 [13] and RTOG 0618 [14]: 60 Gy/3 Fr twice weekly RTOG 0915 [10]: 34 Gy single dose or 48 Gy/4 Fr	–	–	–	–
Liver PTV	HCC size <8 cm	CARO [12] Dose 42–60 Gy/5 Fr	–	–	–	–
	Metastases; less than 5 nos. and 6 cm max diameter	CARO [12] Dose 45–50 Gy/3–5 Fr	–	–	–	–

(continued)

Table 16.2 (continued)

			OAR D_{max} point dose in Gy (total dose)			
Site	Situation	Guideline and PTV dose	One fraction	Three fractions [14]	Five fractions [9, 11]	Seven fractions [9, 11]
OARs	Spinal cord		12.5	18	27.5	31.5
	Oesophagus		13	27		42
	Lung (minus GTV)		V20 < 31%	V20 < 10%	<1500 cc receives ≥12.5 Gy; <1000 cc receives ≥13.5 Gy	
	Liver (minus GTV)		30	60	60	56
	Heart		15	30	≤52.5; <15 cc volume receives >32.5	56
	Trachea and main bronchus		16	30	≤52.5; <4 cc volume receives >18	56
	Brachial plexus		14	24	30–32	35
	Skin		–	24	32	–
	Ribs	Dose to 30 cc of chest wall volume		<30		
	Great Vessels			≤52.5; <10 cc volume receives >47		
	Stomach/ small bowel			12	22	32
	Rectum/ colon			34 Gy to 0.5 cc volume		
	Kidney			≤1/3 volume (sum of left and right) receives ≥15 Gy; V6 < 10%		

even four-dimensional localization of the target volume, and therefore image guidance in set-up verification and treatment delivery is essential. This data is then used to match with the planning image data set, and corrections if required are made, after which the treatment is delivered (Table 16.3).

16.1.8 Summary

- Radiosurgical tumour ablation with high-dose radiation delivered with high accuracy.
- Compared to surgery, it is a minimally or noninvasive procedure with no anaesthesia and can be applied to medically and surgically inoperable patients.

Table 16.3 SBRT/SRT systems available worldwide and their main features

Name of system	Company	Image guidance used	Respiratory tracker used	Field shaping	Remarks
Cyberknife®	Accuray	Dual-fixed X-ray with real-time imaging	Fiducial-based and frameless real-time tracking	Uses circular cones of different dimensions	SRS, SRT, SBRT only
True Beam STx™	Varian	kV-kV imaging, CBCT and RPM™	Exactrac® system using kV imaging and RPM for respiratory movement	By micro-MLCs (5 mm at isocentre) or circular cones	Uses flattening filter-free (FFF) with static and dynamic arcs; 6D couch; allows SRT/SBRT/IGRT/VMAT
Trilogy®	Varian	kV-kV imaging, CBCT; rotating kV imaging for planar views	Respiratory gating with infrared (IR) markers	By micro-MLCs (5 mm at isocentre) or circular cones	Allows SRT/SBRT/IGRT
Synergy S™	Elekta	kV-kV imaging, CBCT; rotating kV imaging for planar views	Airway breathing control (ABC), active breath hold, frames or abdominal compression	By micro-MLCs (4 mm at isocentre) or circular cones	Allows SRT/SBRT/IGRT/VMAT
Axesse™	Elekta	kV-kV imaging, CBCT	4D-CT	By micro-MLCs (4 mm at isocentre) or circular cones	6D couch; allows SRT/SBRT/IGRT/VMAT
Hi-ART™	Tomotherapy	Helical fan beam MVCT imaging	Uses both frame-based and abdominal compression	6 mm wide MLCs with binary movement	Allows SRT/SBRT/IGRT/VMAT
Novalis™	Brainlab	kV-kV imaging	Respiratory gating with infrared (IR) markers	By micro-MLCs (3 mm at isocentre) or circular cones	Allows SRT/SBRT/IGRT but field size restricted to 10 × 10 cm

(continued)

Table 16.3 (continued)

Name of system	Company	Image guidance used	Respiratory tracker used	Field shaping	Remarks
Primatom™	Seimens AG	CT scanner on rails linked to couch	Uses both frame-based and abdominal compression	1 cm leaf MLCs or circular cones	Allows SRT/ SBRT/IGRT
TM2000/ Vero SBRT	Brainlab and Mitsubishi	EPID, dual kV fluoroscopy, CBCT + real-time fluoroscopy	Isocentric and non-isocentric plus dynamic tracking	MLC on orthogonal gimbals in a ring structure	Allows SRT/ SBRT/IGRT

- Benefits relative to radiotherapy: Evidence of improved local control, improved surrounding critical structure sparing and improved radiobiological effects on some tumours.
- High-precision technique with high dose in target volume and rapid fall-off in surrounding tissue.
- Need for image guidance during treatment, taking into account respiratory movements and need for strict quality assurance.

16.2 Adaptive Radiotherapy

Radiotherapy treatment to tumour tissue leads to many anatomic changes during the course of therapy. These may be characterized as:

- Anatomic motion like respiration, peristalsis.
- Treatment-induced changes such as cell death and tumour shrinkage, weight loss or gain, fibrosis of normal tissue.
- Conventional radiotherapy plans were prepared after initial simulation and contouring and remain unchanged during entire course of radiotherapy.
- In the present era of highly conformal precision planned radiotherapy using tight margins for normal tissue sparing and dose escalation, such changes in patient's anatomy either on a daily basis or during course of therapy can lead to missing out on the target volume or inadvertently treating critical surrounding normal structures leading to treatment-related sequelae. Therefore in a patient undergoing radiotherapy, there is always a chance that there may be significant changes in the target volume and regional anatomy during the irradiation course. Hence the treatment plan may be needed to be revised and changed if required.

Therefore this technique called *adaptive radiotherapy* can be described as making changes to an initial radiotherapy plan during the course of radiotherapy because of changes in the target volume or even patient's anatomical contour caused by rapid response in the tumour or patient weight loss or making corrections for patient's internal motions. This change can be retrospective, near real time or even real time, i.e. the changes can be made:

- Offline by a reviewing physician during a check of the CBCT and planning CT image and looking for the corrections made as well as the image fusion results.
- Online or near real time just before delivering therapy by matching again with the cone beam CT. Usually if the correction required for non-stereotactic conformal treatments is below 2 mm, then no action is taken, but if it is between 3–9 mm, then correction in the form of set-up changes may be done. But if correction is around 1 cm or more, then replanning should be done.
- Real-time target volume adaptation during a treatment.

Adaptive radiotherapy can either be a simple application of corrections seen on the couch during set-up verification by fusion of the planning CT and the CBCT/MVCT or even be as complex as the use of modern deformable image registration which can automatically match the newer images with the planning images based on its databank of images, can sum up the new dose distribution and may give a prediction for likely further changes in patient contour during treatment.

16.2.1 Studies on Anatomical Changes During Radiotherapy

A review of inter- and intra-fraction organ motion in prostate cancers was studied by Langen and Jones [15] and found that though the change in position or size was usually of the order of a few millimetres, there were occasions when the change could be more than a centimetre. Abdominal organs such as the liver, pancreas and kidney (especially closely associated with the diaphragm) could however move by more than 1 cm. More studies have found similar displacements and tumour regression causing anatomical changes in many organs and have quantified these changes especially in the lung [16–19], cervix [20], as well as head and neck cancers [21, 22]. In addition to movement, significant shrinkage in tumour volume can cause displacement as observed by Kupelian [16] in a series of 10 lung cancer patients in which the decrease in tumour volume was about 1.2% per day; while in cervix, nearly half of a cohort of 34 patients studied by Mayr et al. [20] regressed during radiotherapy to 20% of their initial volume. Similar observations have been made in head and neck cancers (HNC) (a major focus of adaptive radiotherapy) by Barker et al. [21] who in study of 14 HNC patients on radiotherapy reported a median reduction of 70% in the initial gross tumour volume (GTV). In another study, Lee et al. has reported significant decrease in volume and medial shift in position of the parotid glands during radiotherapy [23]. Martinez et al. [24] have also quantified changes in the prostate PTV volume during IMRT between the initial portal images and through each subsequent week of radiotherapy [25]. They found that the decrease in tumour volume could be as high as 24%, and hence the dose escalation to the GTV varied from 2.5 to 15% with an average of 7.5%.

16.2.2 Clinical Rationale for Adaptive Radiotherapy

Thus with increasing frequency of dose escalation and smaller margins, it becomes necessary for us to correctly deliver the prescribed dose to the intended target volume. As seen previously, in head and neck cancer patients, tumour shrinkage or muscle fibrosis can lead to a medial shift of structures (both PTV and parotid). If the target PTV is not adjusted accordingly, there is high likelihood that there might be increased doses to skin, spinal cord and parotid as well as chance of missing posterior aspects of PTV (Fig. 16.3). Similarly in pelvic tumours being treated by VMAT/IMRT, especially prostate cancers, a CBCT matching is essential to account for daily variation in bladder filling and volume even if bladder-filling protocols are being followed in a department.

Motion and tumour shrinkage make head and neck, thoracic, and abdominal tumour sites good candidates for image-guided adaptive radiotherapy. Mohan and colleagues [26] found a substantial decrease of coverage of the CTV and lymph nodes without adaptation resulting from the changing anatomy though with adaptation, target coverage was maintained. Similarly, Lee and colleagues [27] found a 15% daily variation in the delivered versus planned mean parotid dose of head and neck cancer patients resulting from parotid migration into the high-dose region progressively throughout treatment. Underberg and colleagues [28] in a study of stage I NSCLC found significantly high (>5 mm) shifts of average tumour position compared to bony anatomy in 26–43% of cases. Ramsey and colleagues [29] in a

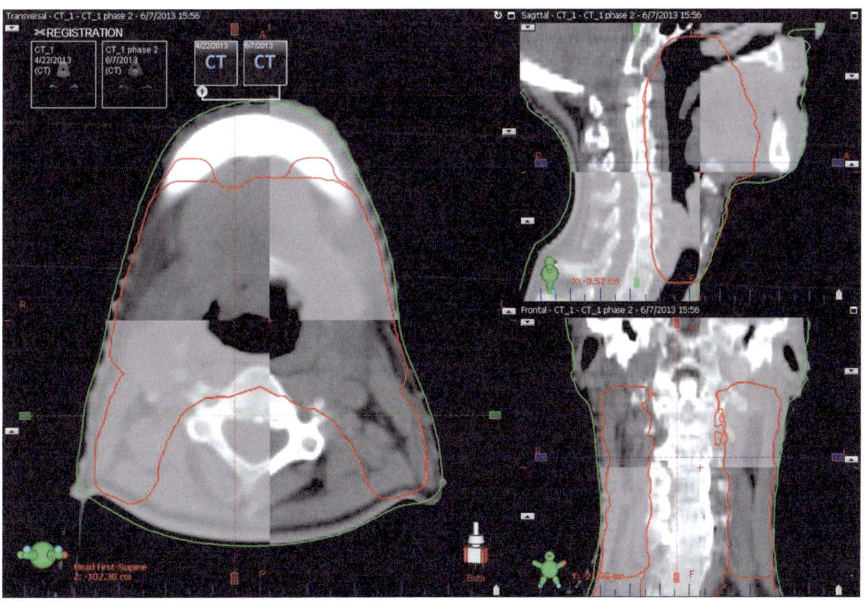

Fig. 16.3 Target PTV adjusted during treatment to prevent missing posterior aspects of PTV and increased doses to skin, spinal cord and parotid

study on lung patients imaged with daily MVCT observed tumour shrinkage of 60–80% through course of treatment and demonstrated a significant (17–23%) reduction in the V20 in the ipsilateral lung. An important consideration when performing image-guided adaptive radiotherapy with X-ray-producing devices is the dose received by the patient. The cost of the use of the X-ray imaging devices must be outweighed by the benefit to the patient of more accurate treatment. To date, very few known prospective randomized trials have compared adaptive radiotherapy with standard of care [30].

16.2.3 Timing of Adaptive Radiotherapy

Image-guided adaptive radiotherapy can be done offline, online and real time. But as time between interventions is reduced from offline through to real-time adaptation, the reliance on automated processes is increased. The increased potential for anatomic conformality offered by adaptation also increases the error risk of adaptive processes and careful human operator oversight is necessary.

A key tool for image-guided adaptive radiotherapy is deformable image registration that allows dose and contour information to be transferred between images, substantially reducing workload. As the timescales for adaptation decrease, the computation time of deformable image registration must correspondingly decrease. Adaptive radiotherapy is also useful in compensation of uncertainties, including organ deformation and inter-fraction organ motion as well as dosimetric errors incurred in previous fractions [26, 31–34].

16.2.3.1 Image Registration

This is the process in which one set of imaging data is fused with another set over a common coordinate template. It is done by realigning or changing the coordinates of one data set to match those of the other so that both sets can exactly be superimposed on each other. Deformable registration involves modelling of voxel-dependent distortion. Advantages of using adaptive radiotherapy include (1) better definition or redefinition of changing target volumes [35], (2) image enhancement [36, 37], (3) delineation or even copying of organ contours from one image set to another [38], (4) dose calculation in organs with inter- or intra-fraction volume changes [39–42] and (5) 4D image reconstruction [43, 44].

Therefore image registration broadly refers to the process of applying one set of images over another to better delineate the target volumes and OAR; and this process can be done manually, matching of image sets by matching prominent landmarks, matching the surface anatomical contours on each data set and matching by imaging intensity patterns or even mutual information-based registrations. Deformable image registration is a rapidly evolving area and intense efforts are being made from to increase its acceptability and visibility with newer versions of planning systems now providing this software.

16.2.3.2 Offline Adaptive Radiotherapy

Offline adaptation means that the imaging and treatment sessions are separate. Head and neck cancers are amenable to offline adaption because tumour shrinkage is significant. The rationale for offline image-guided adaptive radiotherapy is that the substantial shrinkage of the tumour throughout the course of therapy is observed between the anatomy at the time of the original CT scan and the cone beam CT scans acquired during treatment; and hence target volumes can be adjusted and replanned accordingly (Fig. 16.4). Care must be taken with adaptation, as this process is based on imaging and interpretation of the images has a large interobserver variability [45–47].

Also questions arise for how to adapt the CTVs, in which by definition there is suspected but no image-visible disease. Some studies report that there should be no change in target contours made initially. Only check is to be made for any significant loss of normal tissue due to weight loss or fibrosis and targets realigned accordingly. Others argue that after tumour shrinkage to protect underlying normal tissue, it may be necessary to recontour target volumes. The debate is still going on between both groups, but no guidelines have been framed.

The imaging system used for offline adaptive radiotherapy is typically either a conventional CT scanner or an in-room CT scanner. The adaptation can be triggered by a protocol (e.g. after 20 and 40 Gy delivered dose), by clinical observations of masks not fitting, weight loss or other surface changes or by changes observed on an in-room imaging system.

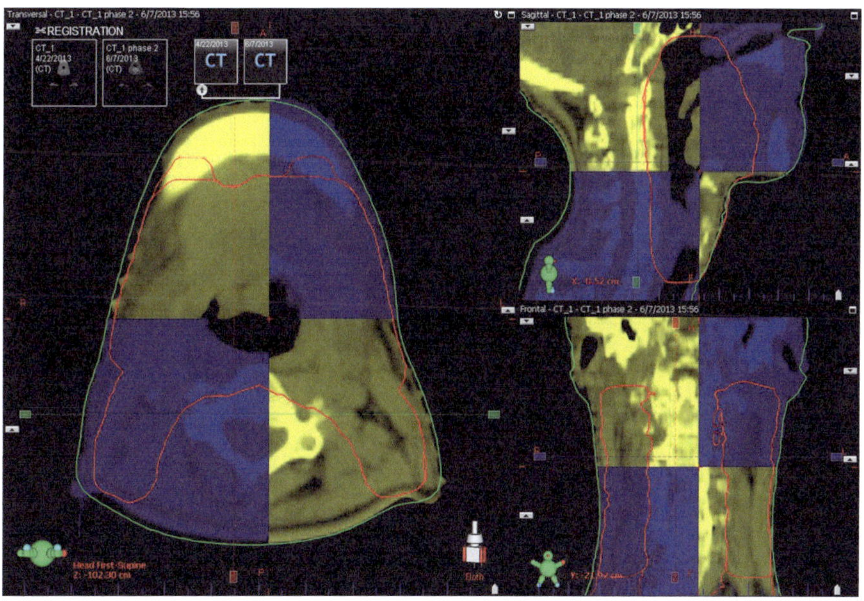

Fig. 16.4 Image registration and matching

16.2.3.3 Online Image-Guided Adaptive Radiotherapy

Online adaptation means that the imaging session and treatment session occur in the treatment room within a given treatment fraction. Head and neck cancer is particularly amenable to online adaptation, because variable neck flexion can be significant and change the position of the lower neck and supraclavicular node targets with respect to the primary tumour and upper-neck nodal targets from that planned. Involved field prostate radiotherapy is also amenable to online adaptation because the prostate can move independently of the treated pelvic nodes, and therefore the two targets are in different geometric locations from each other to that planned.

The imaging system for online image-guided adaptive radiotherapy is typically an in-room CT scanner, which can be a fan beam or cone beam kilovoltage or megavoltage imaging system. To avoid additional geometric errors, it is important to minimize the time between the imaging procedures and treatment completion.

16.2.3.4 Real-Time Image-Guided Adaptive Radiotherapy

Real-time adaptation means that the imaging session and treatment session take place at same time. Abdominal and thoracic tumours are particularly amenable to online adaption as respiration-induced tumour motion is significant. Other than real-time image-guided adaptive radiotherapy, there are other options to manage intra-fraction motion, particularly respiratory-induced motion which has been described in previous section on stereotactic radiation. A review and use guidelines for these methods are given in the AAPM Task Group 76 report [48].

Real-time image-guided adaptation is a complex form of adaptation, requiring more imaging, faster decision-making and even more reliance on the system for guidance, plan changes and fidelity of delivery to moving targets. Desirable characteristics of the ideal imaging system for real-time adaptive therapy are:

(a) Volumetric
(b) High spatial resolution
(c) High-temporal resolution
(d) High degree of reproducibility
(e) Fast acquisition of images and transfer of the same treatment console to planning station for matching and replanning if required
(f) No physical or electronic interference with treatment delivery
(g) Noninvasive
(h) No or as little as possible imaging dose
(i) Can optimize and compute dose
(j) Reduces treatment time
(k) Cheap, with low operational costs

Desirable characteristics of the ideal radiation delivery system for real-time adaptive therapy are:

(a) Integrates all sources of imaging information
(b) Integrates all sources of uncertainty

(c) Optimizes in real time using all available degrees of freedom
(d) Modifies delivery appropriately

Delivery systems under investigation for real-time adaptation to tumour motion include the CyberKnife robotic treatment system [49, 50], the multileaf collimator [51–53] and the couch compensation system [54–56]. Proton and heavy-ion treatment systems [57, 58] are also being investigated for real-time adaptation. A system's reaction time depends on a number of factors like detection time for change in target position, processing speed of position data, communication with beam-alignment system and repositioning of either the beam or patient.

16.2.4 Summary

- Adaptive radiotherapy is a dynamic pattern of radiotherapy delivery which caters to changes in the target volume and patient's anatomy caused by tumour regression, weight loss or changes in tumour position. It can be practised retrospectively offline, in near real time just before patient's treatment delivery as a quality check or in real time as target volume matching on the treatment couch.
- Adaptive radiotherapy can thus track changes in the target volume and critical OAR volume during radiotherapy as well as inter-fraction movement and is also useful in compensation for uncertainties during radiotherapy.
- Newer forms of adaptive radiotherapy use deformable image registration for transferring changed anatomic contours and dose between sets of images along with automatic treatment planning and deformable dose summation.

References

1. Blomgren H, Lax I, Naslund I, et al. Stereotactic high dose fraction radiation therapy of extracranial tumors using an accelerator. Clinical experience of the first thirty-one patients. Acta Oncol. 1995;34:861–70.
2. Hamilton AJ, Lulu BA, Fosmire H, et al. Preliminary clinical experience with linear accelerator-based spinal stereotactic radiosurgery. Neurosurgery. 1995;36:311–9.
3. Timmerman RD. An overview of hypofractionation and introduction to this issue of seminars in radiation oncology. Semin Radiat Oncol. 2008;18:215–22.
4. Barendsen G. Dose fractionation, dose rate and isoeffect relationships for normal tissue responses. Int J Radiat Oncol Biol Phys. 1982;8:1981–97.
5. Brenner DJ. The linear-quadratic model is an appropriate methodology for determining isoeffective doses at large doses per fraction. Semin Radiat Oncol. 2008;18:234–9.
6. Kirkpatrick JP, Meyer JJ, Marks LB. The linear-quadratic model is inappropriate to model high dose per fraction effects in radiosurgery. Semin Radiat Oncol. 2008;18:240–3.
7. Ch'ang HJ, Maj JG, Paris F, et al. ATM regulates target switching to escalating doses of radiation in the intestines. Nat Med. 2005;11:484–90.
8. Lax I, Blomgren H, Naslund I, et al. Stereotactic radiotherapy of malignancies in the abdomen. Methodological aspects. Acta Oncol. 1994;33:677–83.

9. Bezjak A, Paulus R, Gaspar LE, Timmerman RD, Straube WL, et al. Efficacy and toxicity analysis of NRG Oncology/RTOG 0813 Trial of stereotactic body radiation therapy (SBRT) for centrally located non-small cell lung cancer (NSCLC). Int J Radiat Oncol Biol Phys. 2016;96(2 Suppl):S8.
10. Videtic GMM, Hu C, Singh AK, et al. NRG Oncology RTOG 0915 (NCCTG N0927): a randomized phase II study comparing 2 stereotactic body radiation therapy (SBRT) schedules for medically inoperable patients with stage I peripheral non-small cell lung cancer. Int J Radiat Oncol Biol Phys. 2015;93(4):757–64.
11. Benedict SH, Yenice KM, Followill D, Galvin JM, et al. Stereotactic body radiation therapy: the report of AAPM Task Group 101. Med Phys. 2010;37(8):4078–101.
12. Sahgal A, Roberge D, Schellenberg D, Purdie TG, et al. The Canadian Association of Radiation Oncology scope of practice guidelines for lung, liver and spine stereotactic body radiotherapy. Clin Oncol (R Coll Radiol). 2012;24(9):629–39.
13. Timmerman RD, Hu C, Michalski J, Straube W, et al. Long-term results of RTOG 0236: a phase II trial of stereotactic body radiation therapy (SBRT) in the treatment of patients with medically inoperable stage I non-small cell lung cancer. Int J Radiat Oncol Biol Phys. 2014;90(1 Suppl):S30.
14. Timmerman RD, Paulus R, Pass HI, Gore E, et al. RTOG 0618: Stereotactic body radiation therapy (SBRT) to treat operable early-stage lung cancer patients. J Clin Oncol. 2013;31(15 Suppl):7523.
15. Langen KM, Jones DT. Organ motion and its management. Int J Radiat Oncol Biol Phys. 2001;50:265–78.
16. Kupelian PA, Ramsey C, Meeks SL, et al. Serial megavoltage CT imaging during external beam radiotherapy for non-small-cell lung cancer: observations on tumor regression during treatment. Int J Radiat Oncol Biol Phys. 2005;63:1024–8.
17. Bosmans G, van Baardwijk A, Dekker A, et al. Intra-patient variability of tumor volume and tumor motion during conventionally fractionated radiotherapy for locally advanced non-small-cell lung cancer: a prospective clinical study. Int J Radiat Oncol Biol Phys. 2006;66:748–53.
18. Britton KR, Starkschall G, Tucker SL, et al. Assessment of gross tumor volume regression and motion changes during radiotherapy for non-small-cell lung cancer as measured by four-dimensional computed tomography. Int J Radiat Oncol Biol Phys. 2007;68:1036–46.
19. Siker ML, Tome WA, Mehta MP. Tumor volume changes on serial imaging with megavoltage CT for non-small-cell lung cancer during intensity-modulated radiotherapy: how reliable, consistent, and meaningful is the effect? Int J Radiat Oncol Biol Phys. 2006;66:135–41.
20. Mayr NA, Magnotta VA, Ehrhardt JC, et al. Usefulness of tumor volumetry by magnetic resonance imaging in assessing response to radiation therapy in carcinoma of the uterine cervix. Int J Radiat Oncol Biol Phys. 1996;35:915–24.
21. Barker JL, Garden AS, Ang KK, et al. Quantification of volumetric and geometric changes occurring during fractionated radiotherapy for head-and-neck cancer using an integrated CT/linear accelerator system. Int J Radiat Oncol Biol Phys. 2004;59:960–70.
22. Hansen EK, Bucci MK, Quivey JM, et al. Repeat CT imaging and replanning during the course of IMRT for head-and-neck cancer. Int J Radiat Oncol Biol Phys. 2006;64:355–62.
23. Lee C, Langen KM, Lu W, et al. Evaluation of geometric changes of parotid glands during head and neck cancer radiotherapy using daily MVCT and automatic deformable registration. Radiother Oncol. 2008;89:81–8.
24. Martinez AA, Yan D, Lockman D, et al. Improvement in dose escalation using the process of adaptive radiotherapy combined with three-dimensional conformal or intensity-modulated beams for prostate cancer. Int J Radiat Oncol Biol Phys. 2001;50:1226–34.
25. Yan D, Lockman D, Brabbins D, et al. An off-line strategy for constructing a patient-specific planning target volume in adaptive treatment process for prostate cancer. Int J Radiat Oncol Biol Phys. 2000;48:289–302.
26. Mohan R, Zhang X, Wang H, et al. Use of deformed intensity distributions for on-line modification of image-guided IMRT to account for interfractional anatomic changes. Int J Radiat Oncol Biol Phys. 2005;61:1258–66.

27. Lee C, Langen KM, Lu W, et al. Assessment of parotid gland dose changes during head and neck cancer radiotherapy using daily megavoltage computed tomography and deformable image registration. Int J Radiat Oncol Biol Phys. 2008;71:1563–71.
28. Underberg RW, Lagerwaard FJ, van Tinteren H, et al. Time trends in target volumes for stage I non-small-cell lung cancer after stereotactic radiotherapy. Int J Radiat Oncol Biol Phys. 2006;64:1221–8.
29. Ramsey CR, Langen KM, Kupelian PA, et al. A technique for adaptive image-guided helical tomotherapy for lung cancer. Int J Radiat Oncol Biol Phys. 2006;64:1237–44.
30. Bentzen SM. Randomized controlled trials in health technology assessment: overkill or overdue? Radiother Oncol. 2008;86:142–7.
31. Paganetti H, Jiang H, Trofimov A. 4D Monte Carlo simulation of proton beam scanning: modelling of variations in time and space to study the interplay between scanning pattern and time-dependent patient geometry. Phys Med Biol. 2005;50:983–90.
32. Wu Q, Liang J, Yan D. Application of dose compensation in image-guided radiotherapy of prostate cancer. Phys Med Biol. 2006;51:1405–19.
33. de la Zerda A, Armbruster B, Xing L. Inverse planning for adaptive radiation therapy using dynamic programming. Paper presented at annual meeting of ASTRO, Philadelphia; 2006.
34. Lu W, Chen ML, Olivera GH, et al. Fast free-form deformable registration via calculus of variations. Phys Med Biol. 2004;49:3067–87.
35. Xing L, Thorndyke B, Schreibmann E, et al. Overview of image-guided radiation therapy. Med Dosim. 2006;31:91–112.
36. Thorndyke B, Schreibmann E, Maxim P, et al. Enhancing 4D PET through retrospective stacking. Med Phys. 2005;32:2096.
37. Li T, Schreibmann E, Thorndyke B, et al. Radiation dose reduction in 4D computed tomography. Med Phys. 2005;32:2094.
38. Lu W, Olivera GH, Chen Q, et al. Automatic re-contouring in 4D radiotherapy. Phys Med Biol. 2006;51:1077–99.
39. Keall P. 4-Dimensional computed tomography imaging and treatment planning. Semin Radiat Oncol. 2004;14:81–90.
40. De la Zerda A, Armbruster B, Xing L. Inverse planning for adaptive radiation therapy using dynamic algorithm. Int J Radiat Oncol Biol Phys. 2006;66:S123–4.
41. Keall PJ, Joshi S, Vedam SS, et al. Four-dimensional radiotherapy planning for DMLC-based respiratory motion tracking. Med Phys. 2005;32:942–51.
42. Langen KM, Meeks SL, Poole DO, et al. The use of megavoltage CT (MVCT) images for dose recomputations. Phys Med Biol. 2005;50:4259–76.
43. Li T, Thorndyke B, Schreibmann E, et al. Model-based image reconstruction for four-dimensional PET. Med Phys. 2006;33:1288–98.
44. Li T, Schreibmann E, Yang Y, et al. Motion correction for improved target localization with on-board cone-beam computed tomography. Phys Med Biol. 2006;51:253–67.
45. Van de Steene J, Linthout N, de Mey J, et al. Definition of gross tumor volume in lung cancer: inter-observer variability. Radiother Oncol. 2002;62:37–49.
46. Fiorino C, Vavassori V, Sanguineti G, et al. Rectum contouring variability in patients treated for prostate cancer: impact on rectum dose-volume histograms and normal tissue complication probability. Radiother Oncol. 2002;63:249–55.
47. Hermans R, Feron M, Bellon E, et al. Laryngeal tumor volume measurements determined with CT: a study on intra- and interobserver variability. Int J Radiat Oncol Biol Phys. 1998;40:553–7.
48. Keall PJ, Mageras GS, Balter JM, et al. The management of respiratory motion in radiation oncology report of AAPM Task Group 76. Med Phys. 2006;33:3874–900.
49. Schweikard A, Shiomi H, Adler J. Respiration tracking in radiosurgery. Med Phys. 2004;31:2738–41.
50. Willoughby TR, Kupelian PA, Pouliot J, et al. Target localization and real-time tracking using the Calypso 4D localization system in patients with localized prostate cancer. Int J Radiat Oncol Biol Phys. 2006;65:528–34.

51. Webb S, Binnie DM. A strategy to minimize errors from differential intrafraction organ motion using a single configuration for a "breathing" multileaf collimator. Phys Med Biol. 2006;51:4517–31.
52. Webb S. Quantification of the fluence error in the motion-compensated dynamic MLC (DMLC) technique for delivering intensity-modulated radiotherapy (IMRT). Phys Med Biol. 2006;51:L17–21.
53. Papiez L, Rangaraj D. DMLC leaf-pair optimal control for mobile, deforming target. Med Phys. 2005;32:275–85.
54. D'Souza WD, Naqvi SA, Yu CX. Real-time intra-fraction-motion tracking using the treatment couch: a feasibility study. Phys Med Biol. 2005;50:4021–33.
55. Qiu P, D'Souza WD, McAvoy TJ, et al. Inferential modeling and predictive feedback control in real-time motion compensation using the treatment couch during radiotherapy. Phys Med Biol. 2007;52:5831–54.
56. Wilbert J, Meyer J, Baier K, et al. Tumor tracking and motion compensation with an adaptive tumor tracking system (ATTS): system description and prototype testing. Med Phys. 2008;35:3911–21.
57. Bert C, Saito N, Schmidt A, et al. Target motion tracking with a scanned particle beam. Med Phys. 2007;34:4768–71.
58. Grozinger SO, Rietzel E, Li Q, et al. Simulations to design an online motion compensation system for scanned particle beams. Phys Med Biol. 2006;51:3517–31.

17 Intraoperative Radiotherapy

Intraoperative irradiation therapy (IORT) as the name implies means delivery of irradiation at the time of an operation, either by using electrons (IOERT), high-dose-rate brachytherapy (HDR-IORT) or orthovoltage. This includes delivery such as irradiation either during or immediately after surgery, with or without external beam irradiation therapy (EBRT) and chemotherapy. IORT aims to achieve higher effective doses of irradiation to the tumour bed after displacing away surgically the dose-limiting normal tissues [1–3].

17.1 Rationale for Intraoperative Irradiation

17.1.1 Influence of Dose on Local Control

Various studies done on animal models have shown that the dose required to control or cure a cancer cell type increases with increase in the tumour volume; and a dose which would be otherwise effective against a small tumour volume may not be effective in controlling a larger volume disease. Similar principles were espoused by Fletcher [4] in his studies on human tumours in breast cancer wherein 60–70% cases with subclinical nodal or chest wall disease could be controlled with doses of 30–35 Gy, 85% with 40 Gy and 95% with 45–50 Gy at 2.0 Gy fractions. But for gross tumours with bigger volumes, the dose required to achieve 70% local control (LC) could be as high as 90 Gy.

Fletcher and Shukovsky [4] and Tepper [5] have extensively studied the effect of volumes in the dose required to control squamous cell carcinomas of the head and neck and have reported that doses of 30–40 Gy produce LC in 60–70% of patients for microscopic disease in lymph nodes compared to more than 90% control at doses of 50 Gy in conventional fractions. Tepper has stated that in locally advanced head and neck cancers, doses of less than 45 Gy produce less than 20% LC while doses of up to 60 Gy give 50% control. Effective local control (more than 80%) is achieved only with higher dose of 75.5 Gy [5].

A. Mukherji, *Basics of Planning and Management of Patients during Radiation Therapy*, https://doi.org/10.1007/978-981-10-6659-7_17

17.1.2 Effect of Complications on Local Tumour Control

Patients having locally advanced abdominal or pelvic malignancies are usually not good candidates for radical surgery with negative margins, and in these cases, the use of external beam radiotherapy (with or without chemotherapy) is generally considered. However in the pelvis and in the abdomen, it is usually not possible to exceed doses of 50–54 Gy in conventional fractions because of the many surrounding critical organs with tolerance much less than the curative doses required. Dose required for tumour control after surgery with microscopic residual disease is about 60 Gy and even higher if gross disease is left behind. Small or large bowel problems resulting from increased RT dose lead to complications such as fistulae, perforations which usually require re-surgery.

Many alternatives to the use of external beam radiotherapy in these cases have been studied. In many gynaecological cancers, there is now extensive use of interstitial and intracavitary brachytherapy to boost doses above 45–50 Gy to nearly an equivalent dose of 80–85 Gy. This is because these organs are accessible from the perineum. However many abdominal and retroperitoneal cancers do not offer such possibilities. In these cases, external beam radiotherapy (EBRT) to doses of 45–50 Gy is given preoperatively (at 1.8 Gy per fraction) and then IORT as boost dose subsequently during surgery immediately after resection in the open wound. Dose-limiting organs are moved away from the beam by surgical mobilization or shielding. This approach allows an increase in local control or LC with a lower risk of complications than with an EBRT-only approach.

17.1.3 Effect of Local Control on Distant Metastases

It has also been seen through several studies that good local control of the primary disease also results in control of distant metastases, and these metastases are affected by both tumour size and stage. In studies done on fibrosarcoma cell lines in the C3H/Sed mouse, Ramsey et al. reported increased rates of distant metastases with 12 mm compared to 6 mm tumour size and primary versus recurrent tumours [6]. These findings where further corroborated by Suit et al. [7] who reported that larger (12 mm) isotransplants of C3H mouse mammary tumours after irradiation had higher distant metastases as well as less local control.

17.2 Techniques of IORT

EBRT with IORT: Early studies on the use of intraoperative electrons (IOERT) in Japan and the US have used 20–40 Gy electrons as a single modality. But since then, other investigators have mainly used this method as a boost in combination with preoperative radio−/chemoradiotherapy and maximal surgical resection.

Potential advantages of use of combined EBRT-IORT when compared to the use of IORT alone are:

(a) Improvement in local-regional control (LRC) as a higher dose can be delivered to the tumour and regional lymphatics with better cell kill due to dose fractionation (*Refer* Chap. 7) along with less damage to surrounding normal tissues. Addition of the boost dose by IORT allows for increased effective dose with less tissue morbidity and decreased overall treatment time, thus preventing repopulation.
(b) The volume of tissue receiving boost dose is significantly reduced because of direct tumour visualization and appositional treatment with IORT which also prevents dose to surrounding normal structures by mobilizing them out of the beam or using direct shielding.

17.2.1 Use of Boost Techniques

Traditionally the initial EBRT field includes a 2–5 cm margin beyond the gross tumour volume plus regional nodal areas that are at risk for subclinical disease and is treated to a dose of 45–50.4 Gy in conventional (1.8–2.0 Gy) fractions. Further boost dose (by IORT) is delivered to bring gross disease dose to 65–80 Gy with EBRT or brachytherapy.

Such combined treatment techniques have yielded good long-term results especially in breast, gynaecological, as well as head and neck cancers where good LC is achieved with relatively low morbidity to dose-limiting normal tissues. Patients with head and neck and breast lesions require interstitial techniques or fractionated outpatient electrons or a conformal EBRT boost; gynaecologic lesions are treated with an intracavitary technique or conformal boost with additional brachytherapy. Thoracic or pelvic lesions can safely receive boost dose by IMRT or VMAT techniques. It is in the case of abdominal or retroperitoneal cancers where dose escalation by traditional means cannot be meaningfully executed that IOERT or HDR-IORT is used.

17.3 Patient Selection and Evaluation

Patient Selection Guidelines: Cases planned for IORT should be discussed between the surgeon and the radiation oncologist as well as other stakeholders in a multidisciplinary meet which may also determine the treatment modality sequencing. All patients should be explained of their expected line of management, expected results and complications, and an informed consent should be taken.

General criteria to guide patient selection include:

1. Cases where surgery alone may not achieve acceptable local control with high chance of at least microscopic residual disease.
2. Surgery is not contraindicated or precluded because of any existing medical condition.
3. Standard adjuvant radiotherapy doses by EBRT technique which would otherwise ensure adequate local control would be more than the surrounding normal tissue tolerance and not possible to deliver by even conformal radiotherapy.

4. Facilities are available to provide IORT at the time of the planned surgery.
5. The IORT-plus-EBRT technique will involve direct visual noting of tumour bed/ or unresected tumour and irradiating it while removing critical structures away from portal.
6. There is no evidence of distant metastases or peritoneal seeding; except in cases which are either very slow growing or have excellent response to chemotherapy.

Patient Evaluation: It is essential before treatment that the patient undergoes a full evaluation and investigation for full staging and mapping of the extent of disease which would include history, examination, routine investigations, imaging, tumour markers (CEA/CA 19.9/CA-125) and even physiological imaging (PET) where required. It is essential to rule out unresectability or distant metastases before surgery. Modalities such as CT or MRI help identifying presence of absence of resection planes or spread into adjacent or parietal structures and help determine sequence of therapy (whether surgery up front or preoperative radio-/ chemotherapy followed by surgery and IORT). Extra-regional spread to nodes or liver is determined, or findings on CT/MRI suggest surrounding organ involvement.

17.4 Treatment Sequencing, Dose and Technique

Sequencing of Surgery, EBRT and IORT: It is essential to have a multispecialty consultation involving a surgeon, radiation oncologist, radiologist, pathologist and medical oncologist to discuss the optimal therapy required as well as sequencing of the various modalities. Surgery should be preferentially done before radiotherapy wherever possible, though in locally advanced cases it is better to first give EBRT or chemotherapy followed by surgery and then boost irradiation. Resection is generally found possible in oesophagogastric, colorectal, gynaecologic and renal cancers as well as abdomino-pelvic sarcomas but less feasible with biliary and pancreatic cancers.

As explained before, in locally advanced lesions, pre-op EBRT of 45–50 Gy with or without chemotherapy followed by surgery after 3–5 weeks may be better than surgery and IORT followed by EBRT. This may be due to:

- Patients with very aggressive disease who develop metastases during EBRT need not undergo surgery and can be treated by palliative chemotherapy thereafter.
- Pre-op EBRT may cause tumour shrinkage, and though the extent of resection is still the same, there is less morbidity with better margins and even the possibility of achieving a gross total resection.
- Risk of tumour cell implantation in case of surgery first is avoided.
- Giving radiotherapy before surgery has the advantage that the free radicals produced by radiotherapy are able to use the intact vascular supply having better oxygenation and thus achieve better tumour cell kill.

17.4.1 Technique

External Beam Radiotherapy: The usual preoperative EBRT dose is 45–54 Gy over 5–6 weeks in conventional fractions delivered using ≥10 MV photons by conformal radiotherapy techniques (3D-CRT or IMRT) for pelvic lesions, while for extra pelvic lesions, non-resected or residual disease with 3–5 cm margin is treated to a dose of 40–45 Gy after which the field is reduced with 2–3 cm margins and given a further boost of 5–10 Gy to a total dose of 45–54 Gy. Concurrent chemotherapy is given with external irradiation using 5-FU/capecitabine or cisplatin-based regimens especially in locally advanced disease. Patients who have received prior irradiation and have a local recurrence can be treated by re-irradiation. These patients receive either full treatment by conformal EBRT (IMRT) to a dose of about 70–80% of previous full dose wherever technically possible (head and neck, sarcomas, pelvis), or they may receive low-dose preoperative EBRT doses of 20–30 Gy in conventional fractions, preferably with concurrent chemotherapy followed by surgery and boost IORT. Correct immobilization, beam selection, treatment delivery and quality assurance help in minimizing side effects.

IORT: After surgical exploration and maximal resection, the radiation oncologist joins the surgeon in the operating room to determine whether IORT is indicated and feasible, based on a review of surgical-pathologic findings. The site of the IORT treatment field is determined and marked with sutures or clips. If treatment machine is in the radiation oncology department, the patient is transferred there after temporary closure of incisions and placed on the linear accelerator table in the radiation oncology department for IOERT treatment. If the institution has a mobile X-band accelerator that can be brought to the operating room, the IOERT applicator is immobilized in position with a retractor.

Field size selected includes tumour bed or unresected disease with a margin of ·-1 cm. The operating room table is then shifted adjacent to the IOERT machine, and the gantry angle of the mobile accelerator is adjusted to cover the applicator. The IORT team exits the room and IOERT is delivered, while the patient and anaesthesia equipment are monitored. After delivery of radiotherapy, the operating room table is then shifted back to the original location for surgical reconstruction and closure of incisions. The IOERT energy and dose are dependent on the amount of residual disease remaining after maximal resection and on the EBRT component.

17.4.2 Dose

- When an R0 or R1 resection has been accomplished, 6 or 9 MeV electrons would provide adequate depth dose.
- In R2 resection or unresectable disease, 9–12 MeV electron energies or higher are required to ensure adequate depth dose coverage.
- Previously untreated patients having received preoperative EBRT doses of 45–54 Gy require 10–20 Gy IORT; microscopic residual disease or less, 10–12.5 Gy; and gross residual disease, 15–20 Gy.

- Patients who have received radiation before and have local disease recurrence are usually treated to an IORT dose of 15–20 Gy if they have received re-irradiation by EBRT to a dose of 20–30 Gy preoperatively. If they have not received any pre-op EBRT, then IORT dose can be increased to 25–30 Gy, but there is higher risk of nerve intolerance.

The biologic effectiveness of single-dose IORT is considered equivalent to 1.5–2.5 times the same total dose of fractionated EBRT [8]. Thus the EQD2 or the 2 Gy equivalent dose for a combination of EBRT plus IOERT when 45–50 Gy has been given by EBRT would amount to 60–70 Gy2 for 10 Gy IOERT, 75–87.5 Gy2 with a 15 Gy boost and 85–100 Gy2 with 20 Gy IOERT.

Delivery: IORT is given with IOERT (electrons), HDR-IORT (brachytherapy) or orthovoltage machines. HDR-IORT is not ideal if thickness of residual disease exceeds 0.5 cm. If both electrons and brachytherapy are feasible, electrons are chosen because of shorter set-up and treatment times, better depth dose and more homogeneous dose distribution.

IOERT is delivered with rigid Lucite or metal applicators; hence, locations may be anatomically challenging, and HDR-IORT with malleable flab applicators may be preferable, in such locations. Most abdominal sites are usually easily treated with IOERT approaches using either flat or 15° bevel applicators.

For pelvic lesions, the availability of 30° bevel applicators usually allows successful approximation of the IOERT applicator to the tumour bed whether treated through the abdominal incision or the perineal incision after abdominal-perineal resection.

Dose-Limiting Structures and Sequelae: Peripheral nerve is the main dose-limiting normal tissue for intraoperative electron beam radiotherapy (IOERT) in the pelvis or retroperitoneum [9–16] and anatomical locations of peripheral nerve tissue where if adjacent to or involved by tumour can make it difficult to displace from the RT field without causing damage. Structures such as ureter and bile duct are affected by the dose delivered, but they are not dose limiting [9, 13, 14, 17] as even if strictures occur post-radiotherapy, stents can be inserted to overcome obstruction and preserve renal or liver function. Hence it is advised not to compromise on dose if there is risk of involvement of these structures in irradiated field. In an analysis of 146 patients with ureter in the IOERT field, the risk of subsequent obstruction was found to be most in patients receiving more than 15 Gy IOERT dose [18].

A study of nerve and ureteral tolerance to IOERT was done in 51 patients who had received IOERT as part of treatment of locally advanced primary or recurrent pelvic malignancies [9]. Treatment consisted of initial EBRT followed by maximal resection and an IOERT boost with 9–18 MeV electrons. Sixteen patients (32%) developed grade 1 to 3 peripheral neuropathy. Pain was severe (grade 3) in only 3 (6%). Neuropathy incidence by IOERT location was in pelvic sidewall in 15 of 32 (47%), presacral area in 1 of 12 (8%) and central pelvis in 0 of 6 (0%). In another analysis in 187 patients with locally advanced colorectal cancer treated by IOERT regimens [14, 15], there was again dose-dependent incidence of peripheral neuropathy with doses of 10–12.5 Gy causing grade 2 to 3 neuropathy in 5% while doses above ≥15 Gy causing an incidence of 19%.

17.5 Summary

- Thus intraoperative irradiation therapy (IORT) tries to achieve higher effective doses of irradiation by delivering the radiation dose immediately after surgery with dose-limiting structures surgically displaced away from the tumour bed. The dose given by IORT is thought to be biologically 1.5–2.5 times in terms of EQD2 EBRT value.
- IORT is given with IOERT (electrons), HDR-IORT (brachytherapy) or an orthovoltage machine. HDR-IORT is not ideal if thickness of residual disease exceeds 0.5 cm.
- If both electrons and brachytherapy are feasible, electrons are chosen because of shorter set-up and treatment times, better depth dose and more homogeneous dose distribution.
- IOERT is delivered with rigid Lucite or metal applicators, and where locations are anatomically challenging, and HDR-IORT with malleable flab applicators may be preferable.
- Most abdominal sites are usually easily treated with IOERT approaches using either flat or 15° bevel applicators.
- Peripheral nerve is the principal dose-limiting normal tissue for IOERT in the pelvis or retroperitoneum. The anatomic location of peripheral nerve tissue often makes it adjacent to or involved by tumour and even when uninvolved is usually difficult to displace from RT field without damage. IOERT doses of ≥15 cause significant peripheral neuropathy.

References

1. Gunderson LL, Tepper JE, Biggs DJ, et al. Intraoperative +/– external beam irradiation. Curr Probl Cancer. 1983;7:1–69.
2. Johnstone PA, Sindelar WF, Kinsella TJ. Experimental and clinical studies of intraoperative radiation therapy. Curr Probl Cancer. 1994;18:249–92.
3. Gunderson LL, Willett CG, Harrison LB, Calvo F. Intraoperative irradiation: techniques and results. Totowa: Humana; 1999. p. 1–550.
4. Fletcher GH, Shukovsky LJ. The interplay of radiocurability and tolerance in irradiation of human cancers. J Radiol Electrol. 1975;56:383–400.
5. Tepper J. Clonogenic potential of human tumors: a hypothesis. Acta Radiol Oncol. 1981;20:283–8.
6. Ramsay J, Suit HD, Sedlacek R. Experimental studies on the incidence of metastases after failure of radiation treatment and the effect of salvage surgery. Int J Radiat Oncol Biol Phys. 1988;14:1165–8.
7. Suit HD, Sedlacek RS, Gillette EL. Examination for a correlation between probabilities of development of distant metastasis and of local recurrence. Radiology. 1970;95:189–94.
8. Okunieff P, Sundararaman S, Chen Y. Biology of large dose per fraction radiation therapy. Totowa: Humana; 1999. p. 25–46.
9. Shaw EG, Gunderson LL, Martin JK, et al. Peripheral nerve and ureteral tolerance of intraoperative radiation therapy: clinical and dose response analysis. Radiother Oncol. 1990;18:247–55.
10. Kinsella TJ, DeLuca AM, Barnes M, et al. Threshold dose for peripheral neuropathy following intraoperative radiotherapy (IOERT) in a large animal model. Int J Radiat Oncol Biol Phys. 1991;20:697–701.

11. LeCouteur RA, Gillette EL, Powers EL, et al. Periopheral neuropathies following experimental intraoperative radiation (IORT). Int J Radiat Oncol Biol Phys. 1989;17:583–90.
12. Gillette EL, Powers BE, Gillette SM, Gunderson LL, Willett C. Peripheral nerve tolerance: experimental and clinical. In: Gunderson LL, Willett CG, Harrison LB, Calvo FC, editors. Intraoperative irradiation: techniques and results. Totowa: Humana; 1999. p. 165–74.
13. Sindelar WF, Tepper JE, Kinsella TJ. Late effects of intraoperative radiation therapy on retroperitoneal structures, intestine and bile duct in a large animal model. Int J Radiat Oncol Biol Phys. 1994;29:781–8.
14. Gunderson LL, Nelson H, Martenson J, et al. Locally advanced primary colorectal cancer: intraoperative electron and external beam irradiation? 5-FU. Int J Radiat Oncol Biol Phys. 1997;37:601–14.
15. Gunderson LL, Nelson H, Martenson J, et al. Intraoperative electron and external beam irradiation with or without 5-fluorouracil and maximum surgical resection for previously unirradiated, locally recurrent colorectal cancer. Dis Colon Rectum. 1996;39:1379–95.
16. Haddock MG, Miller RC, Nelson H, Gunderson LL. Intraoperative electron irradiation for locally recurrent colorectal cancer. ISIORT 2008 Proceedings. Rev Cancer. 2008;22:50.
17. Gillette EL, Gillette SM, Vujaskovic Z, et al. Influence of volume on canine ureters and peripheral nerves irradiated intraoperatively. In: Schildberg FW, Willich N, Kramling H, editors. Intraoperative radiation therapy—proceedings 4th international IORT symposium, Munich, 1992. Verlag Die Blaue Eule; 1993. p. 61–3.
18. Miller RC, Haddock MG, Petersen IA, Gunderson LL, Furth AF. Intraoperative electron-beam radiotherapy and ureteral obstruction. Int J Radiat Oncol Biol Phys. 2006;64:792–8.

18 Particle Beam Therapy: A Quick View

18.1 Proton Beam Therapy

In recent years, proton beam therapy has increasingly interested both researchers and clinicians due to their desirable characteristics of definite range, high-LET beams and Bragg peak. Protons like any other heavy charged particle continuously interact with their travelling medium and deposit energy in large clusters, the size of which increases with decreasing energy of beam, as they traverse through a medium until they come to a stop. These beams deposit the greatest amount of energy near the end of their range. As a result the beam profile of a proton beam has very typical features of definite range and rapid fall-off (Fig. 18.1). The peak of highest dose is called the Bragg peak.

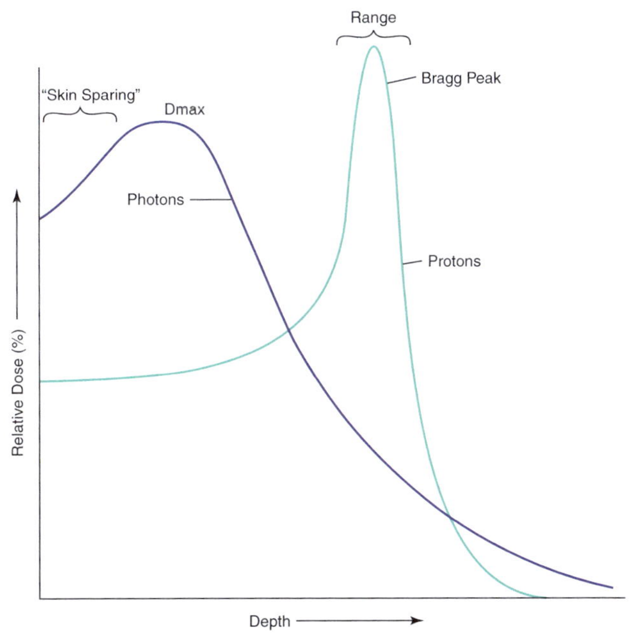

Fig. 18.1 Profile of a proton beam

A. Mukherji, *Basics of Planning and Management of Patients during Radiation Therapy*, https://doi.org/10.1007/978-981-10-6659-7_18

However the biggest disadvantage of proton beams is the very narrow range of the Bragg peak (in mm), which is insufficient to encompass deep-seated tumours. This requires the Bragg peak to be extended over a larger volume and is called spread-out Bragg peak (SOBP, Fig. 18.2) which has a lower dose at the entrance, a flat region of spread-out peak and a rapid fall-off at the distal edge. A therapeutically useful beam can be produced by:

1. Modulating the energy of the narrow monoenergetic beam and scattering it laterally to cover the target volume. This technique is called passively scattered proton therapy (PSPT). This produces the classical SOBP that requires custom shaping with a block or aperture to conform the lateral edges of the beam to target shape and a range compensator to conform the distal edge of dose distribution to the target volume.
2. Scanning the narrow (pencil) beams of a sequence of energies magnetically. In this method, clinical objectives are met by optimizing the intensities of the many thin proton "pencil beams" at a matrix of points in the target. This is called intensity-modulated proton therapy (IMPT). In both methods, generally two or more fields are used per treatment fraction.

The clinical result of this phenomenon of definite range, sharp cut-off and Bragg peak is a greater sparing of normal tissues and reduced tissue integral doses. This allows protection of critical adjacent normal tissue with dose escalation as in base of skull and spinal tumours.

Physical Properties: The primary interactions of protons with medium through which they travel are (1) Coulomb interactions with electrons, (2) Coulomb interactions with nuclei (3) and nuclear interactions. Protons lose most of their energy as they pass through a medium by interactions with atomic electrons, and these then

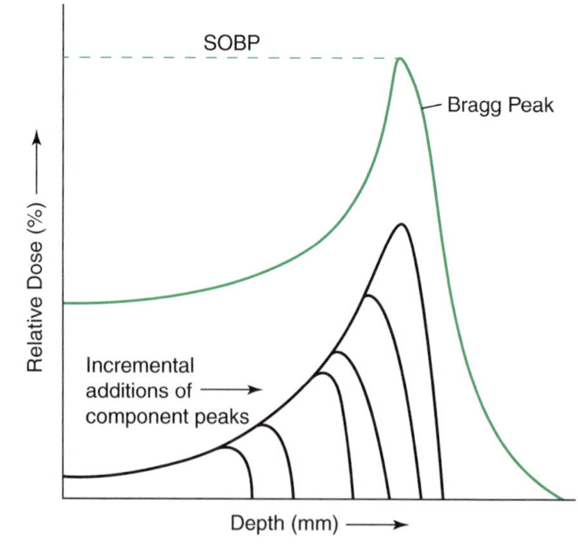

Fig. 18.2 Spread-out Bragg peak (SOBP)

travel very short distances from the path of the proton while ionizing other atoms and molecules and depositing energy which increases inversely with square of the velocity. This leads to the formation of the characteristic Bragg peak. When protons pass near nuclei, they suffer small deflections by Coulomb repulsion without losing significant energy. But multiple such deflections can result in significant lateral dispersion of protons and form the width of the beam penumbra.

Protons also suffer elastic and nonelastic scattering with nuclei when they traverse media. In the case of interactions with atomic nuclei, the protons transfer a large part of their energy to the nuclei and the traverse a bigger angle. In elastic nuclear scattering, the target nucleus recoils, while in nonelastic scattering, either the target nucleus may be left in an excited state, a nucleon exchange or transfer may occur, or it may disintegrate into smaller fragments. These nucleons or other fragments are absorbed within a short distance in the medium, and these reactions might also lead to the release of neutrons. These travel larger distances with more penetration requiring greater amount of protection and cause significant radioactive contamination [1–3].

Biologic Properties: Various experiments have suggested that relative biologic effectiveness (RBE) of protons is 1.1 relative to cobalt-60 radiation. But LET of protons increases as they slow down, and consequently the RBE increases with increasing depth [4, 5]. Even this LET distribution, and the RBE, in a passively scattered beam going through a compensator undergoes scattering leading to spectral changes. And in IMPT, individual pencil beams meeting inside target volume create different distribution of LET compared to a monoenergetic beam with known lateral beam edges and range. In passively scattered beams, such variation in LET and energy deposition patterns can lead to higher dose near the end of the range and different from that planned. Therefore aiming the beams towards a normal critical structure is avoided.

18.1.1 Beam Generation

Protons of energies in the range of 70–250 MeV are needed for cancer treatment. Protons for radiotherapy are accelerated using a cyclotron or a synchrotron. Cyclotrons are more compact, have higher beam intensity and produce a continuous stream of protons. After accelerating the protons to a maximal level, clinically desired energies are produced by introducing mechanical degraders into the beam line before it enters the treatment room.

Synchrotrons accelerate pulses of protons to the desired energy levels which are then extracted and transmitted by the beam line to the treatment room for delivery. The accelerator then goes through deceleration and reset steps and starts the next cycle. Synchrotrons have greater energy flexibility, smaller energy spread and lower power consumption.

The narrow beam of protons produced by the accelerator has a relatively small initial energy and angular spread. After extraction from the accelerator, the beam is directed magnetically through the beam line to the gantry and into the treatment head or "nozzle". In PSPT, protons of a few discrete initial energies for required treatment depth are directed into the gantry of which one is used for a given beam. The beam energy can be further reduced in fine steps using range shifters which are thin slabs of water-equivalent material. For scanning beam applications, energies entering the nozzle are much larger in number and at finer steps. A single proton accelerator can supply protons for gantries in multiple rooms.

Therapeutic Proton Beams: Proton beams entering the nozzle are focused, circularly symmetric thin pencil beams which later get spread out as they pass through the tissue medium. To be clinically useful, such distributions must be spread out laterally and longitudinally, hence the term SOBP, which is achieved by either passively scattering protons with rotator wheel or actively scanning with magnets.

1. **Passively Scattered Proton Beams**
   Conventionally, this is the technique most commonly employed, with a rotating range modulation wheel (RMW) used to produce protons of a sequence of energies up to a maximum. The RMW is like a propeller placed in the path of protons with multiple banks of steps of a range of thicknesses. As the wheel rotates, the proton beam passes through different thickness of the material and is slowed down to different energies. The thinnest step corresponds to the deepest penetration, and the thickest one corresponds to the most proximal Bragg peak. SOBPs of in-between widths may be achieved by turning the incident beam off and on repeatedly at predetermined angles during the wheel's rotation. The advantage of extracting field-size-specific energy protons is in generating fewer neutrons. Present gantry designs contain two scatterers of high-atomic-number materials to spread the beam laterally and flatten it within the region of interest. The first scatterer is usually built into the RMW like a primary collimator in photon machine; the second scatterer acts like a flattening filter in photon beam machines. Scatterers and RMWs reduce the maximum range of protons which then depends on the degree of spreading.
2. **Scanned Beams**
   Magnetic scanning of thin pencil beams provides greater flexibility and control for optimum conformal proton dose distributions. Also elimination of mechanical beam shaping saves the time required for the insertion of these devices and eliminates the need to enter the treatment room between fields. Protons in a pencil beam incident on a patient or phantom are very nearly monoenergetic and are distributed essentially as a narrow bell curve of position relative to the pencil beam's centre.

The high-dose region at the end of the range of a pencil beam is often referred to as the spot. The spot size is important for scanned proton beam therapy as it affects the width of the penumbra and limits the adjustment of dose possible to achieve optimum IMPT dose distributions. Recent designs of proton therapy systems are considering multileaf collimators to reduce the penumbra width but at the cost of some increase in neutron dose. It is important to reduce the spot size by improving focusing and reducing the material in the path of the incident beam or by reducing the drift space between the point where the protons enter the nozzle and the isocentre. The treatments with scanning beams are also referred to as spot scanning treatments. The lateral position of the spot is controlled by two orthogonal magnets, and the range of the spot is controlled by changing the energy of the incident pencil beams.

Scanned beam treatments are delivered using either raster scanning or discrete spot scanning (DSS). In the case of raster scanning, the pencil beam is moved continuously while its intensity is varied. In DSS, the pencil beam is stopped, specified dose is delivered, irradiation is then turned off and the pencil beam is moved to the next spot.

18.1.2 Proton Therapy Planning Algorithm

18.1.2.1 Simulation

Patient simulation is performed on a CT simulator with one or more well-defined imaging protocols [6]. For protons, the CT Hounsfield units (HUs) must be converted to proton stopping power ratios [7]. These factors may reflect the various imaging conditions. Patient's positioning for simulation has to reproduce exactly the patient's positioning for treatment. One approach to address this issue is to digitally remove the imaging couch before treatment planning and replace it with the digitally reconstructed image of the treatment couch.

18.1.2.2 Field Shaping

To conform the dose distribution laterally to the shape of the target volume, a brass aperture, of sufficient thickness (2–8 cm) to absorb incident protons of highest energy, is used. Brass is a compromise material as it produces fewer neutrons with apertures sufficiently compact and manageable. To achieve sharp beam boundaries, the field aperture is positioned close to the patient. Multileaf collimators are also used to shape the lateral field boundaries.

Dose distribution is conformed to the distal shape of the target; the SOBP of the passively scattered beam is shaped further by using a range compensator made of a nearly water-equivalent material such as Lucite. The air gap between the patient and the compensator is minimized to reduce the penumbra by moving the snout close to the patient.

Compensator thickness calculation is done on a point to point basis using water-equivalent material. SOBP width for a passively scattered beam is designed to be constant across the entire field, and passive scattering provides no control over dose distribution proximal to the target.

For scanning beams, proximal and lateral field shaping is achieved by limiting the positions of the spots to within the target regions only. Compensators are not required as the energy of spots can be varied to achieve dose distribution and ensuring no dose beyond target volume. This principle is used in delivering "patched" fields where, in case of a target volume that cannot be encompassed by a beam from one direction (called "**through beam**"), complete coverage can be obtained by another "patch" field that can cover the volume from another aspect (Fig. 18.3). In case of these patched fields, only binary modulation (full dose or no dose) is possible.

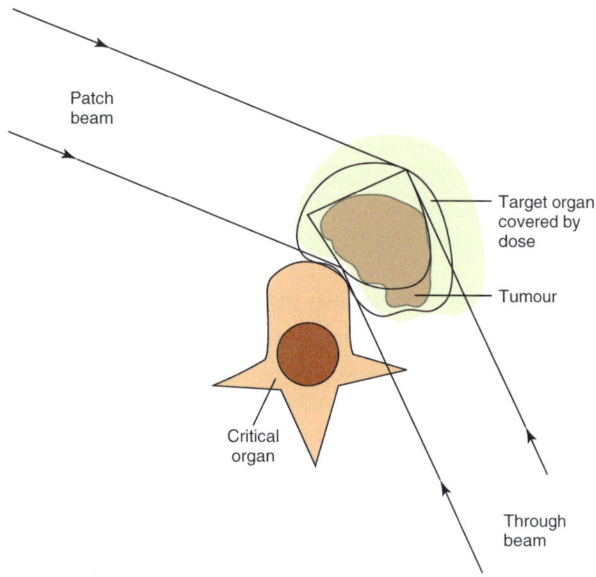

Fig. 18.3 Use of "Patch Beams"

18.1.2.3 Target Volume Definition

Conventional target volumes as described in ICRU reports 50 and 62 need to be reconsidered for proton therapy planning because of the specific physical properties of protons. In case of passively scattered proton therapy (PSPT), distal and proximal margins need to be added to CTV to cater for uncertainty in range to ensure coverage along the path of each beam. These margins have been estimated to be about 3% of depth of the target. Lateral margins depend on the anatomic variations orthogonal to the beam direction. Aperture margin is determined by adding width of the penumbra to the lateral margin.

18.1.2.4 Proton Treatment Planning

The objective of treatment planning is to determine the configuration and parameters of beams that will lead to an optimum dose distribution and include the number and directions of proton beams. In the PSPT mode, for each beam, parameters also include distal and proximal margins, lateral margin, beam energy (or the maximum proton range), modulation width and the characteristics of the aperture, compensator and range shifter. Energy and modulation width are subsequently used to select the modulator and its parameters and the second scatterer. For scanned beam treatments, the parameters include the intensities and energies of the spots and their spacing. Hence in the parlance of *photon* beam planning, PSPT mode proton beams are forward planned, while scanned beams are inverse planned.

The plans are evaluated using dose distributions and dose-volume histograms. Uncertainties in proton beam planning are due to uncertainty in range, inter- and intra-fractional variations in anatomy, the approximate values of the Hounsfield units and proton stopping powers in tissues and the approximations in models to compute dose distributions, especially in the presence of complex heterogeneities.

Smearing: Positioning uncertainties and changes in inhomogeneities in the path of a proton beam affect the depth of penetration and the conformity of the dose distribution to the distal and proximal edge. Hence compensators are smeared to prevent misalignment with patient's anatomy [8]. This process involves decreasing the width of the higher thickness regions of the compensator to allow protons to penetrate more deeply. Smearing and margins for range uncertainty ensure coverage of the target and account for lateral scatter but results in higher dose to distal normal tissues. Respiratory motion can lead to target underdosing or normal tissue overdosing [9]. In such cases, compensators are prepared from the maximum intensity projection image of the ITV in which each voxel within the ITV is set to its maximum intensity in any one of the phases [9]. Another method devised by Engelsman et al. [10] uses the 4D CT where one compensator is designed for each phase of the 4D CT. The union of all the compensators represents the final composite compensator. It is highly desirable that gated or breath-hold treatments be used for proton therapy if the intra-fractional motion exceeds 0.5 cm.

In the case of scanned beam and intensity-modulated proton therapy, positions of the spots are predetermined being automatically placed at specified intervals of positions lateral to the beam direction and at predefined steps of energy longitudinally. Computer-aided optimization techniques are used to determine the intensities of individual spots composing the incident proton beams to achieve specified clinical objectives. In IMPT, various techniques have been described. In the simplest type, each beam is optimized independently to achieve a uniform dose to the target while minimizing dose outside the target volume. This is called single-field uniform dose (SFUD) approach. Since each beam is optimized, uncertainties can be identified and corrected. This method is preferred in present-day practice. In a more advanced form of IMPT (3D IMPT), the optimization process simultaneously optimizes intensities of all spots from all beams to achieve the best possible approximation of dose distribution that balances the specified dose and dose-volume objectives for the target volume and critical normal structures. Thus in "intensity-modulated proton therapy" (IMPT), the final dose distribution (not the fluence) is the result of the contribution from different fields, each delivering an inhomogeneous dose distribution in the target. IMPT dose distributions are based on the assumption that anywhere within the target a homogeneous dose may be achieved by the sum of (highly) modulated fields.

Another method called "distal edge tracking" is described where the spots for each of a number beams are placed only at the distal edge of the target. This approach requires a much smaller number of spots but is most vulnerable to range uncertainties. Targets that move because of respiration are planned either (a) with *high-speed raster scanning* and fast energy changes, (b) by *repainting* where each energy layer is scanned multiple times to smear the interplay effect or by (c) *respiratory gating*.

18.1.2.5 Treatment Plan Evaluation

The main difference between protons and photons is the effect of various uncertainties on the depth of penetration of protons. Beam-specific distal and proximal margins to account for range uncertainty are assigned to ensure target coverage. Also smearing, anatomic variations and other uncertainties may create a situation where the DVH may not correctly represent the real dose delivery.

Initially while evaluating plans, the oncologist has to ensure that, for each beam, the distance between the lateral edge of the CTV and the prescription isodose surface is equal to at least the lateral margin (analogous to CTV → PTV margin in photon beam RT). Similarly, the distal and proximal CTV edges should be within prescription isodose surface by distal and proximal range uncertainty margins. Smearing may cause the computed dose distribution to have apparent hot and cold streaks and other dose inhomogeneities within and outside the target volume. Motion would remove these effects, and hence editing of compensator should not be done.

In another method of plan evaluation in presence of respiratory motion, multiple dose distributions for a given plan are computed for the nominal image and for each of the images obtained by plus and minus anteroposterior (AP), lateral and supero-inferior (SI) displacements of the body, plus and minus variations in CT numbers and, if applicable, end-inhale and end-exhale. A "worst-case" dose distribution is then prepared by assigning inside the CTV the minimum dose on any of the plans and outside the CTV the maximum dose on any of the plans. The resulting dose distributions and dose-volume histograms, representing the worst-case scenario, are then used to evaluate the plan. But this method requires calculating large number of situations and may not be very feasible [11–13]. In proton beams, one can therefore report doses as a probability of CTV coverage rather than as discrete dose-volume quantities for PTV and OARs as seen in photon beam planning. Hence the doses for target volume are reported as a probability of whether or not the minimum dose in the CTV is above or below a designated threshold for plan acceptance.

18.1.2.6 Dose Calculations

Dose distributions are used to predict the outcome of treatments and toxicities. In current scenario, semiempirical pencil beam models are used for dose calculations for both passively scattered and intensity-modulated proton therapies [14–16].

The treatment planning system usually provides the treatment parameters [17]. For passive scattering, however, the TPS may or may not provide the monitor units (MUs). For scanning beams, the TPS must provide the MUs per spot as well as the spot location and energy. The proton TPS generates both dose distribution and parameters for apertures and compensators. Usually, the limited number of beams is used for proton treatments, as acceptable treatment plans can be generated with two or three beams. Care must be taken in choosing a gantry angle for treatment planning. The beam should not intercept the edge of the couch or patient's positioning device, as this will result in change in beam characteristics before the beam reaches the patient. Beam directions that involve complex heterogeneities should be avoided.

18.1.2.7 Treatment Set-Up and Delivery

Daily images are taken to ensure that the isocentre is in the correct location relative to the patient. In-room X-ray units provide a beam's eye view as well as an imaging system perpendicular to the nozzle. These images are acquired as digital radiographs. The couch can then be translated to place the isocentre in the correct position within the patient. A second set of images may then be taken to confirm the couch movement. The actual treatment time (the beam-on time) is relatively short, generally less than 1 min per field.

18.1.2.8 Patient-Specific, Machine-Specific Quality Assurance and Treatment Safety

Many current proton delivery systems do not have multileaf or adjustable collimators, and patient-specific beam defining devices must be constructed. The designs of both the apertures and the compensators are created in the treatment planning system. Quality assurance is performed on the physical devices themselves after they have been constructed to confirm the appropriate shapes and thicknesses.

Proton delivery systems require the determination of the number of MUs to deliver the prescribed dose. Determination of MUs for passively scattered beams can be done by using patient dose distribution as input to calculate a "verification plan" in a water phantom. A representative point in the verification plan is chosen to correspond to a point in the target volume where the dose is relatively uniform. Measurements can then be performed in a water phantom to determine the MUs required, delivering the prescribed dose. SOBP is however known to affect MU determination as the smaller the SOBP, the fewer the MUs required for delivering the dose [18].

Daily pretreatment quality assurance tests should include standard output checks, safety features like treatment room door interlock and alignment between the proton beam and the X-ray systems. Proton facilities generally have a room-sweeping alarm, which is activated before the treatment door is closed and should be tested every day. Periodic (weekly, monthly, quarterly, annual) safety and quality assurance tests should be performed to insure proper operation of the proton delivery system.

18.2 Carbon Ion Therapy

Use of charged particles was first suggested in 1946 by physicist Robert Wilson [19], while Cornelius Tobias of the University of California, Lawrence Berkeley National Laboratory, was instrumental in clinical use of charged-particle beams [20, 21]. The rationale for using charged-particle beams of carbon ions for radiotherapy is the result of dose distribution of these high-LET radiations due to their deposition along Bragg peak, thus giving required depth coverage and sparing of surrounding tissues [20]. But application of this spread Bragg peak charged-particle therapy of cancer was only made possible clinically with the increasing use of CT scanning in the 1970s. CT scans allowed rapid, accurate determination of the beam path through varying tissue densities in a patient.

18.2.1 Radiobiology of Charged Particles

1. **Biophysical Aspects**: The carbon ion beams better have dose localization and depth-dose distribution advantages over lighter protons. Carbon ions being high-LET particles are biologically more damaging primarily because they cause more severe, less reparable damage per unit track length than low-LET radiations. Carbon ions also have better Bragg peak characteristics compared to pro-

ton beams with a sharper and steeper dose gradient as well as lateral fall-offs which are useful for treating deep-seated tumours with significant sparing of surrounding normal structures.

2. **Relative Biologic Effectiveness and Relation with Tumour Oxygenation**: RBE is defined as the ratio of absorbed doses of the beam to be tested compared to that produced by a 250 kV beam. Grey-equivalent (GyE) dose is the dose of a particle modality that yields an equivalent biologic response to a dose of mega-voltage X-ray or cobalt-60 gamma rays. For 160- to 230-meV proton beams, the RBE is considered to be approximately 1.1 to 1.2, and for heavier particles (helium, carbon, neon, silicon), the RBE ranges from 1.2 to 4.5. This difference in the RBE of carbon ions gives a decisive advantage compared to photons and protons especially for tumours that have a low radiosensitivity and where the tumour is surrounded by more radiosensitive normal tissues. In studies, short-course hypofractionation is likely to increase the therapeutic ratio in carbon ion therapy. At the National Institute of Radiological Sciences (NIRS) in Chiba, Japan, hypofractionated carbon ion therapy has been used with significant reduction of overall treatment time for many tumours [22, 23]. Carbon ions being high-LET radiations do not have a high dependence on the extent of tumour oxygenation with OER values between 1.6 and 1.7 and usually cause direct DNA damage. Cell-survival dose response curves for carbon ions show absent or very narrow shoulder indicating decreased repair to DNA injury. This is attributed to the dense pattern of ionization at the end of the range of high-LET radiations.
3. **Decreased Radioresistance and Increased Reoxygenation:** This is still a field of ongoing study. Studies have shown that most tumours have significant numbers of hypoxic cells that are preferentially killed with high-LET irradiations. Carbon ions have also been shown to increase the gene expression of SPHK1 (related to cell growth and proliferation control) in human oral squamous cell carcinoma which is not seen with X-rays [24]. Carbon ion irradiation has been shown experimentally to accelerate the reoxygenation of murine fibrosarcoma compared with X-ray irradiation [25]. This suggests that high-LET radiations can be effective in hypofractionated treatment schedules.
4. **Nondependence on Cell Cycle Phase:** High-LET radiation because of increased frequency of DNA hits causes more irreparable damage than photons and has less dependence on whether DNA is coiled or uncoiled. Thus they affect cells irrespective of their cycle phase. This is of advantage in both fast-growing tumours with a large proportion of cells in the S phase and slowly proliferating tumours with a large fraction of cells in G1 or G0.
5. **Risk of Carcinogenesis and Other Late Radiation Effects**: In high-LET carbon ion therapy, there is a risk of enhanced late sequelae, like undesirable tissue fibrosis, vascular damage, central nervous system (CNS) toxicities, genomic instability and secondary cancers. However this susceptibility to incidence of second malignancies varies in different genetic set-ups even within the same species. Sprague-Dawley rats were found to be more susceptible to carbon ion-induced mammary carcinomas but without the common H-ras and Tp-53 mutations seen with low-LET radiation-induced tumours [26].

Early Clinical Studies with Heavy Ions: Clinical studies with charged-particle therapy, including carbon ions, were carried out from 1975 to 1992 at the Lawrence Berkeley National Laboratory (LBNL) [27, 28] in collaboration with the Medical Center at the University of California. These particles (like helium) deposit a small amount of high LET with clinical effects similar to protons [29–31]. Carbon ions were used for the first time in the treatment of human tumours at LBNL in 1977. A few patients with advanced tumours were treated with carbon ions in phase I studies at LBNL in 1977 and 1978. Subsequently, neon ions were preferred over carbon ions because of their greater potential for high-LET advantage. From 1978 to 1992, 433 patients at LBNL were treated with neon ion therapy, of which 299 received at least 10 Gy (about 30 GyE). These clinical studies showed that neon and carbon ions could be delivered safely, providing careful treatment planning and delivery occurred, with evidence of beneficial effect especially in slow-growing tumours [22, 32–34]. But increased late tissue reactions involving CNS and GIT were noted [35], and further study on silicon and argon ions was halted.

With the increasing integration of new technologies in imaging and beam-delivery techniques, as well as the designing of facilities with smaller footprint and energy requirements for operation [36], there is slowly a shift in focus towards providing individually tailored image-guided dose plans [31, 37, 38].

Carbon Ion Radiation Therapy in Japan and Germany: Major credit for the current clinical emphasis on carbon ion therapy goes to the NIRS programme in Japan, followed by the GSI programme in Germany. Carbon ion therapy for medical use in a dedicated facility was first available from 1994 in NIRS (Chiba) in Japan. The second carbon ion therapy facility started operations from 1997 in Germany at the GSI, University of Heidelberg [39, 40]. A third carbon ion therapy facility started at the Hyogo Ion Beam Medical Center facility in Harima, Japan, in 2004 [41]. Later more facilities are planned or under construction in Italy, France, Germany, Austria, the United States and Japan.

18.2.2 Treatment Techniques

1. **Passive Beam Delivery**: This method was started at the NIRS, Chiba, Japan, and is performed using modulators, collimators and compensators. The advantage is in a simple treatment planning algorithm; but the major disadvantage is that a significant amount of the dose is also delivered along the entrance path which includes nontarget normal tissue. Inter-fractional and intra-fractional movements are addressed by adding a safety margin to ensure that the clinical target volume (CTV) is fully covered during treatment.
2. **Active Beam Delivery**: This technique has been developed at GSI, Germany, using the raster scan method. Focused pencil beams produced in a synchrotron are deflected laterally by two magnetic dipoles, while the energy of the incoming beam is varied during the treatment. Thus 3D intensity-modulated carbon ion therapy can be achieved, and the dose distribution tailored to any irregular tumour shape without adding passive absorbers, compensators or collimators [42]. The

dose distribution can also be conformed to the proximal edge of the target volume, and normal tissue that resides along the entrance channel of the beam can thus be spared. For delineating the target volume, adding a safety margin around the CTV is not sufficient, because movement of the target during the scanning process can cause regions already irradiated to again move into the path of the beam, whereas regions that have not been irradiated can escape the path of the beam.

3. In both the above techniques, patient immobilization and daily reproducibility is a must for achieving high spatial accuracy with particle beams.
4. Precision head and body immobilization systems, stereotactic target localization and image guidance with pretreatment correction of even small patient set-up deviations are used at modern particle therapy centres.
5. At present, carbon ion RT is delivered with fixed-beam lines. The charged-particle therapy facility at the Heidelberg University is the first to be equipped with a rotating gantry for proton and carbon ion radiotherapy.

References

1. Hall EJ. Intensity-modulated radiation therapy, protons, and the risk of second cancers. Int J Radiat Oncol Biol Phys. 2006;65:1–7.
2. Hall EJ. The impact of protons on the incidence of second malignancies in radiotherapy. Technol Cancer Res Treat. 2007;6:31–4.
3. Brenner DJ, Hall EJ. Secondary neutrons in clinical proton radiotherapy: a charged issue. Radiother Oncol. 2008;86:165–70.
4. Paganetti H. Significance and implementation of RBE variations in proton beam therapy. Technol Cancer Res Treat. 2003;2:413–26.
5. Paganetti H, Niemierko A, Ancukiewicz M, et al. Relative biological effectiveness (RBE) values for proton beam therapy. Int J Radiat Oncol Biol Phys. 2002;53:407–21.
6. Engelsman M, Mazal A, Jaffray D. Patient positioing and set-up verification for planning and treatments. In: Delaney T, Kooy H, editors. Proton and charged particle radiotherapy. Philadelphia: Lippincott, Williams & Wilkins; 2008.
7. Schaffner B, Pedroni E. The precision of proton range calculations in proton radiotherapy treatment planning: experimental verification of the relation between CT-HU and proton stopping power. Phys Med Biol. 1998;43:1579–92.
8. Urie M, Goitein M, Wagner M. Compensating for heterogeneities in proton radiation therapy. Phys Med Biol. 1984;29:553–66.
9. Kang Y, Zhang X, Chang JY, et al. 4D proton treatment planning strategy for mobile lung tumors. Int J Radiat Oncol Biol Phys. 2007;67:906–14.
10. Engelsman M, Rietzel E, Kooy HM. Four-dimensional proton treatment planning for lung tumors. Int J Radiat Oncol Biol Phys. 2006;64:1589–95.
11. Goitein M. Calculation of the uncertainty in the dose delivered during radiation therapy. Med Phys. 1985;12:608–12.
12. Goitein M, Abrams M. Multi-dimensional treatment planning: I. Delineation of anatomy. Int J Radiat Oncol Biol Phys. 1983;9:777–87.
13. Goitein M, Abrams M, Rowell D, et al. Multi-dimensional treatment planning: II. Beam's eye-view, back projection, and projection through CT sections. Int J Radiat Oncol Biol Phys. 1983;9:789–97.
14. Schaffner B, Pedroni E, Lomax A. Dose calculation models for proton treatment planning using a dynamic beam delivery system: an attempt to include density heterogeneity effects in the analytical dose calculation. Phys Med Biol. 1999;44:27–41.
15. Schaffner B. Proton dose calculation based on in-air fluence measurements. Phys Med Biol. 2008;53:1545–62.

16. Hong L, Goitein M, Bucciolini M, et al. A pencil beam algorithm for proton dose calculations. Phys Med Biol. 1996;41:1305–30.
17. Bussiere MR, Adams JA. Treatment planning for conformal proton radiation therapy. Technol Cancer Res Treat. 2003;2:389–99.
18. Kooy HM, Schaefer M, Rosenthal S, et al. Monitor unit calculations for range-modulated spread-out Bragg peak fields. Phys Med Biol. 2003;48:2797–808.
19. Wilson RR. Radiological use of fast protons. Radiology. 1946;47:491–8.
20. Tobias CA, Anger HO, Lawrence JH. Radiological use of high energy deuterons and alpha particles. Am J Roentgen Radium Ther Nucl Med. 1952;67:1.
21. Tobias CA, Alpen E, Blakely E, et al. Radiobiological basis for heavy ion therapy. Treatment of radio-resistant cancers. North Holland: Elsevier Biomedical Press; 1979.
22. Tsujii H, Mizoe J, Kamada T, et al. Overview of clinical experiences on carbon ion radiotherapy at NIRS. Radiother Oncol. 2004;73(S2):41–9.
23. Tsujii H, Mizoe J, Kamada T, et al. Clinical results of carbon ion radiotherapy at NIRS. J Radiat Res. 2007;48:A1–13.
24. Higo M, Uzawa K, Kawata T, et al. Enhancement of SPHKl in vitro by carbon ion irradiation in oral squamous cell carcinoma. Int J Radiat Oncol Biol Phys. 2006;65(3):867–75.
25. Ando K, Koike S, Ohira C, et al. Accelerated reoxygenation of a murine fibrosarcoma after carbon ion irradiation. Int J Radiat Biol Phys. 1999;75(4):505–12.
26. Imaoka T, Nishimura M, Kakinuma S, et al. High relative biologic effectiveness of carbon ion radiation on induction of rat mammary carcinoma and its lack of H-ras and TP53 mutations. Int J Radiat Oncol Biol Phys. 2007;69(1):194–203.
27. Castro JR, Chen GTY, Blakely EA. Current considerations in heavy charged particle radiotherapy. Radiat Res. 1985;104(2):s263.
28. Linstadt D, Castro J, Phillips T. Neon ion radiotherapy. Results of the phase I-II clinical trial. Int J Radiat Oncol Biol. 1991;20:761.
29. Castro JR, Char DH, Petti PL, et al. 15 years' experience with helium ion radiotherapy for uveal melanoma. Int J Radiat Oncol Biol Phys. 1997;39:989–96.
30. Castro JR, Collier JM, Petti PL, et al. Charged particle radiotherapy for lesions encircling the brain stem or spinal cord. Int J Radiat Oncol Biol Phys. 1989;17(3):477.
31. Evans PM. Topical review: anatomical imaging for radiotherapy. Phys Med Biol. 2008;53:R151–91.
32. Lillis-Hearne PK, Castro JR. Indications for heavy ions: lessons from Berkeley. In: Linz U, editor. Ion beams in tumor therapy. New York: Chapman & Hall; 1995. p. 133.
33. Schoenthaler R, Castro JR, Petti PL, et al. Charged particle irradiation of sacral chordomas. Int J Radiat Oncol Biol Phys. 1993;26(2):291–8.
34. Castro JR, Saunders WM, Tobias CA, et al. Treatment of cancer with heavy charged particles. Int J Radiat Oncol Biol Phys. 1982;8(12):2191–8.
35. Castro JR. Results of heavy ion radiotherapy. Radiat Environ Biophys. 1995;34:45–8.
36. Peggs S, Satogata T. A survey of hadron therapy accelerator technologies. In: IEEE Proceedings of PAC07, Albuquerque; 2007. p. 115–9.
37. Kramer M, Jakel O, Haberer T, et al. Treatment planning for heavy-ion radiotherapy: physical beam model and dose optimization. Phys Med Biol. 2000;45:3299–317.
38. Kanematsu N, Yonai S, Ishizaki A, et al. Computational modeling of beam-customization devices for heavy-charged particle radiotherapy. Phys Med Biol. 2008;53:3113–27.
39. Kraft G. Tumor therapy with heavy charged particles. Prog Particle Nucl Phys. 2000;45:S473–544.
40. Kraft G. Tumor therapy with heavy ions. Darmstadt: Verein zum Forderung der tumortherapie mit Schwerenionen e.V.; 2007.
41. Abe M. Charged particle radiotherapy at the Hyogo ion beam medical center: characteristics, technology and clinical results. Proc Jpn Acad Ser B. 2007;83:6.
42. Haberer T, Becher W, Schardt D, et al. Magnetic scanning system for heavy ion therapy. Nucl Instrum Methods Phys Res A. 1993;330:296–305.

Part III

Use of Other Agents with Radiation

19 Using Concurrent or Sequential Chemotherapy and Biomolecules

19.1 Introduction

In recent years in many sites, adding chemotherapy either concurrently or before/after radiation therapy is being increasingly practiced with evidence showing better responses and survival rates. This practice has been started to obtain not only improved treatment results with increased tumour response and/or survival with some increase in normal tissue toxicity. The rationale for this concept of combined radiation therapy and chemotherapy described by Steel and Peckham was explained by four mechanisms by which combined modality therapy could improve therapeutic outcome: spatial cooperation, toxicity independence, protection of normal tissue and enhancement of tumour response [1]. A further revision of these radiation-drug interactions and their varying mechanisms was described by Bentzen et al., which was based on clinical investigations, and incorporated the rapid emergence of molecular targeted agents [2].

Combination of chemotherapy and radiotherapy results in some advantages which may not be achieved effectively with the use of a single modality. These advantages include optimizing or maximizing cell kill within the toxicity range that can be tolerated by the host, offering a more broad-based coverage and thus eliminating or limiting any resistant cell line in a tumour cell population, as well as preventing or slowing development of any new drug-resistant cell lines. A few terms need to be introduced in the context of the use of combination of chemotherapy and radiotherapy.

Spatial cooperation refers to the combination of chemotherapeutic drug with radiation, which in effect combines systemic action with locoregional effect. This mechanism entails delivering full doses of radiotherapy and chemotherapy preferably given sequentially to bring down acute reactions and toxicity. Examples include combination of chemotherapy or hormone therapy with radiation therapy in breast or prostate cancer. The disadvantage of sequential therapies is a prolongation of the overall treatment times, which may affect response because of accelerated cellular repopulation [3, 4].

A. Mukherji, *Basics of Planning and Management of Patients during Radiation Therapy*, https://doi.org/10.1007/978-981-10-6659-7_19

Cytotoxic enhancement is the ability of the drug to add to the damage caused by radiation and produce a greater effect on the local tumour than would be expected from simple addition of cell killing activity of each modality and is caused by the introduction or repair of radiation-induced DNA damage. Addition of drugs like 5-fluorouracil into cancer cell DNA has been shown to cause an increase in the radiation-induced DNA damage [5]. Other processes which are targeted by chemotherapy during the interval between exposures to fractionated radiotherapy include tumour cell repopulation, reoxygenation and cellular redistribution, and this effect is called **temporal modulation** [6].

Toxicity independence is the phenomenon of non-overlap of the effects of the systemic effects from chemotherapy and the local sequelae of irradiation. Therefore a combination of chemotherapy and radiation therapy could theoretically make it possible to deliver intensive combined treatment regimens without unacceptable toxicity, even if the anticancer effects of the two modalities overlapped. But in practice, many clinical studies have in fact shown that combined chemo-radiation actually caused an increase in radiation-related side effects [7–9], because of induced cellular repopulation.

Biologic cooperation means either the targeting of specific cell lines or application of different mechanisms for achieving either tumour cell kill or delayed cancer regrowth [2]. An example of such biologic cooperation would be the use of hypoxic tumour cell-killing drugs like misonidazole, tirapazamine or mitomycin C supplementing the effect of irrradiation, which affects well-oxygenated cells [10]. Biologic cooperation by combined modality therapy is helpful because radiation is effective against the well-oxygenated periphery of the tumour, while other drugs can act on the hypoxic centre. This effect is also seen in the use of anti-angiogenic agents with irradiation, where these agents cause a normalization of tumour blood vessels, reducing tumour hypoxia and showcasing biologic cooperation between these drugs and irradiation [11].

Pathways contributing to radiosensitization by chemotherapeutic or molecularly targeted agents include initial induction of radiation-induced DNA damage, DNA damage repair, modulation of cell cycle kinetics, tumour microenvironment and cell repopulation.

19.2 Initial Radiation Damage

The critical mechanism of radiation injury is damage to DNA. Radiation induces several types of lesions, including single-strand breaks (SSBs), double-strand breaks (DSBs), base damage and formation of intermolecular crosslinks. The most common types of lesions caused by radiation are SSBs which are however readily repaired, while DSBs are the primary contributor to cell death if left unrepaired. Chemotherapeutic agents influencing initial radiation-induced damage are the halogenated pyrimidines leading to incorporation of their halogenated thymidine analogues into the DNA during S phase which then cause strand breaks. Tumour cells are supposed to be more susceptible to radiation-induced damage as they may be cycling more rapidly than normal cells in surrounding tissues so that more drug could be incorporated into tumour DNA, resulting in "selective" radiosensitization. The most appropriate tumours are those with a high growth fraction or labelling index and a tumour site in which normal tissues are not proliferating rapidly (e.g. high-grade gliomas or large, unresectable sarcomas).

19.3 DNA Damage Repair

Immediately following radiation-induced DNA damage, a repair process is initiated, which includes DNA damage recognition, chromatin relaxation, formation of multiunit repair protein complexes at sites of DNA damage, DNA DSB repair and finally repair protein dissolution and chromatin restoration. This entire repair process of DNA DSBs is rapid with a majority of base pairs being repaired within 6 h.

Radiosensitization is caused by the interaction of chemotherapeutic drugs with irradiation and the effects of this interaction on DNA repair. Examples include fludarabine (a potent inhibitor of DNA primase, DNA polymerase-α and ribonucleotide reductase), as well as nucleoside analogues like gemcitabine which modulates repair of radiation-induced DNA and chromosome damage by inhibiting ribonucleotide reductase.

19.4 Cell Cycle Kinetics

In general, the G2 or M phases of the cell division phase are the most sensitive to damage by irradiation, while cells in the S phase are the most resistant. This variation in radiosensitivity during the cell cycle can be potentially exploited when designing effective chemo-radiation therapy strategies. An example is the use of taxanes to cause cell cycle arrest in G2M phase. Also the S phase of the cell cycle though more resistant to radiation is particularly sensitive to drugs such as fludarabine or gemcitabine which belong to the class of nucleoside analogues. Hence a combination of these agents with radiation can lead to preferential targeting of cells in radioresistant phases of the cell division process thus leading to enhancement of irradiation effects.

Certain drugs can activate or modulate the G2-M checkpoint, which basically is the point of cell division where there is formation of tubules and the separated uncoiled chromatids are positioned along the equatorial plane of the cell before being pulled to opposite poles. This checkpoint identifies cells which require DNA repair before progression into mitosis and therefore helps protect against radiation-induced cell death [12]. Cells accumulate DNA during the S phase, representing the intermediate region, and finally, cells in G2 and M have the most quantitative DNA per cell. This checkpoint can be modulated by chemotherapeutic agents to achieve radiosensitization.

19.5 Tumour Vasculature and Oxygenation

The surrounding microenvironment of a tumour plays a critical role in its continued growth and may also influence therapeutic response, the most important of which is the presence of oxygenation and vasculature. A tumour to maintain constant growth and division requires effective delivery of nutrients and oxygen which can be maintained by proper blood supply. However since by definition a tumour is an aberrant and uncontrolled expansion of differentiating or undifferentiated tissue, such growth would require the formation of new blood vessels, the process of which is mediated by a cytokine called vascular endothelial growth factor (VEGF). Thus in a tumour there will be areas which are near to a blood vessel and areas which would be further away. Additionally, tumour blood vessels are commonly irregular and tortuous and have blind ends, arteriovenous shunts, incomplete endothelial linings and basement membranes, leading to areas of poor oxygenation within a tumour. Therefore there are regions within a tumour distant from the supporting vasculature or because of defective vascularization within a tumour, where subpopulations of hypoxic cells develop. These populations being not oxygenated are therefore not susceptible to oxygen-mediated free radical damage caused by irradiation and hence are likely to play an important role in radiation resistance [13]. Another accepted principle of such tumour resistance is that hypoxia modulates tumour phenotype and angiogenesis through up-regulation of mediators like hypoxia-inducible factor (HIF-1) [14]. This fact is made use of by drugs which selectively target hypoxic cells (tirapazamine and mitomycin) and are used as radiosensitizers. In addition there are drugs with pro-angiogenic properties which can restore both the abnormal structure and the function of tumour vasculature and are used to counteract the hypoxic tumour environment causing reoxygenation and increasing the effectiveness of conventional radiation or chemotherapy [11].

19.6 Cell Repopulation

Both radiation therapy and chemotherapy are typically administered in multiple and spaced doses. In radiation therapy, dividing a total dose into multiple daily doses or fractions over a period of time helps allow recovery from sublethal radiation-induced damage and allow repopulation of normal tissues. However repopulation of surviving tumour cells can also occur during this interval, increasing tumour burden. In addition, the rate of repopulation may increase during a protracted course of therapy, a phenomenon termed accelerated repopulation, which may further limit the effectiveness of therapy [4]. In fact, Withers and colleagues [15] demonstrated that there was an increased requirement of dose to achieve tumour kill and which was significant from the fourth week of the irradiation course. This was attributed to accelerated repopulation in squamous cell cancers of the head and neck. Thus to account for this "repopulation" by tumour cells, an added dose was thought to be required which has been calculated at between 0.5 and 1 Gy/day of prolonged treatment [4]. Apart from altered fractionation schedules, another approach to reduce accelerated repopulation is to integrate chemotherapeutic agents into the course of radiation treatment given concurrently with radiation therapy and hence mitigate cellular repopulation.

19.7 Sequencing of Chemotherapy and Radiotherapy

The sequencing of chemotherapy and radiation therapy when indicated together can depend on the site, disease stage and treatment plan. This sequencing could be neoadjuvant wherein the chemotherapy is given before definitive therapy (either radiation or surgery) and concurrent wherein both radiation and chemotherapy are given at the same time or after the course of radiation therapy. Induction chemotherapy is also given before starting radiotherapy, differing from neoadjuvant therapy as induction is not followed by definitive treatment. The need for induction chemotherapy is disease debulking and systemic sterilization. It is started early to treat any suspected disseminated disease foci and thus helps decrease the number of tumour clonogens as well as improves the oxygenation of surviving cells, allowing for better penetration of ionizing radicals from radiotherapy and thus better tumour control. Additionally after this induction chemotherapy, any decrease in the size of the tumour would help in better normal tissue sparing while planning and delivering radiation therapy. Though theoretically this reason for the use of induction chemotherapy may sound ideal, in practice, the results have not been good and in fact inferior to concurrent chemo-radiation. This is because after chemotherapy, the surviving tumour cells undergo accelerated repopulation and may also be more resistant to further chemotherapy or even irradiation.

Concurrent chemotherapy means giving both chemotherapeutic drugs and irradiation together in the same treatment course. Such an approach tries to address both micro-metastatic spread and the bulk of the tumour, as explained previously, by utilizing interactions between the free radicals generated by irradiation and cell damage brought about by the chemotherapeutic drugs without exceeding tolerance doses of either. However it is important to understand the pharmacokinetics of the chemotherapeutic drugs as well as their mode of action and interaction with radiation-induced free radicals so that drug-radiation scheduling would enable enjoying maximum tumour sensitization and minimize toxicity to normal tissues. While this has been the theoretical principle behind concurrent chemo-radiation, in clinical practice, concurrent chemo-radiation while having delivered increased local tumour response as well as survival benefit has however been associated with increased tissue toxicities. Concomitant boost radio-chemotherapy is based on the principle of counteracting accelerated repopulation. Chemotherapy in an adjuvant setting implies administration of the regime after completion or radiation therapy. In this setting the chemotherapy is given along with irradiation to account for tumour micro-metastases in the regional lymphatics or tumour bed when the post-operative histopathology review reveals high-risk features such as involved margins, nodal spread, perinodal or soft tissue invasion or even high tumour grade. Addition of maintenance chemotherapy can add to response but at cost of increased treatment time and toxicities.

19.8 Preparation and Administration of Chemotherapy

The administration of chemotherapeutic agents should be done by personnel who are trained in the handling of chemotherapeutic drugs, as many of these drugs can cause severe tissue reactions and acute as well as long-term sequelae. During the preparing and handling of chemotherapeutic agents, the caregivers should follow some basic precautions. These include:

Preparation of drugs: The drugs should be prepared with staff taking personal protection measures like gloves, plastic aprons, face masks, eye shields and head caps to avoid contamination of skin and mucosal surfaces of workers in case of any accident causing a drug spillage. The drugs should be mixed with correct solvents as use of incorrect solvents may lead to precipitation and spoilage of the active drug or formation of reactive products which could be harmful to the body (Table 19.1).

Table 19.1 Solvents for a few commonly used chemotherapy drugs and duration of infusion

Drug	Solvent	Infusion time	Cumulative dose
Doxorubicin	NS	90 min	450–550 mg/m^2
Epirubicin	NS	60–90 min	720–900 mg/m^2
Paclitaxel	NS/5D with codon set	3 h, 24 h	NA
Docetaxel	NS/5D	2 h	NA
Cisplatin	NS/5D	30 min–2 h	Relative limit 600 mg/m^2
Carboplatin	5D	1 h	NA
Oxaliplatin	5D	2 h	NA
Vincristine	Bolus/NS	Bolus to 10 min	24–25 mg/m^2
Vinblastine	Bolus/NS	IV push	NA
Mitomycin C	Bolus/NS	IV push	60 mg/m^2
Actinomycin D	Bolus/NS	15–30 min	NA
5FU	Bolus/NS/5D	Bolus/1–2 h/4–6 h/22 h/46 h/96 h	NA
Gemcitabine	NS	30 min	NA
Etoposide	NS	1 h	NA
Topotecan	NS/5D	15 min	NA
Bleomycin	Bolus/NS	Bolus	400 units
Cyclophosphamide	Bolus/NS	Bolus to 1 h	NA
Ifosfamide	NS	NA	NA
Irinotecan	NS	90 min	NA
Cladribine	NS	2 h	NA
Fludaribine	Bolus/NS	IV push	NA
Bortezomib	Bolus/NS	IV push	NA
Pemetrexed	5D	10 min	NA
Methotrexate	Bolus/NS	Bolus to 12 h	NA
Liposomal doxorubicin	NS	1 h	NA
Bendamustine	NS	30 min	NA
Cytarabine	Bolus/NS	1–3 h (for high dose)	NA
Vinorelbine	NS	IV push	NA
L-Asparaginase	Bolus/NS	IV/IM push	NA

It is extremely important for the clinician to write for every administration of chemotherapy, the complete prescription including the drug to be used, its dose for that day (expressed clearly in SI units, e.g. microgram should be written as mcg and not μg) and the full protocol for the order and type of administration of IV fluids, pre- and post-medication as well as any adjuvant drugs which need to be given. These all should be written as a flow chart with the time duration for each infusion mentioned alongside the drug and daily dose. If the dose of any drug being used is less than a value of 1, then it should be written with zero followed by decimal point and then the dose figure (e.g. 0.5 mg and not .5 mg) because if the zero before a decimal is not written, the drug handler in a situation of heavy patient load or hurry might miss the decimal and thus may give many times the prescribed dose. The IV sets and bags being used for drug administration should be used correctly for each drug given with due precautions for the type of agent (e.g. PVC bags and sets not used for taxanes, photosensitive drugs like dactinomycin covered with black paper during administration).

Instructions regarding management of extravasation also should be mentioned in the chemotherapy administration areas, and personnel should receive training in handling extravasation reactions. Written instructions for reaction handling should include the type of drug likely to cause reactions, which pack to be used based on the chemotherapy drug type, antidotes to be given based again on drug type and an emergency contact number of clinician to call in case of emergency. In all cases the drug administration room should be equipped for rapid intubation in case of laryngeal oedema, management of drug-induced anaphylaxis and subsequent monitoring, and as mentioned before, the staff should be trained to handle chemotherapy-related emergencies.

Site of insertion: It is important to identify upfront the most appropriate and safe site for insertion of an IV cannula to deliver chemotherapy. It is better to have a functioning central venous access device or even a peripheral venous access device such as a chemoport in cases there is difficulty in achieving venous access or a patient has had an axillary dissection (for breast cancer) or multiple insertions are required over a short period of time. Cannulation should not be done on the limb where lymphedema is present and on the side where a mastectomy has been done, though this observation is more of a general practice principle than a recommendation. The following are among the conditions of the cannulation site: The most favourable sites for cannulation in case of peripheral IV administration are the large veins in the forearm. Cannulation should be avoided over joints, over the inner wrist and the lower extremities. Additionally veins in the antecubital fossa or on the dorsum of the hand, particularly for vesicant drugs, should not be used for cannulation as extravasation at these sites of even small amounts of vesicant drugs can cause painful contractures.

Cannula: Winged steel infusion devices ("butterfly" needles) have steel needles which are inserted into the veins kept there. Thus these are at high risk of puncturing through and hence should not be used for infusions of drug solutions and definitely not for vesicant drugs which if extravasated will cause extensive tissue damage. Flexible cannulae should be used for such infusions so that the plastic needle does not damage the vessel. For infusion of vesicant drugs of longer duration (e.g. 12–24 h) inside of peripheral cannulae which can easily go through the veins during patient movements, it is better to use a central venous access.

Procedures: After inserting a cannula into the vein, it is a standard practice to check for the blood flow (which can be seen by the backflow of the blood into the infusion well of the cannula) and then flush with 10 mL normal saline to see if there is tissue extravasation. Flushing with 10–20 mL of saline solution between different drug infusions also should be done to avoid tissue extravasation of any chemotherapeutic drug. Post infusion, the return of the blood back into the infusion well of the cannula (flashback) is a sign of vessel patency and should be always checked before any new drugs are administered and regularly throughout the bolus infusion. It is important to monitor the cannula site during the infusion for any sign of extravasation or tissue induration such as swelling, pain or redness and a slow infusion rate. Bolus dosages of vesicant drugs should always be administered concurrently with a fast-running IV fluid infusion.

19.9 Avoiding Prescribing Errors

Antineoplastic drugs are known to have generally narrower therapeutic ratios with severe reactions caused by overdosages or lack of response or even development of drug resistance due to under-dosages. The doses for each patient cannot be a fixed quantity but depend on the body surface area calculated from the patient's weight and height, while the patient's renal and hepatic parameters may influence drug excretion and hence its bioavailability and duration as well as severity of action.

Errors in prescribing and administration of antineoplastic drugs can occur at any stage from prescription to preparation to its administration. The most important step in avoiding errors in drug delivery is to implement a protocol of proper, clear, legible and internationally accepted prescription format. Thus standardizing prescribing vocabulary should be an essential part of induction training and routine practice in any institute. Some pertinent points to avoid making errors during prescription of chemotherapy schedules (Fig. 19.1) are:

- Always write complete drug name and not abbreviations as we do not know if the nursing staffs preparing the drug solution or injection are conversant with such acronyms or abbreviations. For example, cisplatin or vincristine or etoposide should always be written as such and not as CDDP or VCR/Oncovin or VP-16.
- The use of numbers with drug names like 6-mercaptopurine or 5-fuorouracil should be avoided and written as fluorouracil or mercaptopurine.
- SI units of dosage should be clearly written in their internationally accepted symbols. For example, microgram dose should be written as mcg and *not* µg because if the writing is not clear, µg can be mistaken as mg thus leading to a thousand-fold overdosages.
- The clinician has to write for every administration of chemotherapy the complete prescription including the drug to be used and its dose for that particular day expressed clearly in SI units.
- If the dose is less than a value of 1, then it should be written with zero followed by decimal point then the dose figure (e.g. 0.5 mg and not .5 mg). Trailing decimals after an integral value should not be used if it is 0. For example, 8 mg

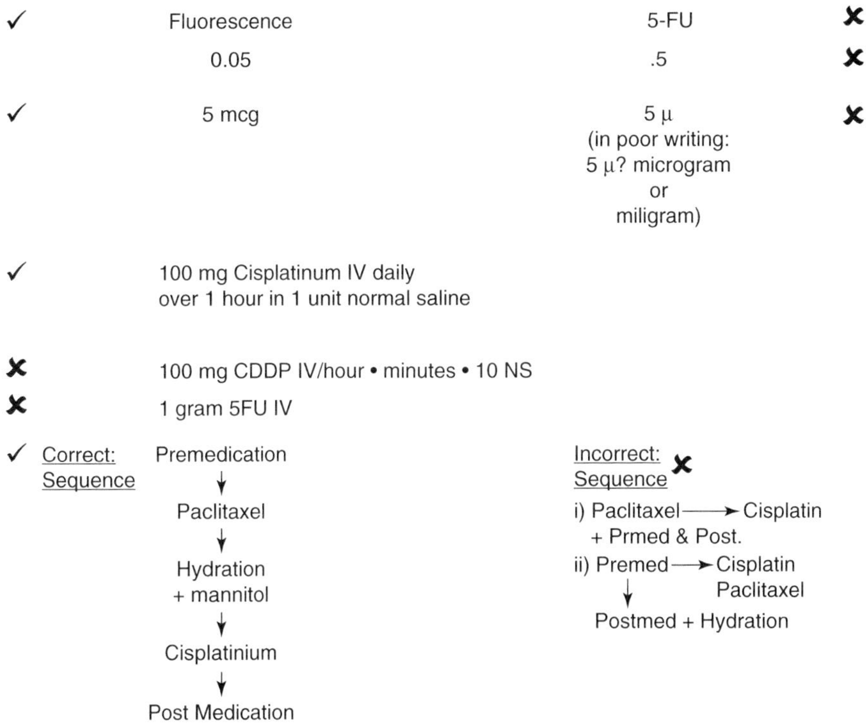

Fig. 19.1 Common chemotherapy drug prescribing errors

should not be written as 8.0 mg as the decimal can sometimes be missed and 80 mg given.

- The full prescription in order of administration of IV fluids, pre- and post-medication and adjuvants should be written as a flow chart; the time duration for each infusion should be mentioned alongside the dose. The drug order should include all pre- and post-medications in the order they are to be administered.
- Duration of a drug infusion should be written clearly in words. The use of short forms such as 5-FU 1200 mg continuous i.v. over days 1–4 is an example of a *wrong* prescription order and should be correctly written as fluorouracil 1200 mg IV continuous infusion over 22 h daily for 4 days over day 1–4 of chemotherapy. On the other hand, writing CDDP 100 mg i.v. over day 1–4 can mean either giving that dose daily each day for 4 days or dividing that dose over 4 days. Hence it should be correctly written as cisplatin 100 mg IV infused over 1 h daily in divided doses over 4 days (day 1–4) or even as 25 mg each day for 4 days.
- Another alternate method of avoiding errors can be to use preprinted forms with drug names, mode of administration, solvent fluid, duration of infusion and number of days in order of administration as either check boxes of fill in blanks with space for writing special instructions.
- It is important to correctly write the duration of infusion for each chemotherapy drug as response or reactions may change with duration of infusion (**see** Table 19.1).

- It is also important to write and administer the chemotherapy drugs in the order in which they are to be infused. Error in such infusions can lead to unwanted reactions. For example, cisplatin should be infused always after paclitaxel as if infused before it may lead to increased toxicity due to decreased excretion. Thus drug-to-drug interactions have to be kept in mind before administration.

19.10 Management of Drug Extravasation

Extravasation is the accidental release and subsequent infiltration of the chemotherapy solution into subcutaneous or subdermal tissues surrounding an intravenous or intra-arterial administration site. Some chemotherapy drugs can cause severe tissue reactions, while others may not have any effects and thus can be divided into "vesicant", "irritant" and "non-vesicant" depending on their ability to cause tissue destruction or ulcers (vesicants), painful indurations with no further tissue damage (irritants) and no reactions at all (Table 19.2). Some vesicant drugs are further classified into two groups: DNA binding and non-DNA binding. Estimates of chemotherapy-induced extravasation reactions vary between 0.01 and 7% in various publications [16–19]. An extravasation should be suspected in the presence of one or more of the following signs and symptoms:

- The patient complains of immediate burning, stinging, or discomfort or pain at the injection site which may differ from the throbbing pain or cold numbness that some chemotherapy drugs might induce on being injected.

Table 19.2 Tissue reaction properties of various chemotherapy drugs and biomolecules

Vesicant drugs	Irritant drugs	Non-vesicant drugs
Alkylating agents Mechloretamine, bendamustine	**Alkylating agents** Carmustine, streptozocin, ifosphamide, dacarbazine, melphalan	Arsenic trioxide, asparaginase, bortezomib, bleomycin, cladribine, gemcitabine, cytarabine, etoposide, fludarabine, methotrexate, pemetrexed, thiotepa, cyclophosphamide
Anthracyclines Doxorubicin, daunorubicin, epirubicin and idarubicin	**Anthracyclines** Liposomal doxorubicin, liposomal daunorubicin and mitoxantrone	
Antibiotics Mitomycin C, actinomycin D and mitoxantrone	**Topoisomerase inhibitor II** Etoposide, teniposide	
Vinca alkaloids Vincristine, vinblastine, vindesine, vinorelbine	**Topoisomerase inhibitor I** Irinotecan, topotecan	
Taxanes Paclitaxel, docetaxel	**Platins** Cisplatin, carboplatin, oxaliplatin	
Others Trabectedin	**Others** Ixabepilone, fluorouracil	

- A swelling with redness, blistering or induration is seen at the site of drug administration which may increase in size with increasing amount of drug solution infused.
- No blood return is obtained. This is not a sign of extravasation if found in isolation.
- A resistance is felt on the plunger of the syringe of a bolus drug.
- There is absence of free flow of the infusion. If in any doubt, treat as extravasation.

Various patient and procedure-related risk factors have been postulated in the occurrence of extravasation reactions. The most common reasons for extravasation reactions could be either a change in the consistency of the venous wall or due to errors of cannulation. Patient-dependant factors include either small or fragile or even sclerosed veins (such as in drug users), elderly patients or those with co-morbid conditions such as altered or impaired circulation due to Raynaud syndrome, advanced diabetes, severe peripheral vascular disease, lymphedema or superior cava syndrome. Other factors include patients with bleeding disorders, obesity or sensory impairment. Patients and especially children who are poor in communication or comprehension may not also adequately understand the importance of proper positioning advice or early warning signs of extravasation. Prolonged infusion periods frequently are at increased risk of extravasation. Physician-related reasons include untrained or inexperienced staff, multiple attempts at cannulation, unfavourable cannulation site, bolus injections with high flow pressure, choice of equipment, inadequate dressings or poor cannula fixation and poorly implanted central venous access device.

General measures: If an extravasation is suspected, the cannula should never be removed immediately, and general and specific measures should be started (Fig. 19.2). These include:

- Stopping further injection/infusion and disconnect the intravenous tubing from the cannula.
- One should then try and withdraw as much of the drug as possible using the existing cannula or central venous access device.
- One should not flush the area through the cannula with saline or water in an attempt to dilute the extravasated drug as it will lead to wider distribution of the vesicant drug over a larger area and may lead to more extensive tissue damage.
- The extent of extravasated tissue should be marked on the skin with an indelible pen for assessment of response later. A photograph also may be taken as soon as possible.
- If appropriate, the peripheral cannula can be removed, but one should not remove the central venous access device.
- Then the extravasation kit should be used, and depending on the drug extravasated, hot or cold packs as well as extravasation reaction antidotes like hyaluronidase/DMSO/dexrazoxane/1% hydrocortisone cream are used.
- The decision to use or not an appropriate pack (hot or cold) and further treatment is decided according to the chemotherapy drug used and standard departmental

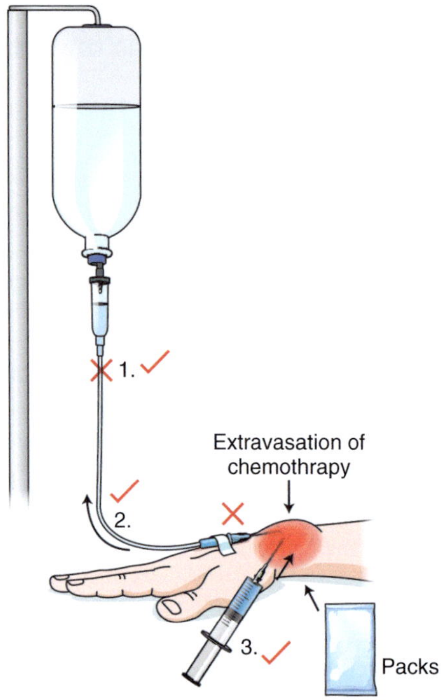

Dont's ✗

1. Immediately remove cannula
2. Press the swelling
3. Use warm compress for all swellings
4. Flush area with saline

Do's ✓

1. Stop infusion
2. Withdraw max. extravasated drug from same cannula
3. Donot flush the area with saline
4. Infiltrate area with dexa
5. Remove cannula
6. Apply hot/cold packs
7. Flushout tissue drug
8. Use specific antidote

Fig. 19.2 Managing extravasation reactions

procedures. There are definite lists available of chemotherapy drugs and their extravasation antidotes and pack type to be used (Table 19.3).

- In case of neutral drugs, for which neither a cold pack nor a hot pack is required, one should aspirate as much fluid as possible and then remove the peripheral cannula. No further treatment may be required.
- After having managed for the specific drug extravasation, the caregiver then should provide symptomatic treatment to the patient as well as document the incident in the patient's notes. A flush-out technique can be considered to remove remaining drug solution in the tissue.

Table 19.3 List of packs and antidotes for extravasation of various chemotherapy drugs

Drug	Pack	Required antidote
Cabazitaxel, docetaxel, oxaliplatin, paclitaxel, vinblastine, vincristine, vinorelbine, vindesine	Warm	Hyaluronidase
Bortezomib, bleomycin, cladribine, cyclophosphamide, cytarabine, eribulin, fludaribine, gemcitabine, ifosfamide, melphalan, pemetrexed, pentostatin	No pack	None
Daunorubicin, doxorubicin, epirubicin	Cold	DMSO if <5 mL extravasation else dexrazoxane
Amsacrine, bendamustine, carmustine, carboplatin, cisplatin, dacarbazine, etoposide, fluorouracil, idarubicin, irinotecan, methotrexate, ralitrexed, streptozocin, topotecan	Cold	Hydrocortisone cream
Liposomal daunorubicin, liposomal doxorubicin, dactinomycin, mitomycin C, mitoxantrone	Cold	DMSO

19.10.1 Instructions on Use of Antidotes

1. **In cytotoxics requiring warm pack**: Inject 1500 IU hyaluronidase (mixed in 1 mL sterile water) via pin cushion s/c injections in 0.1–0.2 mL volumes around the site. Then apply a warm pack to aid absorption of hyaluronidase. Warm pack should remain in situ for 2–4 h.
2. **In cytotoxics requiring cold pack**: Apply cold pack for 15–20 min 3–4 times a day for up to 3 days. Apply hydrocortisone 1% cream thrice daily, as long as redness persists. Once opened, cream must be labelled with patient details. Other options depending on the drug being administered include using cold pack + DMSO or dexrazoxane. If extravasation of doxorubicin, idarubicin, epirubicin or daunorubicin occurs (5 mL or more peripherally or any volume via a CVAD) then stop cold pack, do not apply DMSO and consider use of dexrazoxane.
3. **Use of DMSO (98% dimethyl sulfoxide)**: DMSO is a specific anti-extravasation drug for anthracyclines and antibiotic chemotherapy drugs and has to be applied within 10–25 min of the extravasation. First the extravasated tissue and a margin of surrounding induration should be marked with a marker after which a thin layer of DMSO is applied over this area and allowed to dry. Care should be taken that healthy skin is not treated with DMSO as this may cause blister formation. After this 1% hydrocortisone cream and 30 min of cold compression is applied and this sequence of treatment should be repeated every 2 h for the first 24 h; after which the frequency is decreased to 6 hourly each DMSO alternating with 1% hydrocortisone for the next 7 days.
4. **Use of dexrazoxane**: Dexrazoxane is a DNA topoisomerase II drug that protects against tissue damage with certain anthracyclines: doxorubicin, epirubicin, daunorubicin and idarubicin. Side effects include nausea (very common) and neutropenia/thrombocytopenia (common). It MUST ONLY be prescribed in the following circumstances: If there is a suspected peripheral extravasation of 5 mL or more of doxorubicin, epirubicin, daunorubicin or idarubicin, OR there is an

extravasation of doxorubicin, epirubicin, daunorubicin or idarubicin via the central venous route.

Post-immediate counter extravasation measures: The patient should be encouraged to start gentle movements of the affected limb. Further follow-up would depend on the type of drug and volume extravasated as well as site of extravasation, and decided by a practitioner with experience of extravasation management. Prescription of analgesia as required.

Flush-out technique: In case of a "large" volume extravasation of a vesicant or exfoliant, urgent saline flush-out of the extravasation area, as soon as possible, ideally within 2 h and no later than 24 h after extravasation, should be done. Unfortunately there is no definition of "large" in literature as it is often dependent on the size and age of the patient, as well as the nature of the drug. For anthracycline extravasation, the flush-out technique should not be used in combination with dexrazoxane.

Even after this immediate anti-extravasation treatment, many times there is significant drug left in the tissue which may cause tissue necrosis, ulceration [20] and attendant pain. Many times, there is fresh formation of granulation tissue and closure of wound, but if this does not start within 10 days, then surgical debridement should be considered. Surgical procedures are usually performed on patients in whom there is a severe reaction with ulceration and necrosis or in whom the initial anti-extravasation steps have not been performed, and these procedures include wide local excision of dead tissue followed by reconstruction using a temporary biological dressing and/or skin grafting after the wound is clean [19].

19.11 Side Effects of Chemotherapy

As with radiotherapy, administration of chemotherapeutic agents is also associated with side effects or accompaniments as they are now called. These effects are usually due to the action of these cytotoxic agents on tissues which have a rapid turnover other than tumour tissue such as bone marrow, hair follicles and gastrointestinal mucosa, and especially in tissues where the drug is concentrated. The side effects of chemotherapy are also seen at the sites where these drugs are absorbed, metabolized and excreted. These effects or sequelae can be mild to life threatening and are classified based on the system affected. These effects are influenced by the integrity of body tissues as well as bioavailability and local site concentration of the drug. This means that concurrent radiation-induced tissue damage, lower excretion of drug, higher levels of active drug, pre-existing cardiac/renal/hepatic dysfunction and lower patient general condition can all lead to greater severity of reactions. Many of these effects are enumerated in the following table (Table 19.4).

GI effects are some of the commonest reactions to chemotherapy and are followed in prevalence by features of bone marrow suppression or alopecia. In some patients vomiting can be so much that these patients avoid or become fearful of any chemotherapy and may even result in break in treatment schedule adversely affecting response to therapy. In view of this, it is imperative for cancer care providers to firstly prevent treatment-induced emesis from occurring and if it has set in, to control it at the earliest.

High risk factors for chemotherapy-induced nausea and vomiting include female gender, especially ladies with a history of uncontrolled vomiting during pregnancy,

Table 19.4 Common side effects of chemotherapeutic drugs

System	Common side effects	Pertinent points
GI tract	Nausea, vomiting, loss of appetite, taste changes (dysguesia), constipation, loose stools, oral mucositis, electrolyte disturbance, GI perforations/ulcers/strictures	• Vomiting can lead to break in treatment sequence intensity or even in compliance • Increased diarrhoea or mucositis can lead to serious systemic effects such as electrolyte disbalance or malnutrition • Drugs such as capecitabine, 5-fluorouracil (in high dose or in combination with leucovorin or oxaliplatin), irinotecan, methotrexate and topotecan commonly implicated
Bone marrow	Neutropenia, anaemia, thrombocytopenia, pancytopenia and fibrosis in severe cases Thrombocytopenia is a dose-limiting side effect in agents like carboplatin, gemcitabine, carmustine and lomustine	• Decrease in blood counts can lead to patients at high risk of infections or bleeding • Anaemia can interfere with treatment and increase morbidity and decrease response
Mucosa of oral cavity/upper alimentary tract	Oral mucositis, ulcers, strictures, total denudation	• Can cause reduced oral intake affecting quality of life and therefore treatment compliance and results
Hair	Reversible alopecia, altered hair texture and lustre	• Psychologically one of the most devastating side effect of chemotherapy for the patient • Can affect psychologically by affecting self-confidence and self-esteem as well as effect on social acceptance • Patients require counselling
Sexual function	• Gonadal dysfunction, resulting in sterilization or decreased fertility • In men, reduction in sperm counts seen during chemotherapy, which can be temporary or prolonged • In women, chemotherapy can cause destruction of oocytes, leading to ovarian failure and premature menopause	• High risk of early menopause with increasing age • Patients should be informed of the potential risk of sterility from the planned cytotoxic therapy • Semen cryopreservation should be offered to all male patients interested in having children after the completion of cytotoxic therapy • Patients are advised to wait 6 months after the end of therapy before attempting to conceive • If fertility is preserved, there is high probability of having healthy children

(continued)

Table 19.4 (continued)

System	Common side effects	Pertinent points
Skin/nails	Erythema, brittleness or dryness, desquamation, decreased sensitivity, urticarial or vesicular eruptions, ulcerations. Also seen are venous discolourations or phlebitis, hand-foot syndrome (Fig. 19.3a, b), radiation recall dermatitis or even tissue necrosis after extravasation	• Results in fluid loss, increased risk of infections, increased pain and poor compliance to therapy
Musculoskeletal	Dysplasias, decrease in function, increased fracture rates, neuropathies, osteopathies	• Poor quality of life can result in poor survival
Cardiac	Endocarditis, myocarditis, cardiomyopathies, conduction defects, pericardial effusions, valvular dysfunctions	• Known to affect quality of life and even survival • Some drugs especially anthracyclines have synergistic effects with irradiation to worsen damage caused to tissue
Renal, urologic	Nephritis, acute tubular necrosis, cystitis, leakage nephropathies, haematuria, proteinuria, dyselectrolyturia, renal shutdown, haemolytic uremic syndrome and in severe cases uremia	• Important to avoid renal damage as it can have cascading effect on the heart, liver and circulatory system as well as on haemoglobin production and immunity

younger patients, patients who do not drink alcohol regularly and those who have had a history of poor emetic control during any previous cancer treatment. Three types of nausea and vomiting are known to occur in patients receiving chemotherapy: acute, delayed and anticipatory. *Acute emesis is defined as that happening within the first 24 h of therapy (usually within 1–2 h)* [21]. It is found to be most severe during the first 4–6 h of initial therapy and is related to the emetogenic potential of the drug. Therefore it is important for the treating doctor to have knowledge of the emetogenic potential of the anticancer drug being administered so that appropriate anti-emetic treatment can be started at the earliest. *Delayed emesis has been defined as occurring 24 or more hours after chemotherapy and may last from 1 to 7 days* [21] and is usually found to occur after administration of anticancer drugs like cisplatin, carboplatin, cyclophosphamide, ifosphamide and doxorubicin. Delayed or residual emesis can occur even after the successful control of any acute symptoms by prophylactic use of anti-emetics [21]. *Anticipatory emesis is defined as the experiencing of nausea and/or vomiting before receiving another chemotherapy*

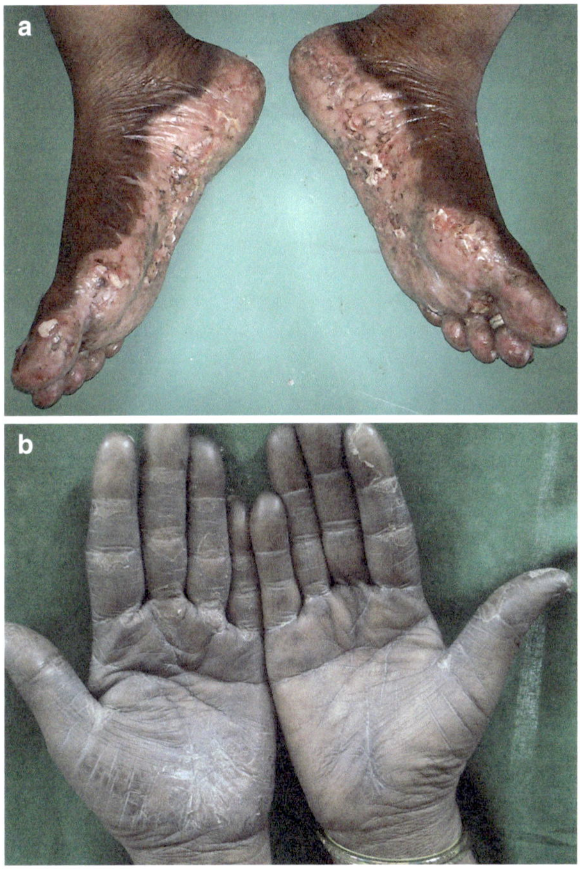

Fig. 19.3 (**a**) Grade 2 Hand-foot reaction in patient receiving concurrent Capecitabine with radiotherapy. (**b**) Grade 1 Palmar reactions in patient receiving concurrent Capecitabine with radiotherapy

treatment and is a conditioned response to a previous episode of poor emetic control caused by inadequate anti-emetic therapy [21]. It can also be fashioned by associated environmental stimuli. *Breakthrough emesis is defined as occurrence of nausea or vomiting despite optimal prophylactic pretreatment and/or delayed therapy* [21]. Steps taken to control chemotherapy-induced nausea and vomiting include proper and prompt use of correct anti-emetics especially in patients who have been chemo-naïve, understanding of the rules of anti-emetic therapy and a proper knowledge of the classification of anticancer drugs based on their emetogenic potential and finally proper assessment of the need for anti-emetic therapy for each patient undergoing chemotherapy [21].

Another common GI side effect is increased frequency of motions and diarrhoea which if not controlled and treated will lead to dehydration and fluid as well as electrolyte loss with their respective ill effects. Diarrhoea can be either early onset (within 24 h) or late onset (3–11 days post-therapy). Early-onset diarrhoea is often preceded by diaphoresis and/or abdominal cramping and can be controlled by the administration of atropine [21].

Oral mucositis is also a common accompaniment of chemotherapy, and the lesions appear within 5–7 days after chemotherapy, which take about 2 weeks to heal after completion or stopping of therapy [21]. It results in increased risk of local infection and local pain. Inflammation of the oral and oropharyngeal mucosal lining causes pain and discomfort, difficulty in speech and swallowing and can compromise oral nutritional and fluid intake. Therefore in these situations, the primary aim is maintain if possible the integrity of the mucosa and if the mucositis has already set in then to limit its severity, prevent secondary infection, provide pain relief and maintain dietary intake. Interventions to maintain health and limit mucosal damage in these patients include avoiding foods with high spice/acid or salt content or very hot or cold food which could inflame further the damaged mucosa, using foods which have a smooth texture like liquids or semi-solids or blending the food and ensuring that the food has a bland taste and is at room temperature as well as taking extra calories with powdered milk or dietary supplements. Fruit juices can be given as they are soothing to the mucosa especially if administered as smoothies (with yoghurt) and provide extra calories. The aim is to ensure intake of a high-protein and high-calorie diet with required amount of fluids.

Bone marrow toxicities are also a major accompaniment of chemotherapy and include anaemia, thrombocytopenia and neutropenia [21]. It has been seen that the white blood cells and among these specifically the neutrophil counts usually drop to their lowest levels towards the end of the first week and mostly by day 14 of chemotherapy. The nadir or the lowest point is thought to occur on day 14 after which the counts slowly are expected to rise over a week's time back to initial values. However during this time, the low level of neutrophils puts the patient at high risk of acquiring severe life-threatening infections. At highest risk are those with absolute neutrophil count (ANC) below 100 cells/mm^3 or with prolonged neutropenia of more than 7 days. While in all patients, the goals of therapy (which will be outlined in Chap. 26, Part IV) are to prevent or combat life-threatening infections and avoid or manage complications; development of a febrile episode in a neutropenic patient represents a life-threatening emergent situation. This does not mean that afebrile patients are not at risk, as some patients with very low counts may not have even sufficient neutrophils to mount an inflammatory response to an infection. All patients should receive empiric antibiotic therapy till culture samples reveal specific sensitivity patterns which can guide further antibiotic therapy. Additionally universal precautions, such as using clean and disposable gloves for each separate patient, avoiding contact as well as barrier nursing care, need to be followed for all patients. Washing hands frequently and thoroughly is considered the single most important measure in preventing infection.

Anaemia can be caused both by direct effects of cytotoxic drugs and host factors such as reduced nutritional intake, existing anaemia caused by chronic disease or blood loss from the disease or any iatrogenic procedure as well as marrow suppression or even decreased erythropoietin production caused by previous chemotherapy or irradiation. Packed red cell transfusion is the preferred line of management for acute anaemia or blood loss. Human recombinant erythropoietin administration is another treatment option. Reduction in platelet counts following chemotherapy (thrombocytopenia) puts the patient at increased risk of bleeding, and clinical symptoms include easy bruising, petechiae, purpura, gum bleeding and hypermenorrhoea. A platelet count below 50,000 cells/mm^3 denotes an increased risk of developing small vessel bleed, and when counts drop below 10,000 cells/mm^3, there is threat of patient having life-threatening bleeding.

Bleeding in patients at moderate to severe risk can be prevented or controlled by steps such as avoiding intramuscular injections or trauma, limiting the patient's activity and hence such risks, avoiding drugs interfering with platelet function and avoiding tissue trauma by physical activities such as blowing hard or sneezing. In case bleeding starts, one should apply pressure for at least 5 min with a pressure bandage for all IV injections, venipunctures and bone marrow procedures. Razor blades should be avoided to prevent tissue trauma, rather electric razors can be used for shaving. Platelet transfusions are indicated at counts below 20,000 cells/mm^3.

19.12 Characteristic Toxicities of Some Commonly Used Chemotherapeutic Agents

See Table 19.5.

19.13 Guidelines for Chemo Dose Adjustments Due to Hepatic or Renal Derangement

The liver or the kidney is the site of metabolism and excretion of a majority of anticancer drugs. Any condition or tumour extension leading to a derangement of the function of the liver or the kidney can adversely affect drug metabolism and/or excretion. This can translate into either decreased circulating levels of the drug due to decreased conversion from prodrug to active drug or in an increased circulating level due to decreased excretion and leading to more toxicity. The table below (Table 19.6) lists various commonly used chemotherapy drugs which require adjustments in dose in situations of hepatic or renal dysfunctions.

19.14 Role of Biomolecules

In recent years, research in cell cycle physiology, signaling and binding pathways and cell kinetics has led to the identification of many receptors, enzymes or growth factors that may either have a direct causal role or indirectly help in the development of resistance in cancer cells to irradiation or other cytotoxic agents and therefore may serve as targets for action by or enhancement of radio-response or

Table 19.5 Characteristic toxicities of chemo and monoclonal agents

Chemotherapeutic agent	Characteristic side effect (may not be the most common)
Asparaginase	Hypersensitivity reactions, pancreatitis
Doxorubicin	Myocarditis and pancarditis, radiation recall
Bleomycin	Interstitial fibrosis of lung
Bevacizumab	GI perforation and delayed wound healing
Epirubicin	Cardiotoxicity
Paclitaxel	Anaphylactic reaction, peripheral neuropathy
Docetaxel	Capillary leak syndrome
Cisplatin	Nephro- and ototoxicity
Cetuximab	Hypersensitivity
Carboplatin	Myelosuppression especially thrombocytopenia
Chlorambucil	Myelosuppression, pulmonary fibrosis
Oxaliplatin	Cold-induced peripheral neuropathy
Vincristine	Neurotoxicity (peripheral)
Vinblastine	Neurotoxicity, acute pulmonary oedema
Mitomycin C	Haemolytic-uremic syndrome, interstitial pneumonitis
Actinomycin D	Phototoxicity, radiation recall
5FU	Oral and GI mucositis, diarrhoea
Capecitabine	Hand-foot syndrome
Dacarbazine (DTIC)	Flu-like syndrome
Gemcitabine	Thrombocytopenia
Etoposide	Myelosuppression, second malignancies
Erlotinib	Interstitial lung disease and fibrosis
Geftinib	Malar rash
Imatinib	Fluid retention
Topotecan	Haematuria
Rituximab	Infusion reactions, pemphigus, tumour lysis syndrome
Cyclophosphamide	Haemorrhagic cystitis
Ifosfamide	Haemorrhagic cystitis
Irinotecan	Diarrhoea, myelosuppression
Cladribine	Immunosuppression and opportunistic infections
Fludaribine	Immunosuppression and opportunistic infections
Bortezomib	Peripheral sensory neuropathy, fatigue, orthostatic hypotension
Pemetrexed	Skin rash
Methotrexate	Myelosuppression, renal or cerebral dysfunction, chemical arachnoiditis
Liposomal doxorubicin	Cardiotoxicity, hand-foot syndrome
Dasatinib	Bleeding complications
Cytarabine	Cerebellar ataxia, lethargy, Ara-C syndrome (hypersensitivity to cytarabine with rash, conjunctivitis, bone pain)
Vinorelbine	GI reactions, SIADH
Temozolamide	Aplastic anaemia, pneumocystis carinii pneumonitis
Procarbazine	Flu-like syndrome, CNS toxicities
Trastuzumab	Cardiotoxicity
Mercaptopurine	Hepatotoxicity, immunosuppression

Table 19.6 Dose adjustment of few commonly used chemotherapy drugs with hepatic and renal function

Drug	Dose adjustment with hepatic function	Dose adjustment with renal function
Asparaginase	No adjustment required	Omit if creatinine clearance (CrCl) <60 mL/min
Bleomycin	No adjustment required	No dose reduction if CrCl >60 mL/min Dose reduced by 25% if CrCl 10–60 mL/min Dose reduced by 50% if CrCl <10 mL/min
Capecitabine	No adjustment required	Dose reduced by 25% if CrCl 30–50 mL/min Omit if creatinine clearance (CrCl) <50 mL/min
Carboplatin	No adjustment required	No dose reduction if CrCl >60 mL/min Dose modified according to AUC
Chlorambucil	No adjustment required	No adjustment required
Cisplatin	No adjustment required	No dose reduction if CrCl >60 mL/min Dose reduced by 50% if CrCl 30–60 mL/min Omit if creatinine clearance (CrCl) <30 mL/min
Cladribine	No adjustment required	NA
Cyclophosphamide	Dose reduced by 25% for bilirubin 3–5 mg/dL or SGOT >180 mg/dL Dose omitted if bilirubin >5 mg/dL	No dose reduction if CrCl >50 mL/min Dose reduced by 50% if CrCl 10–50 mL/min Omit if creatinine clearance (CrCl) <10 mL/min
Cytarabine	No formal recommendation	No formal recommendation; dose reduction may be required
Dacarbazine	No adjustment required	No formal recommendation; dose reduction may be required
Dactinomycin	Dose reduced by 50% for bilirubin >3 mg/dL	NA
Daunorubicin	Dose reduced by 25% for bilirubin 1.5–3 mg/dL Dose reduced by 50% if bilirubin >3 mg/dL	Dose reduced by 50% if serum creatinine >3 mg/dL
Docetaxel	Omit if bilirubin >1.5 mg/dL, SGOT >60 mg/dL or alkaline phosphatase >2.5× upper limit of normal	No adjustment required

(continued)

Table 19.6 (continued)

Drug	Dose adjustment with hepatic function	Dose adjustment with renal function
Doxorubicin	Dose reduced by 50% for bilirubin 1.5–3 mg/dL Dose reduced by 75% if bilirubin 3.1–5 mg/dL Omit if bilirubin >5 mg/dL	No adjustment required
Liposomal doxorubicin	Dose reduced by 50% for bilirubin 1.5–3 mg/dL Dose reduced by 75% if bilirubin 3.1–5 mg/dL Omit if bilirubin >5 mg/dL	No adjustment required
Etoposide	Reduce dose by 50% if bilirubin 1.5–3 mg/dL or SGOT 60–180 mg/dL Omit if bilirubin >3 mg/dL or SGOT >180 mg/dL	No dose reduction if CrCl >50 mL/min Dose reduced by 25% if CrCl 10–50 mL/min Dose reduced by 50% if creatinine clearance (CrCl) <10 mL/min
5-FU	Omit if bilirubin >5 mg/dL	No adjustment required
Fludaribine	No adjustment required	No formal recommendation; dose reduction may be required
Gemcitabine	No adjustment required	No adjustment required
Hydroxyurea	No adjustment required	Dose reduced by 80% if CrCl <10 mL/min
Ifosfamide	No adjustment required	NA
Imatinib	Dose reduced by 25% if bilirubin <1.5 mg/dL or SGOT <2.5 times upper limit normal Omit if bilirubin >3 mg/dL or SGOT >2.5 times upper limit normal	No adjustment required
Irinotecan	No formal recommendation; dose reduction may be required	No adjustment required
Lomustine	No adjustment required	No adjustment required
Melphalan	No adjustment required	No adjustment required; caution advised in presence of renal dysfunction
6-Mercaptopurine	No adjustment required	No recommendation; caution advised in presence of renal dysfunction
Methotrexate	Dose reduced by 25% if bilirubin 3.1–5 mg/dL or SGOT >180 mg/dL Omit if bilirubin >3 mg/dL	No dose reduction if CrCl >60 mL/min Dose reduced by 50% if CrCl 30–60 mL/min Omit if creatinine clearance (CrCl) <30 mL/min

Table 19.6 (continued)

Drug	Dose adjustment with hepatic function	Dose adjustment with renal function
Mitomycin-C	No adjustment required	No dose reduction if CrCl >60 mL/min Dose reduced by 25% if CrCl 10–60 mL/min Dose reduced by 50% if creatinine clearance (CrCl) <10 mL/min
Mitoxantrone	Dose reduced by 25% if bilirubin >3 mg/dL	No adjustment required
Oxaliplatin	NA	NA
Paclitaxel	Omit if bilirubin >5 mg/dL or SGOT >180 mg/dL No recommendations for bilirubin 1.5–3 mg/dL or SGOT 60–180 mg/dL	No adjustment required
Pemetrexed	No adjustment required	Dose reduced if CrCl <60 mL/min
Procarbazine	No formal recommendation; dose reduction may be required	Omit if creatinine clearance (CrCl) <30 mL/min
Rituximab	No adjustment required	NA
Temozolamide	No adjustment required	NA
Topotecan	No adjustment required	No dose reduction if CrCl >60 mL/min Dose reduced by 50% if CrCl 10–60 mL/min Omit if creatinine clearance (CrCl) <10 mL/min
Trastuzumab	NA	NA
Vinblastine	No dose reduction for bilirubin <1.5 mg/dL and SGOT <60 mg/dL Dose reduced by 50% if bilirubin 1.5–3 mg/dL and SGOT 60–180 mg/dL Omit if bilirubin >3 mg/dL or SGOT >180 mg/dL	No adjustment required
Vincristine	No dose reduction for bilirubin <1.5 mg/dL and SGOT <60 mg/dL Dose reduced by 50% if bilirubin 1.5–3 mg/dL and SGOT 60–180 mg/dL Omit if bilirubin >3 mg/dL or SGOT >180 mg/dL	No adjustment required
Vinorelbine	No dose reduction for bilirubin <2 mg/dL Dose reduced by 50% for bilirubin 2–3 mg/dL Dose reduced by 75% if bilirubin 3.1–5 mg/dL Omit if bilirubin >5 mg/dL	No adjustment required

chemo-response. Targets for molecules that have been investigated or are in clinical use include epidermal growth factor receptor (EGFR); cyclooxygenase-2 (COX-2) enzyme; mutated ras; cell cycle checkpoint control proteins such as CHK1; a number of the DNA repair enzymes including DNA-PK, ATM, RAD51, as well as the proteasome; and angiogenic molecules [22]. EGFR, also labelled ErbB1, is a member of the ErbB family of receptor tyrosine kinases which also includes ErbB2 (HER2/neu). On binding to a ligand, the EGF receptor undergoes autophosphorylation and starts a process of signal transduction which plays a role in regulating cell division, proliferation, differentiation, vascularization and death. This receptor is also important for modulating tumour growth and response to chemotherapy and irradiation. The receptor is frequently overexpressed in many types of cancer (e.g. head and neck, lung, colon or gliomas) and is associated with a more aggressive variant of the tumour and tumour resistance to therapy and therefore poor patient prognosis [23, 24].

Therefore any molecules which can cause a blockade of the EGFR or interfere with its signaling kinetics would theoretically block signals enhancing tumour growth or development of tumour resistance to therapy and hence improve response and prognosis [25]. Cetuximab targets the extracellular binding domain inhibiting dimer formation, gefitinib targets the intracellular tyrosine kinase domain, and erlotinib also targets the activity of the tyrosine kinase domain. However the various levels of tumour cell sensitivity to EGFR signaling pathway molecules even from primary tissues which express the EGFR pathway could be due to the formation of various types of dimers between the various ligand molecules and by the autophosphorylation patterns within each ErbB ligand type and can also be further affected by mutations within the EGFR family which would then confer specific sensitivities or resistances.

The COX-2 gene is involved in the production of prostaglandins which are known to positively influence the development and growth of tumours and may have a role in the tumour or normal tissue response to chemotherapy or irradiation [26]. COX-2 is induced by diverse inflammatory stimuli, mitogens and carcinogens, and its expression is up-regulated in many tumours (e.g. colon, pancreatic, prostate, gastric and head and neck cancers) and is associated with more aggressive tumour behaviour with decreased apoptosis, angiogenesis and poor patient prognosis [27, 28]. An expression of specifically COX-2 in tumours enables targeting for cancer therapy, and such agents like celecoxib or rofecoxib have been shown to improve responses in tumour tissue to the effects of chemotherapeutic drugs or irradiation, especially in human colon, breast, lung and prostate cancers [26].

VEGF receptors are critical for vascular integrity, including angiogenesis and endothelial cell survival due to tyrosine kinase activities [29]. VEGF expression induces endothelial cell proliferation by creating a vascular sprout that subsequently organizes into a capillary tube [30], as well as angiogenesis through the formation of a hyperpermeable immature vascular network. VEGF expression is enhanced following radiation, while receptor tyrosine kinases up-regulate VEGF, and COX-2 inhibitors limit the up-regulation of VEGF by prostaglandins. Because radiation can limit the mobilization of angiogenesis inhibitors such as angiostatin, combining radiation with agents that inhibit vascularization has been tried with some success (e.g. role of bevacizumab in metastatic colon cancer or in high-grade gliomas).

Activating mutations in the ras oncogene are found in many tumours including lung, colon, head and neck, glioblastoma and others. These activating mutations drive intracellular signaling pathways with proliferative and survival advantages to tumour cells. The most commonly evaluated pathways include alteration of chromatin, recruiting of repair enzymes to the break site and initiation of cell cycle checkpoint control following DNA damage. Thus there are multiple signaling pathways that can affect tumour cell proliferation, chemo- and radioresistance and overall survival which may be interlinked. Therefore strategies that combine radiation with agents targeting multiple signaling pathways either through the use of multiple agents or with agents acting alone on multiple pathways hold the most promise for improved patient outcome.

References

1. Steel GG, Peckham MJ. Exploitable mechanisms in combined radiotherapy-chemotherapy: the concept of additivity. Int J Radiat Oncol Biol Phys. 1979;5(1):85–91.
2. Bentzen SM, Harari PM, Bernier J. Exploitable mechanisms for combining drugs with radiation: concepts, achievements and future directions. Nat Clin Pract Oncol. 2007;4(3):172–80.
3. Bentzen SM. Repopulation in radiation oncology: perspectives of clinical research. Int J Radiat Biol. 2003;79(7):581–5.
4. Kim JJ, Tannock IF. Repopulation of cancer cells during therapy: an important cause of treatment failure. Nat Rev Cancer. 2005;5(7):516–25.
5. Nishimura Y. Rationale for chemoradiotherapy. Int J Clin Oncol. 2004;9(6):414–20.
6. Harari PM, Huang SM. Head and neck cancer as a clinical model for molecular targeting of therapy: combining EGFR blockade with radiation. Int J Radiat Oncol Biol Phys. 2001;49(2):427–33.
7. Bentzen SM, Overgaard M, Thames HD, et al. Early and late normal-tissue injury after postmastectomy radiotherapy alone or combined with chemotherapy. Int J Radiat Biol. 1989;56(5):711–5.
8. Denis F, Garaud P, Bardet E, et al. Late toxicity results of the GORTEC 94-01 randomized trial comparing radiotherapy with concomitant radiochemotherapy for advanced-stage oropharynx carcinoma: comparison of LENT/SOMA, RTOG/EORTC, and NCI-CTC scoring systems. Int J Radiat Oncol Biol Phys. 2003;55(1):93–8.
9. Trotti A, Bentzen SM. The need for adverse effects reporting standards in oncology clinical trials. J Clin Oncol. 2004;22(1):19–22.
10. Peters KB, Brown JM. Tirapazamine: a hypoxia-activated topoisomerase II poison. Cancer Res. 2002;62(18):5248–53.
11. Jain RK. Normalization of tumor vasculature: an emerging concept in antiangiogenic therapy. Science. 2005;307(5706):58–62.
12. Carson CT, Schwartz RA, Stracker TH, et al. The Mre11 complex is required for ATM activation and the G2/M checkpoint. EMBO J. 2003;22(24):6610–20.
13. Gray LH, Conger AD, Ebert M, et al. The concentration of oxygen dissolved in tissues at the time of irradiation as a factor in radiotherapy. Br J Radiol. 1953;26(312):638–48.
14. Semenza GL. Targeting HIF-1 for cancer therapy. Nat Rev Cancer. 2003;3(10):721–32.
15. Withers HR, Taylor JM, Maciejewski B. The hazard of accelerated tumor clonogen repopulation during radiotherapy. Acta Oncol. 1988;27(2):131–46.
16. Larson DL. Treatment of tissue extravasation by antitumor agents. Cancer. 1982;49:1796–9.

17. Bertelli G, Gozza A, Forno GB, et al. Topical dimethylsulfoxide for the prevention of soft tissue injury after extravasation of vesicant cytotoxic drugs: a prospective clinical study. J Clin Oncol. 1995;13:2851–5.
18. Mader I, Fürst-Weger P, Mader R, et al. Extravasation of cytotoxic agents; compendium for prevention and management. 2nd ed. New York: Springer; 2009.
19. Schulmeister L. Extravasation management: clinical update. Semin Oncol Nurs. 2011;27(1): 82–90.
20. Tsavaris N, Komitsopoulou P, Karagiaouris P, et al. Prevention of tissue necrosis due to accidental extravasation of cytostatic drugs by a conservative approach. Cancer Chemother Pharmacol. 1992;30:330–3.
21. Kwong C. Management of side effects from chemotherapy. Hong Kong Anti-Cancer Society. p. 1–7.
22. Mason KA, Komaki R, Cox JD, et al. Biology-based combined-modality radiotherapy: workshop report. Int J Radiat Oncol Biol Phys. 2001;50:1079–89.
23. Liang K, Ang KK, Milas L, et al. The epidermal growth factor receptor mediates radioresistance. Int J Radiat Oncol Biol Phys. 2003;57:246–54.
24. Mendelsohn J, Fan Z. Epidermal growth factor receptor family and chemosensitization. J Natl Cancer Inst. 1997;89:341–3.
25. Milas L, Mason K, Hunter N, et al. In vivo enhancement of tumor radioresponse by C225 antiepidermal growth factor receptor antibody. Clin Cancer Res. 2000;6:701–8.
26. Milas L. Cyclooxygenase-2 (COX-2) enzyme inhibitors as potential enhancers of tumor radioresponse. Semin Radiat Oncol. 2001;11:290–9.
27. Fosslien E. Molecular pathology of cyclooxygenase-2 in neoplasia. Ann Clin Lab Sci. 2000;30:3–21.
28. Masferrer JL, Leahy KM, Koki AT, et al. Antiangiogenic and antitumor activities of cyclooxygenase-2 inhibitors. Cancer Res. 2000;60:1306–11.
29. Petrova TV, Makinen T, Alitalo K. Signaling via vascular endothelial growth factor receptors. Exp Cell Res. 1999;253:117–30.
30. Pepper MS, Montesano R, Mandriota SJ, et al. Angiogenesis: a paradigm for balanced extracellular proteolysis during cell migration and morphogenesis. Enzyme Protein. 1996;49:138–62.

20 Use of Radiosensitizers and Radioprotectors

The success of radiotherapy depends upon the relative damage suffered by normal tissues and tumours from ionizing radiation. Dose response relationship for tumour cure and normal tissue damage is shown in Fig. 20.1, and the separation between the two curves is an indicator of success of radiotherapy. Radioresistant tumours are the ones which cannot be cured by the dose that causes maximum acceptable level of damage in normal tissues. The radioresistance of tumours can be due to a variety of causes such as intrinsic radioresistance of tumour cells, hypoxia and ability to recover from potentially lethal damage or rapid tumour cell repopulation. One of the approaches is to use tumour radiosensitizers and normal tissue radioprotectors to shift apart the tumour response and normal tissue dose response curves (Fig. 20.1). In addition potentially lethal damage repair (PLDR) inhibitors, hyperthermia and high-LET radiations have been used to overcome the problem of radioresistance.

20.1 Sensitizers

Many sensitizers such as electron-attracting compounds, DNA base analogues, chemotherapeutic agents like 5-FU, etc. have been tried in radiotherapy as radiosensitizers. The main purpose of using these drugs is to shift the tumour control probability curve (TCP) to the left and thus increase the gap between tumour control and normal tissue complication probabilities. In other words, the aim of using these classes of drugs is to achieve cure by increasing the damage caused by radiotherapy on the tumour and at the same time trying to minimize damage to normal tissues.

The various drug types which are commonly used as radiosensitizers are:

- **Halogenated pyrimidines**: these are known to sensitize tumour cells differentially, i.e. the cells in tissues which have a faster turnover take-up more of the drug than surrounding normal tissues and will be affected by irradiation more than other tissues.

A. Mukherji, *Basics of Planning and Management of Patients during Radiation Therapy*, https://doi.org/10.1007/978-981-10-6659-7_20

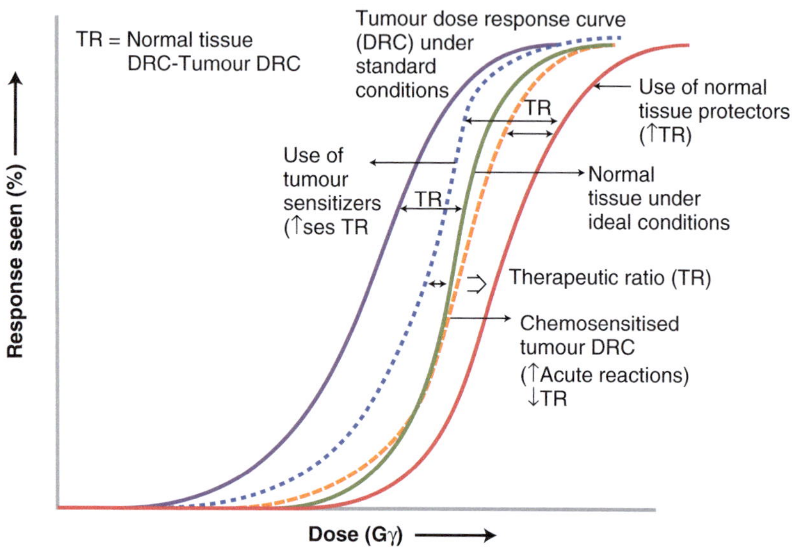

Fig. 20.1 Tumour and normal tissue dose response curves and its relations

- **Hypoxic cell sensitizers**: these agents help in increasing radiosensitivity of cells by enabling the cells to absorb more oxygen.
- **Chemotherapeutic agents**: (like cisplatin, 5FU, paclitaxel, gemcitabine).

Halogenated pyrimidines: The halogenated pyrimidines 5-iododeoxyuridine (5-IDUr) and 5-bromodeoxyuridine (5-BDUr) are structurally similar to normal DNA precursor thymidine, with a halogen in place of the methyl group and are taken up into the DNA chain replacing the base thymidine which results in a *weakening* of the DNA chain, putting these cells at higher risk of damage by gamma rays or ultraviolet light. But these agents are effective as sensitizers only if they have been taken up by the cells for several cell generations so that a significant quantity of the analogue actually is incorporated into the DNA. The extent of radiosensitization increases with the percentage of thymidine bases replaced. The rationale for their use is that tumour cells cycle more rapidly than the normal cells in surrounding tissues, and hence more drug is incorporated in the tumour cell DNA, resulting in "selective" radiosensitization. Iododeoxyuridine is preferred to bromodeoxyuridine because it is an equally effective radiosensitizer compared to the bromide compound but a less effective photosensitizer, so there is less rash.

Hypoxic cell sensitizers and cytotoxins: Most solid tumours have abnormal vasculature with division from arterioles to capillaries and then to venules and veins not proceeding orderly but rather as bunch of ill-formed blood vessels which results in lack of penetration of the tumour tissues by oxygenation and leads to the prevalence of a hypoxic environment inside these solid tumours (Fig. 20.2). This in turn causes resistance to irradiation, as cell killing is dependent on the presence of oxygen for generating free radicals. Drugs which are hypoxic cell radiosensitizers can

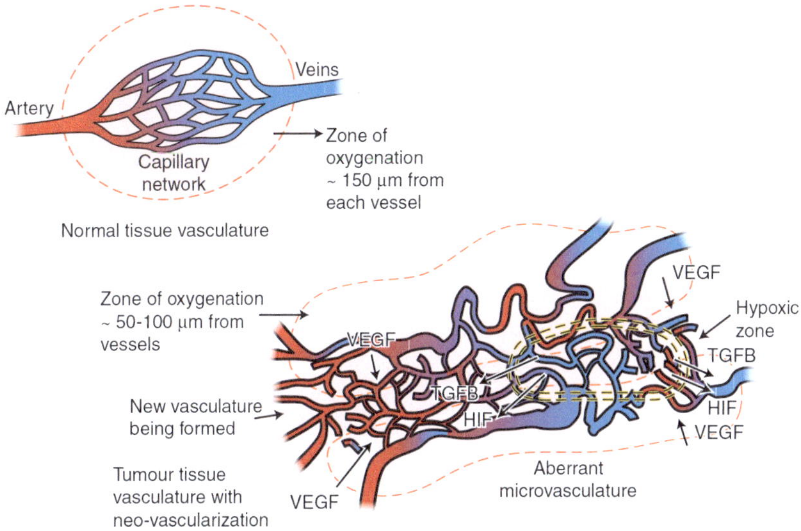

Fig. 20.2 Tumour blood vessels and tissue oxygenation

mimic the radiosensitizing properties of oxygen and can sensitize hypoxic cells but must diffuse throughout the tumour to be effective. Nitromidazoles are a class of drugs with a role as hypoxic cell radiosensitizers. Misonidazole has been the most studied compound from this class and has been found to be capable of sensitizing hypoxic cells in vitro with the process being dose dependent and at the same time spares sensitization of oxygenated cells. But results from clinical use in trials with misonidazole have been disappointing because clinically effective dose of misonidazole was limited by the occurrence of peripheral neuropathy which was influenced by the dose of drug administered. Studies with less toxic drugs such as etanidazole and nimorazole have not resulted in encouraging results, and while nimorazole showed improved tumour control in head and neck cancer, benefit was not seen with etanidazole. A recent meta-analysis of results from 50 randomized trials with more than 7000 patients has shown a small but significant improvement in local control and survival mostly seen in patients with head and neck cancer. Therefore it should be noted that while overall clinical benefits with the use of these drugs have not been noted, it could be more because of faulty case selection as studies have shown that only tumours that are severely hypoxic benefit from such treatment, and therefore case selection should be based on measurements of tumour hypoxia.

Use of bioreductive drugs: The deleterious effect of hypoxia on the radiation response of tumours can be overcome also by using drugs which are toxic under hypoxic conditions, and when complemented by irradiation against aerobic cells, an increase in therapeutic ratio can be achieved. Tirapazamine, a benzotriazine di-*N*-oxide, is such a bioreductive drug and is cytotoxic in an hypoxic environment where it is metabolized to an oxidizing radical causing DNA damage by creating double-strand breaks possibly by interacting with topoisomerases, and in an oxygen-rich environment, this radical converts back by the process of oxidation into the parent compound. Administration of this drug along with cisplatin which is also known to have an increased cytotoxic role in a hypoxic environment can increase its toxicity in tumour tissues. Tirapazamine has been evaluated in clinical trials and shown efficacy in a phase III trial with cisplatin in non-small-cell carcinoma of the lung as well as in patients with cancers of the head and neck when used in combination with cisplatin and radiation therapy. Tirapazamine in these studies was shown to be safe for the patients and resulted in disappearance of tumour hypoxia as assessed with F18-MISO PET scans.

Chemotherapeutic agents: These may influence the radiation survival curve by principally three pathways. They can affect tumour tissue by (a) displacing the cell survival curve downwards by cell kill caused by the drug alone, (b) causing a straightening of the shoulder on the radiation survival curve which would imply a loss of ability to repair radiation-induced damage in the presence of the drug and (c) change in slope of the exponential part of the radiation survival curve, i.e. drug sensitization or radioprotection (Fig. 20.1). It is seen that most chemotherapeutic drugs or molecules employ the first two mentioned pathways of influencing effects (survival curves) in which the sublethal damage caused by these agents may be independent or overlapping. A change in slope of the dose response curve defines radiation sensitizers or protectors, for example, inconsistently for cisplatin and for prolonged exposure to 5-FU after radiation. An improvement in therapeutic index, i.e. a widening of the gap between the TCP and NTCP curves when cytotoxic drugs or irradiation is being used, means that there should be more damage to tumour cells compared to normal tissues. Combined treatment with radiation and drugs leads to therapeutic advantage wherein irradiation is used to provide effective treatment for sites of bulky disease or primary tumour, and drugs are used to treat sites containing smaller numbers of cells or microscopic disease (**spatial cooperation**). It is important for us to note that such combined use of irradiation and drugs in view of high risk of increased side effects would make sense only if the therapeutic advantage is greater on the tumour than the surrounding normal tissue and higher than with individual use of each modality in a sequential manner.

As discussed in the previous chapter, anticancer drugs given *concurrently during* the course of fractionated radiation have been shown to be more effective than the use of various combinations sequentially delivered. Concurrent treatments inhibit repopulation during fractionated radiotherapy. A therapeutic advantage with concurrent chemo-radiation is achieved only in cases where rate of repopulation is greater for the tumour cells than for normal tissues. Greater specificity is seen with drugs that inhibit specifically the proliferation of tumour cells, such as hormonal agents (tamoxifen, antiandrogens) used concurrently with radiation in breast or prostate cancer treatment.

20.2 Radioprotectors

An alternative strategy is to protect the normal tissues by using radioprotective compounds, which will reduce normal tissue reactions, and higher dose could be delivered to the tumour. One compound that has been used extensively over the last three–four decades is *S*-2(3-amino-propylamino) ethyl phosphorothioic acid (amifostine), and being phosphorylated it is less toxic than the parent thiol compound. The main limitation of this drug is the severe side effects of hypotension. Amifostine has been shown to concentrate in the bone marrow and lining of intestinal epithelium and provides excellent protection to these tissues, while most tumours do not take up amifostine (except hepatoma). Sparing of CNS and lung is very poor because the CNS does not take the drug, and in the lung the high oxygen status reduces the effectiveness of radioprotectors.

As will be described in the next section on radiation sequelae in this book, many drugs or compounds can protect against radiation-induced damage to cells in culture, either by scavenging radiation-produced radicals, such as dimethyl sulfoxide (DMSO) or the superoxide dismutase enzymes (SODs), or by donating a hydrogen atom back to a radical site created on a macromolecule such as DNA, including the nonprotein sulfhydryls, glutathione and cysteine. But these drugs or agents have a vital shortcoming, namely, the short in vivo half-life of radiation-induced radicals. Because of this short half-life of the free radicals, any agent which is designed to act against their effects needs to be present in the target tissue at the time of the irradiation and theoretically therefore may be equally effective for both tumour and normal cells in vitro. Radioprotection specificity in vivo depends on preferential absorption into the normal tissue of such agents compared to tumour tissue.

Gene therapy can also be used for radioprotection with a viral vector designed to increase the expression of oxygen radical scavenger molecules such as manganese superoxide dismutase (MnSOD). This can provide protection for normal lung and oral mucosa in rodents without effect on the tumour growing in same tissue. Viral vectors can be effectively adsorbed through the mucosa or lung surface but cannot penetrate effectively into the tumour. A similar approach is suggested for managing subcutaneous fibrosis in patients by direct injections of SOD/α-tocopherol into the fibrotic region or with the use of steroids. Animal-based studies especially in rodents have demonstrated that tissues which have higher levels of expression of angiotensin-converting enzyme (ACE) in the lung and kidney after irradiation can be protected specifically by the use of drugs which block ACE activity or block directly the action of angiotensin II and thus prevent radiation-induced fibrosis and nephropathy.

20.3 Inhibitors of Potentially Lethal Damage Repair (PLDR)

It is suspected that in radioresistant tumours like melanomas and some of the sarcomas, PLDR occurs very efficiently. PLDR has been detected in many other tumours in vivo. It has been suggested that PLDR may be primarily responsible for the radioresistance of some of the tumours. Hence, the inhibition of PLDR may result in the improvement of tumour control at least in some cases. However some of the recent investigations have revealed that the nondividing normal tissues (thyroid and mammary) are also capable of PLDR. Hence, the success of PLDR inhibition as a means of improving the local control of tumours depends on the differential between the ability of the tumour and normal tissues to recover from PLD. Some of the drugs used for PLDR inhibition are D-arabinofuranosyladenine (ara-A), 2-deoxy-D-glucose (2-DG), cordycepin, nucleoside analogue 3′-deoxyadenosine (3′dA) and 3′-deoxyguanosine (3′dG). Besides, postirradiation heat treatment has also been shown to inhibit PLDR in vitro. A clear understanding of PLDR in normal as well as individual tumours should alone help to exploit this phenomenon for improvement of radiotherapy.

20.4 Novel Therapies

In recent years the marriage of biotechnology with clinical medicine has led to the evolution of many new classes of biomolecules and compounds which can be specifically designed or customised to target specific biochemical (signalling) pathways or specific processes in tissues which are important for tumour growth such as angiogenesis. A number of such drugs are now coming out into clinical practice for treatment of specific types of cancer (e.g. imatinib for chronic myelogenous leukaemia or gastrointestinal stromal tumours, sorafinib in metastatic renal cell cancers or lapatinib/erlotinib in lung cancers) though only a few such as cetuximab or nimotuzumab have been tested with irradiation. Many more drugs are in the pipeline, and most of these have not yet been extensively tested in combination with radiation. Gene-directed prodrug therapy (GDEPT) uses agents which are activated by radiation vectors containing radiation-inducible promoters and then directly drive production of toxic molecules (e.g. TNF-α) or expression of enzymes which convert prodrugs into active species. These vectors or carrier molecules are programmed to be activated when they have reached the tissue to be irradiated and then activate the prodrugs in the irradiated volume. One of the problems with such an approach is to ensure the distribution of the vector into the tumour cells only so as to cover the entire tumour volume. Bystander effect is also commonly seen in this technique though it is advantageous in this situation as it helps encompass the tumour volume albeit at cost of some normal tissue toxicity.

Bibliography

1. Adams GE. Chemical radiosensitization of hypoxic cells. Br Med Bull. 1973;29:48–53.
2. Adams GE, Clarke ED, Gray P, et al. Structure-activity relationships in the development of hypoxic cell radiosensitizers: 11. Cytotoxicity and therapeutic ratio. Int J Radiat Biol. 1979;35:151–60.
3. Brown JM, Goffinet DR, Cleaber JE, Kallman RF. Preferential radiosensitization of mouse sarcoma relative to normal skin by chronic intra-arterial infusion of halogenated pyrimidine analogs. J Natl Cancer Inst. 1971;47:75–89.

4. Brown JM, Lemmon MJ. Tumor hypoxia can be exploited to preferentially sensitize tumors to fractionated irradiation. Int J Radiat Oncol Biol Phys. 1991;20:457–61.
5. Churchill-Davidson I. The oxygen effect in radiotherapy: Historical review. Front Radiat Ther Oncol. 1968;1:1–15.
6. Hall EJ, Roizin-Towle L. Hypoxic sensitizers: Radiobiological studies at the cellular level. Radiology. 1975;117:453–7.
7. Overgaard J. Clinical evaluation of nitroimidazoles as modifiers of hypoxia in solid tumors. Oncol Res. 1994;6:507–16.

Part IV

Managing Radiotherapy Complications

21 Expected Complications During Treatment

21.1 Acute Reactions or Treatment Sequelae

Acute responses to radiation therapy are defined as events which take place either during the course of therapy or within 1–2 months of completion of therapy. They are usually seen in tissues having cells with high turnover rate like the gastrointestinal mucosa, bone marrow, skin, oropharyngeal and esophageal mucosa. A hierarchical organization exists in such tissues [1–4] with a lesser number of stem cells constituting a highly proliferative compartment of progenitor cells that differentiate into mature, nonproliferative, functional cells. Irradiation may deplete the stem and progenitor cell pools, but nonproliferating, differentiated cells maintain tissue function until they are lost through continuing normal cell turnover.

After irradiation, these depleted stem and precursor cells first recover their own numbers before differentiating to restore function. While some tissues (like jejunal crypts) regenerate quickly, others (like skin) regenerate less quickly but continuously produce some functional cells. Some other tissues like seminiferous epithelium continue in steady state, producing sperm in numbers which can be reduced for months or years in direct proportion to extent of stem cell loss.

The severity of radiation injury depends both on how much is the extent of stem cell depletion as well as the duration of the delay before new functional cells take the place of the stem cells into the differentiated compartment. This severity increases with dose, but if the proliferating compartment does not fall below a critical value, the symptoms are transient and recovery can be complete. Dose fractionation also can lessen the severity of acute effects by allowing regeneration from the stem/progenitor cell compartment during the course of therapy (Chap. 7, Part II). Thus the rate at which acute injury develops and the latent time to the appearance of symptoms are determined by various factors like *dose of radiation given and fractionation schedule, treated volume and organs involved, any concomitant or previous chemotherapy given, previous surgery done having caused tissue damage as*

A. Mukherji, *Basics of Planning and Management of Patients during Radiation Therapy*, https://doi.org/10.1007/978-981-10-6659-7_21

well as the individual radiosensitivity of the tissue and the person being treated. These points can be illustrated by the following examples:

- Blood counts after an irradiation dose demonstrate that leucocyte and platelet numbers having a fast turnover rate drop quickly due to bone marrow suppression from irradiation, whereas anaemia is not immediately seen because red cells turn over slowly.
- Similarly, in the testis, early differentiating spermatogonia are few in number and are selectively depleted by doses which have little effect on cells in the more mature stages of spermatogenesis, and hence sperm counts remain normal for several weeks after exposure, falling steeply only at the time when the progeny of the irradiated spermatogonia would normally have reached the seminal vesicles.
- In the mucosa of the small bowel, mitotic activity is mostly seen in the crypts, while cells lining the villus are usually nonproliferative. Because crypt cells divide rapidly, they are lost within days when irradiated. The villus shows no immediate effect of irradiation, with shortening becoming evident only as programmed shedding of differentiated cells into the lumen continues in the absence of renewal from the crypts. This is why symptoms take about 2 weeks to appear in patients undergoing standard daily doses of abdominal irradiation.

21.2 Subacute Responses

Certain tissues may display subacute reactions several weeks to months after irradiation and reflect the failure of cell repopulation over a longer turnover period of time. Symptoms are generally reversible, although in some instances they may be associated with severe damage and even death. Examples include Lhermitte's syndrome after spinal cord irradiation, somnolence after brain irradiation and subacute pneumonitis within 3 months after the start of lung irradiation. Subacute effects occur most often during the remodelling phase in irradiated tissues and prior to the onset of late effects that are associated with slowly progressing damage. These effects are determined largely by the total dose delivered and the fractionation schedule as well as overall treatment time (basically time-dose relation). Treatment is usually symptomatic and most patients recover over a period of time.

21.3 Late Responses

Late reactions to radiation therapy in normal tissues can be severe, and recovery is often limited. They are generally considered to be the result of the depletion of slowly proliferating well-differentiated cells that are lost from the tissue at a slow rate. These lesions can appear with time in a dose-dependent manner [2] and can take even decades to occur after irradiation and are an increasing problem as patients live longer following cancer therapy. Late-reacting tissues usually contain cells that are usually both functional and able to proliferate on demand [1–3]. The relative inability of late effects tissues to be repopulated from stem cells results in long term and sometimes even irreversible damage to these tissues as a result of radiation with resultant decrease in the quality of life.

The delivered dose has a greater influence on latency of effects, with late injury developing more quickly with dose escalation or fraction size increment. This is because with higher dose per fraction or even total dose escalation, the extent of direct damage increases irrespective of which phase of the mitotic cycle the cell is in, and it leads to rapid onset of apoptosis within a few reproductive cycles [3]. Also as cells die, lethally injured residual target cells are increasingly recruited to the proliferative pool where the cell damage can lead to nonviability causing a cascade of cell death and functional tissue failure. The time required for the development of such injury can be shortened or severity increased by various other factors like surgery, chemotherapy, infection or physical trauma [4], and these can precipitate the onset of late effects in humans.

Late effects can be predicted by the total dose received by a tissue and by the volume of tissue receiving the dose (based on postulations of Emami et al. for 2D radiotherapy and Bentzen et al. in QUANTEC analysis for beam-modulated radiotherapy) [5, 6]. These effects occur after completion of therapy, and hence dose adjustments unlike in acute effects are not possible, underlying the importance of recognizing organ tolerance doses and customizing fields to prevent non-required doses to normal structures as far as possible [5, 7].

Another issue of growing clinical importance is the extent to which these late radiation effects can be reversed with studies showing modification of the observed late reactions by several agents like captopril, an ACE inhibitor, which slows the development of radiation-induced nephritis [8], pneumopathy and lung fibrosis [9] in rats; steroids, which are known to prevent onset of fibrosis and decrease scar tissue formation; and pentoxifylline, alone or with vitamin E [10], which protects against radiation-induced late effects like fibrosis [11, 12].

21.4 Functional Subunits

The tolerance of a tissue to irradiation is determined by the number of cells with regenerative potential and the way they are organized, in addition to their intrinsic radiosensitivity. Tissues are thought of as being composed of functional subunits (FSUs), which are the minimum clonogenic entity required for regeneration of a structure. This can be explained by the following example regarding skin reactions seen during radiotherapy. Epilation is known to occur at lesser doses than desquamation. This is because the number of functional subunits present in a hair follicle is much less than in the basal layer of the epidermis and thus has a much lower regenerative capacity than epidermis.

The concept of functional subunits can also explain why some tissues require tolerance doses as a mean value and why for some tissues, the tolerance dose is limited by a maximal cut-off point dose. This can be explained by the arrangement of FSUs in an organ either in series circuit or as parallel circuit (as in electrical connections). In a series arrangement, loss of even one FSU can lead to a break in the chain of FSUs resulting in loss of function of that organ. On the other hand, in a parallel arrangement, the FSUs are interconnected parallel and sequentially. Thus loss of function by even one or few FSUs can be compensated by the surviving FSUs. For example, in the kidney, each nephron is an FSU [13]. If a tubule is completely de-epithelialized, it is lost permanently because it is not repopulated from adjacent nephrons. But for the kidney to completely loose its function, a large number of nephrons have to be destroyed which is possible only with large dose involving larger volume of the kidney. Therefore, the tolerance dose for the kidney is determined both by the number of tubule cells per nephron and the number of nephrons. Tolerance doses can vary very much among tissues and organs, even if the target cells have the same intrinsic radiosensitivity as radiation-induced damage is a series of random hits by reactive species, and therefore the number of surviving cells per FSU cannot be always predicted. Organs with acinar or alveolar architecture (like the salivary glands, pancreas, sweat glands, testis, mammary epithelium, lung and even liver) resemble the kidney in having structurally defined FSUs, while the target cells in dermis, CNS, various mucosae, gut and epidermis are less restricted by physical barriers, and cellular migration may influence regeneration.

21.5 Volume Effects

Traditionally, whenever larger volumes were required to be treated, the approach has been to either decrease the total dose to normal tissue or to decrease the dose per fraction to allow greater normal tissue repair in between fractions [14]. However with modern radiotherapy techniques, use of beam intensity modulation and image guidance has resulted in more accurate delivery of radiation with greater normal tissue sparing. This has allowed dose escalation to the tumour volume.

The concept of volume effect has assumed importance in normal tissue sparing especially in tissues with serial FSUs like spinal cord, nerve tracts or the small bowel where the loss of one subunit may result in an overt expression of injury, regardless of the state of the other subunits in the series. The probability of injury increases with volume (i.e. the number of FSUs exposed). This volume effect has been demonstrated both for small bowel obstruction [15] and myelitis [16–18]. For example, there is no evidence that cellular radiosensitivity is affected by an increase in treatment volume [19]. Also, no evidence exists for an increased role for vascular damage as volume increases [20].

A classic example of a volume effect is when a patient tolerates a small area of injury better than a large area of the same severity because pain, exudation and infection are worse, healing is slower, and consequential contraction and scarring are more of a problem. The effect of increasing volume is to make the injury more incapacitating, even though the severity of the radiation response is independent of volume treated. Large gradients in dose distribution and heterogeneity develop as volume increases. Without proper planning, a tumour dose may be prescribed at the 80 or 90% level, leading to a 10–25% higher dose in the region of D_{max}. Also, with large fields, large variations in contour may exist. These variations could result in a high-dose region where tissue thickness is less than that measured at the midplane, as in the neck in planning by conventional 2D technique for head and neck cancers where dose is prescribed to midplane at level of mandible and may result in higher doses in the neck where the separation is much less as well as lower doses in the face region. A better alternative would be to take an average of separations at mid-field, upper and lower borders.

This increase in physical dose is further compounded by the biologic effectiveness of each dose per fraction being increased by more than 25%, i.e. the combined effect of increased physical and biological dose. The magnitude of the increase in biological dose will depend on the dose per fraction and the type of normal tissue but will be greatest in late-responding normal tissues with increase in dose per fraction. Since this additional increase in the biologic dose is not evident from physical isodose contours, an increased biologic effect may be wrongly attributed to the large volume being treated.

21.6 Effect of Fractionation in Early and Late Injury

As discussed previously in this chapter, normal tissue damage is of two types, early reaction and late injury. Late-responding normal tissue has a large number of cells in resting phase. Early-responding tissues generally constitute fast-proliferating cells. *The skin, mucosa, interstitial epithelium, bone marrow, colon, testis,* etc. *constitute early-responding tissues, whereas the spinal cord, bladder, lung and kidneys respond very late*. Acutely reacting tissues proliferate to compensate the cell loss in these tissues. Tissues like the skin and mucosa begin to proliferate 2 or 3 weeks after the start of radiotherapy. In late-responding tissues, this type of proliferation occurs only after the end of therapy. As a result, prolongation of therapy could decrease the acute normal tissue reactions without sparing the late damages. However, one of the positive benefits of increasing the intervals between fractions is to allow for adequate reoxygenation. Thus use of hypoxic sensitizers and high-LET radiations to overcome the hypoxic cell radioresistance may have a critical role in shorter schedules. Since it has been observed that use of large fraction in shorter schedules results in unacceptable levels of late injury, large number of smaller dose fractions (hyperfractionation) can effectively bring about cure, while not increasing the late tissue damage. Hyperfractionation may also increase the early tissue damage but not to an unacceptable level. This concept has already been discussed in Chap. 11 Part II and is being rediscussed to point out the advantage of dose fractionation with respect to normal tissue response.

21.7 What Sequelae to Expect and When

Finally in conclusion to this chapter, we discuss the time frame in which various "reactions" to radiotherapy, both early and late, are seen based on consensus guidelines. The first major effect seen in most patients is the gradual thinning out and loss of hair. But unlike chemotherapy, this treatment-induced alopecia is localized to the treatment field and occurs due the sensitivity of the rapidly dividing hair follicles to irradiation. Depending on the dose delivered, this effect can be transient or permanent. There is initially an increase in hair loss beginning at a dose of 15–20 Gy (third or fourth week) which progresses to complete alopecia over treated area over the next 2–3 weeks. Recovery starts usually 2–3 months after completion of therapy.

Skin changes can occur as early as within 2–3 weeks into radiotherapy and either may resolve, remain stable or even progressively worsen over the next 2 weeks. In most cases the skin changes begin as localized erythema and usually proceed to a dry desquamation in most cases after which they gradually resolve over the next 3–4 weeks depending on the size of field, any concurrent chemotherapy used, use of tangential fields or bolus and depth of dose prescription.

In the irradiating head and neck, the major early effect seen is the advent of stomatitis or mucositis. This will be dealt with in detail in the next chapter. Early changes start at the end of the second week of therapy and may worsen or remain stable depending on the treatment technique, dose, number of fields and portals used. Usually in ideal conditions, it is expected to worsen by fourth or fifth week after which it gradually resolves over the next 2–3 months. It is also associated with varying degrees of xerostomia which can complicate the picture by predisposing to increased sensitivity of the teeth, dental caries and even local infections. This effect is also dose dependent and with most modern parotid function saving techniques (like IMRT) is transient and mild to moderate in severity. These effects are further worsened by concurrent chemotherapy.

The first early effects in irradiation of the CNS start usually at the end of the first week to tenth day of therapy with signs of a transient increase in cerebral oedema. This may then lead to a cascade of other symptoms if not treated. The oedema depends on the fraction size and volume being treated. In most cases with effective medical measures, the symptoms subside in the next 1–2 weeks. Towards the end of therapy at 4–5 weeks, patients also exhibit increased somnolence, mild behavioural changes or short-term memory loss which may take up to 2–3 months post-therapy to resolve or even last for a longer time becoming a late effect.

In irradiation of the chest and abdomen, common early effects seen are esophagitis and enteritis which if not controlled can progress to chronic inflammatory lesions and even stricture formation. Esophagitis usually starts after completion of third or fourth week of therapy and can worsen towards the end of treatment. It usually resolves over the next 6–7 weeks about the end of second month post-radiotherapy in many cases but can also develop into a chronic problem. Similarly enteritis starts towards end of fourth or fifth week of therapy and can resolve over the next 4–5 weeks.

Cardiac side effects can occur if the heart or the great vessels are in the treatment field. Most of these effects are typically late effects but can also occur early if tissue tolerances are not respected. These effects are mostly seen after full-organ doses of 35–40 Gy and can lead to thrombosis with resultant transient or even severe and life-threatening pericarditis and tamponade as well as myocarditis. The initial point of disruption is the myocardial capillary pericytes leading to a cascade of events. Another effect of abdominal irradiation is nausea and vomiting which can be due to increased reflux, gastric and enteric stasis, an increased turnover of mucosal cells, decreased gut motility due to peripheral nerve sheath inflammation or even triggering of central pathways by vagal stimulation.

Similarly treatment of pelvic fields can result in cystitis, proctitis or even large bowel effects depending on size of fields, concurrent chemotherapy and any pre-existing disease or postsurgical status. These reactions are generally noted after fourth week and resolve over the next 4–7 weeks.

Late effects of radiotherapy are generally thought to include those starting after 3–4-month post-radiotherapy and may include those early effects which have continued or even advanced further. These include pneumonitis, carditis, strictures, fibrosis of connective or subcutaneous tissues or behavioural changes, and these can lead to physical or functional or psychosocial disabilities. Each of the above reactions will be dealt with in detail in subsequent chapters.

References

1. Michalowski AS. Effects of radiation on normal tissues: hypothetical mechanisms and limitations of in situ assays of clonogenicity. Radiat Environ Biophys. 1981;19:157.
2. Michalowski AS. Post-irradiation modification of normal-tissue injury: lessons from the clinic. Br J Radiol. 1992;24(Suppl):183.
3. Michalowski AS. The pathogenesis and conservative management of radiation injuries. Neoplasma. 1995;42:289.
4. Wheldon TE, Michalowski AS, Kirk J. The effect of irradiation on function in self-renewing normal tissues with differing proliferative organisation. Br J Radiol. 1982;55:759.
5. Turesson I. The progression rate of late radiation effects in normal tissue and its impact on dose-response relationships. Radiother Oncol. 1989;15:217.
6. Lo Y-C, Taylor JMG, McBride WH, et al. The effect of fractionated doses of radiation on mouse spinal cord. Int J Radiat Oncol Biol Phys. 1993;27:309.
7. Gorodetsky R, Mou X, Fisher DR, et al. Radiation effect in mouse skin: dose fractionation and wound healing. Int J Radiat Oncol Biol Phys. 1990;18:1077.
8. Emani B, Lyman J, Brown A, et al. Tolerance of normal tissue to irradiation. Int J Radiat Oncol Biol Phys. 1991;21:109–22.
9. Bentzen SM, Constine LS, Deasy JO, Eisbruch A, Jackson A, Marks LB, Ten Haken RK, Yorke ED. Quantitative analyses of normal tissue effects in the clinic (QUANTEC): an introduction to the scientific issues. Int J Radiat Oncol Biol Phys. 2010;76:S3–9.
10. Rubin P, Casarett GW. Clinical radiation pathology, vol. 1 and 2. Philadelphia: WB Saunders; 1968.
11. Moulder JE, Fish BL, Cohen EP. Treatment of radiation nephropathy with ACE inhibitors. Int J Radiat Oncol Biol Phys. 1993;27:93.
12. Molteni A, Moulder JE, Cohen EF, et al. Control of radiation-induced pneumopathy and lung fibrosis by angiotensin-converting enzyme inhibitors and an angiotensin II type 1 receptor blocker. Int J Radiat Biol. 2000;76:523.
13. Delanian S, Balla-Mekias S, Lefaix JL. Striking regression of chronic radiotherapy damage in a clinical trial of combined pentoxifylline and tocopherol. J Clin Oncol. 1999;17:3283.
14. Dion MW, Hussey DH, Doornbos JF, et al. Preliminary results of a pilot study of pentoxifylline in the treatment of late radiation soft tissue necrosis. Int J Radiat Oncol Biol Phys. 1990;19:401.
15. Koh WJ, Stelzer KJ, Peterson LM, et al. Effect of pentoxifylline on radiation-induced lung and skin toxicity in rats. Int J Radiat Oncol Biol Phys. 1995;31:71.

16. Withers HR, Mason KA, Thames HD. Late radiation response of kidney assayed by tubule cell survival. Br J Radiol. 1986;59:587.
17. Fletcher GH, editor. Textbook of radiotherapy, I, II and III. Philadelphia: Lea & Febiger; 1966, 1973, 1980.
18. Letschert JG, Lebesque JV, Aleman BM, et al. The volume effect in radiation-related late small bowel complications: results of a clinical study of the EROTC Radiotherapy Cooperative Group in patients treated for rectal carcinoma. Radiother Oncol. 1994;32:116.
19. Hopewell JW, Morris AD, Dixon-Brown A. The influence of field size on the late tolerance of the rat spinal cord to single doses of x-rays. Br J Radiol. 1987;60:1099.
20. Schultheiss TE, Stephens LC, Ang KK. Volume effects in rhesus monkey spinal cord. Int J Radiat Oncol Biol Phys. 1994;29:67.
21. van der Kogel AJ. Effect of volume and localization on rat spinal cord. In: Fielden EM, Fowler JF, Hendry JH, Scott D, editors. Proceedings of the 8th International Congress of Radiation Research. London: Taylor & Francis; 1987. p. 352.
22. Withers HR, Taylor JMG, Maciejewski B. Treatment volume and tissue tolerance. Int J Radiat Oncol Biol Phys. 1988;14:751.
23. Withers HR, Peters LJ, Kogelnik HD. The pathobiology of late effects of irradiation. In: Meyn RE, Withers HR, editors. Radiation biology in cancer research. New York: Raven; 1980. p. 439–48.

Management of Oral Mucosal Reactions and Oro-dental Care

22

22.1 Introduction and Pathophysiology

Inflammation of the oral and oropharyngeal mucosal lining as a result of radiation therapy is a frequent and significant accompaniment of radiotherapy. This condition is usually called "mucositis" and can be a major cause of treatment-induced morbidity due to local or somatic pain, difficulty or pain during swallowing as well as change in salivary secretions and taste. These can cause dehydration and malnutrition and may result in a reduced quality of life of the affected patients. The breakdown of the lining mucosa and subsequent ulceration in severe cases can even cause systemic infections, especially in immunocompromised patients [1], and treatment breaks (Chap. 11, Part II). Thus *mucositis can be defined as an inflammatory reaction with ulcerative lesions of the mouth and oropharynx that occur due to radiotherapy and certain chemotherapy regimens* [2]. The term "mucositis" has been differentiated from stomatitis which also affects oral cavity and can be due to many factors, but mucositis specifically refers to radiation- or chemotherapy-induced inflammation of the oral mucosa. Occurrence as well as severity of this mucosal reaction depends both on the type of anticancer treatment received and patient-related factors. Severe oral mucositis is noted in almost all patients of head and neck cancer who receive concurrent chemo-radiation [3]. It may also be seen in up to 40% of patients receiving conventional chemotherapy as well as more than three quarters of patients receiving induction therapy for bone marrow transplantation [4, 5]. A plethora of morbidities associated with oral mucositis include local pain as well as pain associated with swallowing, local and systemic infections, inadequate nutritional intake, loss of weight, dental abnormalities including caries and osteoradionecrosis as well as taste changes and xerostomia.

The pathogenesis of oral mucositis has both direct and indirect components. The direct pathway affects the capability of the basal epithelium to regenerate after injury by causing inhibition of both cellular DNA replication and proliferation/replacement of damaged mucosal cells. Loss of the epithelium's ability to replace cells will result in thinning of the epithelium or mucosal atrophy along with collagen breakdown, and

A. Mukherji, *Basics of Planning and Management of Patients during Radiation Therapy*, https://doi.org/10.1007/978-981-10-6659-7_22

this can finally lead to ulceration of the surface mucosa [6, 7]. The oral and lower gastrointestinal mucosa particularly has a very high cellular turnover and therefore is more labile to suffer damage by irradiation [8]. On the other hand, indirect pathways which can cause mucosal inflammation and injury following irradiation can be because of the effects of inflammatory mediators, loss of protection from salivary secretions as well as occurrence of bacterial, fungal or viral infection on the damaged mucosa. Therapy-induced neutropenia is also attributed as a cause for the development of oral mucosal inflammation.

Based on experimental and radiobiological data, oral mucositis is described to occur in four phases: an *initial inflammatory phase with vascular involvement, an epithelial phase, formation of pseudomembranous slough with local discrete or widespread ulceration and bacteriological infection and a healing phase* [9]. During the initial phase of local inflammation and vascular compromise, irradiation of the tissue already affected by the malignancy leads to generation of free radicals which cause further activation of modified proteins and pro-inflammatory cytokines such as interleukin-1β (IL-β), prostaglandins and tumour necrosis factor-α (TNF-α) by the affected tissues and especially in tissues with high turnover rates. As a result the epithelial, endothelial and connective tissue cells are damaged, either directly or by increased vascular permeability, further increasing local concentration of cytotoxic drugs or free radicals. An associated release of anti-inflammatory cytokines, like interleukin-11, may counteract this early inflammatory response [10].

The initial inflammatory phase is followed after 4–5 days by the epithelial phase and is mediated by the pro-apoptotic as well as cytotoxic effect of radiotherapy on dividing basal cells. The amount of tissue damage that occurs in this phase is directly related to the proliferative rate of the oral epithelium with younger patients having quicker basal cell regeneration rates recovering faster [6, 11–14]. Many factors can modify the course of this inflammatory "oral mucositis" such as epidermal growth factor, keratinocyte growth factor or transforming growth factor-β3 (TGF-β3) [10]. These agents affect cellular turnover, the inflammation produced in the oral epithelium and effector cells for the body's immunological response.

The destruction or breakdown of the epithelial covering of the mucosa is the result of various events which lead up to the ulcerative phase of oral mucositis. This usually takes place after a week or 2 weeks of starting treatment. This loss of the covering epithelium causes exudation of fibrinous fluid from the underlying layers which gradually coalesces to form a pseudomembrane which in case of continuing injury breaks down to expose underlying ulcerative lesions. These changes result in the acute symptoms characteristic of this phase, and the severity is the highest of all four phases. Therefore patients developing this phase of mucositis suffer the greatest impact on their well-being and are most susceptible to infection. The damaged mucosal surfaces are at risk of colonization by bacteria and fungi especially gram-negative organisms and yeast, which may be complicated or worsened by concomitant neutropenia. Such infections could result in severe local infection or life-threatening septicaemia due to release of bacterial metabolites, like endotoxin, resulting in further enhancing tissue levels of inflammatory mediators such as interleukin-1, nitric oxide and TNF-α [9].

The next or the fourth phase is that of local tissue healing usually taking place from day 12 to 16. This recovery process depends very significantly on factors such how fast the damaged epithelium can proliferate, blood cells and bone marrow recovery as well as rejuvenation of the local microbial flora. Also early recovery is inversely related to presence of factors interfering with wound healing, such as infection and mechanical irritation [9, 14].

22.2 Assessing Oral Mucositis

Oral mucositis being a subjective and objective condition with both organic lesions present and functional effects resultant has lacked a definitive technique to appropriately measure and assess the severity and hence guide therapy. In the last two to three decades, health workers and researchers have developed many instruments to document and quantify changes during and after cancer treatment. These involve assessments taken both anatomically in the irradiated tissues and in organ or tissue function, and these instruments or scales could vary from simple 3- or 4-point "toxicity scales" to detailed and specific descriptions/assessments of mucosal events and changes scored for different regions of the oral cavity, oropharynx, larynx and hypo- and nasopharynx [15].

A scoring system to be considered good should have proper content/validity and inter-user or intra-user reproducibility. Standardization of content and its validity can be done with a proper review of literature preferably by a panel of experts which could then be created as a consensus document and validated with field trials. Reproducibility of the scoring system refers to the ability of the scoring system to produce the same results when used by the same person at different points of time or by different people over a period of time at different places. A few of the commonly used mucositis scoring systems are shown in Table 22.1. We can see that

Table 22.1 Descriptions of various scoring systems commonly used for assessing oral mucositis

Grade	RTOG criteria [16]	WHO criteria [17]	NCI-CTC (RT induced) [18]
Grade 0 (none)	None	No symptom	None
Grade 1 (mild)	Soreness and mild pain	Soreness and erythema	Erythema of the mucosa
Grade 2 (moderate)	Patchy mucositis with serosanguinous discharge with moderate pain	Erythema, ulcers; can eat solid food	Patchy pseudomembranous reaction (patches generally ≤1.5 cm in diameter and noncontiguous)
Grade 3 (severe)	Confluent fibrinous reactions with severe pain	Ulcers; requires liquid diet only	Confluent pseudomembranous reaction (contiguous patches generally >1.5 cm in diameter)
Grade 4 (life-threatening)	Ulceration, haemorrhage or necrosis	No possible alimentation	Necrosis or deep ulceration; may include bleeding not induced by minor trauma or abrasion

the various scales commonly used all employ same or similar descriptive terms for each grade of tissue reaction. However these various scales cannot be used interchangeably or be compared to each other. This is because each of these scales uses different terminologies to describe the various presentations of the different grades of mucositis and exhibits a lack of agreement regarding the score attached to a specific sign or symptom complex.

Availability of new treatment techniques and an increased focus on quality of life issues have necessitated the rationale for universally accepted and validated scales to assess all treatment-related adverse events. Therefore scales which are generalized or assess overall simple grading scores based on clinical impressions (such as the WHO oral mucositis scale) have limited applications but are still being widely used because of their easy techniques though they may have widely dispersed interobserver variations. What may look like a grade 3 ulcer to one observer may classify as only advanced grade 2 to another. In recent years, scales have been developed which have combined a description or clinical assessment of mucosal changes noted during therapy with various subjective (e.g. pain) and performance criteria (e.g. speaking, swallowing). An example is the scale developed by Eilers et al. [19] which consists of eight categories such as voice quality; ability to swallow; condition of sites like the lips, tongue, mucous membranes, gingiva and teeth; as well as quality of saliva and which are rated using a 1 (normal) to 3 (definitively compromised) scale.

22.3 Factors Predisposing Towards Mucositis

The use of radiation or chemo-radiation can increase the risk of occurrence of oral mucositis and which is moderated by many factors, which may be both patient and therapy related. Patient-related factors could include age, nutritional status, malignancy, pretreatment oral or dental condition, care during treatment and pretreatment neutrophil counts. On the other hand, therapy-related factors include specific chemotherapeutic drug, dose of radiation, fractionation schedule and technique as well as site of radiation therapy. The use of altered radiotherapy fractionation schedules as well as the use of concomitant chemo-radiation have been shown in many trials to improve patient response and survival and are now recommended. But these modalities are also known to cause higher rates of acute toxicity and, if they become severe enough, can lead to treatment breaks or even noncompliance. Either of these eventualities would adversely affect any benefits achieved from therapy. Studies, such as by Trotti et al. [20], have demonstrated that there is a relationship between higher grades of mucositis and treatment breaks and eventually survival rates. In an analysis of 33 studies by Trotti, ulcerative mucositis was seen in 80% of the 6181 patients studied with grade 3/4 mucositis seen in 39% of all patients, in 43% of patients treated with concurrent chemo-radiation and in 57% of patients treated with altered fractionation radiotherapy schedules.

22.4 Timescale of Occurrence of Mucosal, Dental and Salivary Reactions with Radiotherapy

Patients undergoing radiation therapy report early signs of mucositis in doses between 10 and 20 Gy, while formation of superficial and later, if untreated, deep ulcers starts after delivery of doses between 20 and 30 Gy. *Radiation-induced leukoplakia is one of the earliest changes seen.* As these cells are then shed, the mucosa becomes friable and denuded. Beyond doses of 25 Gy, there is increased oedema and lessening of erythema leading to stretching of the thin mucosal covering and formation of ulcerations (Fig. 22.1). Beyond 30 Gy there is onset of ankyloglossia, and patients find it difficult and painful to even eat or talk. Any ulcerative lesions formed in the mucosal lining during irradiation are usually seen to last for the entire duration of treatment and even for a week or 2 post-therapy. The reactions may worsen or remain stable depending on the treatment technique, dose, number of fields and portals used. Usually in ideal conditions, it is expected to worsen by fourth or fifth week after which it gradually resolves over the next 2–3 months. Towards the end of therapy schedule, pseudomembranes are formed from the fibrinous exudates and which may have coexisting candidal infection. [21]

Salivary glands, especially the parotid glands, are known to be highly sensitive to irradiation with their functions being affected even by lower doses of radiation [2]. Serous acinar glandular cells have been shown in studies to be more readily affected by irradiation than mucinous acinar and ductal cells [22]. This effect is also dose dependent and with most modern parotid function saving techniques (like IMRT) is transient and mild to moderate in severity, and the effects are further worsened by concurrent chemotherapy. There is progressive degeneration of the acinar epithelium and development of interstitial fibrosis which is directly proportional to the dose of irradiation received. Radiation-induced changes in parotid glandular

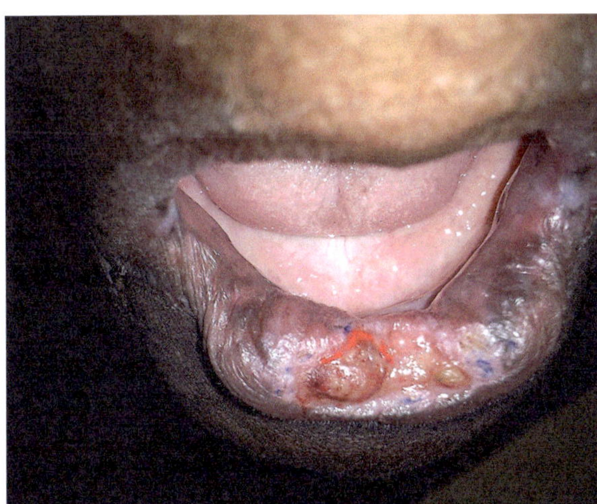

Fig. 22.1 Grade 2 mucosal reaction

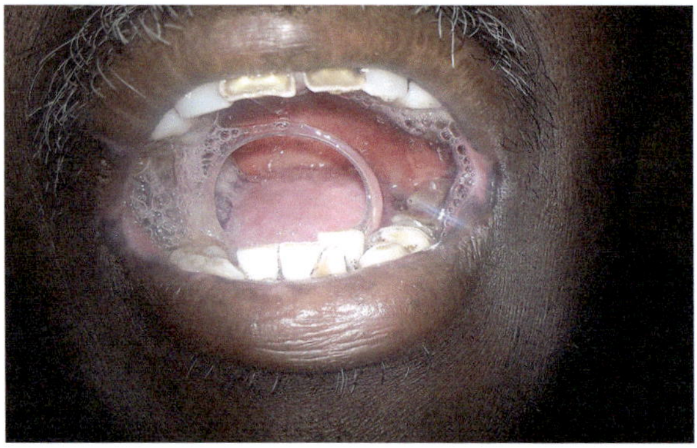

Fig. 22.2 Thickening of salivary secretions during radiotherapy

Table 22.2 RTOG grading system used for assessing salivary reactions [16]

Grade	RTOG criteria
Grade 0 (none)	No change over baseline
Grade 1 (mild)	Mild mouth dryness/slightly thickened saliva/slightly altered taste
Grade 2 (moderate)	Moderate to complete dryness/thick, sticky saliva/markedly altered taste
Grade 3 (severe)	–
Grade 4 (life-threatening)	Acute salivary gland necrosis

tissue have been described to occur in four phases [23]. The first phase (first 10 days of radiotherapy (RT)) at doses of about 10 Gy presents with rapid fall in flow rate of saliva but without changes in amylase secretion or acinar cell density. Later the saliva changes its consistency from a thin watery fluid to a thick ropey discharge-like consistency which sticks to the teeth and mucosa (Fig. 22.2). This results in difficult and painful swallowing and chewing and causes loss of taste and digestion, resulting in poor oral hygiene and predisposing to oral and dental infections. In the next or the second phase (from tenth day of RT to second month), there is a reduction in the amylase secretion in addition to a reduction in the number of functioning acinar cells. There is a third phase (2–4 months post-RT), where however there is no appreciable change in the flow rate, amylase secretion or acinar cell numbers, but the severity of the symptoms gradually increases (Table 22.2). Finally the fourth phase (4–6 months and beyond, post-RT), if not treated before, results in deterioration of gland function caused by increased numbers of acinar cells being produced but with poor tissue differentiation and function. Following irradiation effects on taste buds and saliva, there is also an alteration of taste sensation [24] which could slowly return to normal or near normal at or about 1 year after radiotherapy [25].

Another effect of radiation-induced changes in salivary gland tissue is the formation of radiation-induced dental caries caused by hyposalivation and altered salivary composition leading to dietary changes and which then produces a shift in the oral flora towards cariogenic bacteria (*S. mutans*, *Lactobacillus* species). Therefore prevention of hyposalivation helps in the prevention of radiation caries.

Table 22.3 RTOG grading system [16] used for assessing pharyngeal and laryngeal reactions

Grade	RTOG criteria (pharynx)	RTOG criteria (larynx)
Grade 0 (none)	No changes	No changes
Grade 1 (mild)	Mild dysphagia/odynophagia, require soft diet	Mild or intermittent hoarseness/cough/erythema of mucosa not requiring antitussive
Grade 2 (moderate)	Moderate dysphagia/odynophagia, requires liquid diet	Persistent hoarseness but able to vocalize/referred ear pain/sore throat, patchy fibrinous exudate requiring antitussive
Grade 3 (severe)	Severe dysphagia/odynophagia with dehydration or weight loss requiring NG feeding/IV fluids or hyperalimentation	Whispered speech, throat pain or referred ear pain, confluent fibrinous exudate, marked arytenoid oedema requiring narcotic analgesic
Grade 4 (life-threatening)	Complete obstruction/ulceration/perforation/fistula	Marked dyspnoea, stridor or haemoptysis with tracheostomy or intubation required

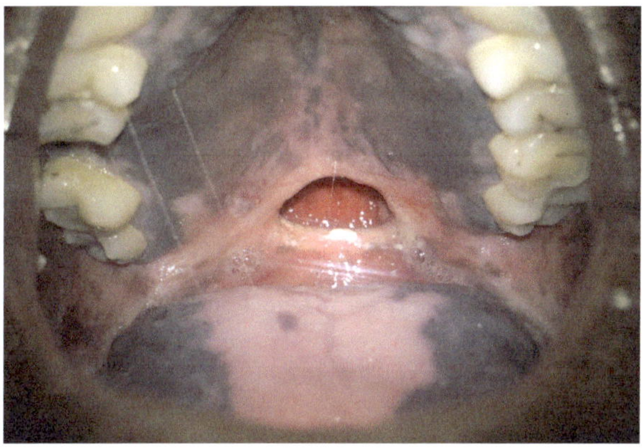

Fig. 22.3 Pigmentation changes with oro-pharyngeal fistula after tumor regression

Late effects of radiotherapy on the oral mucosa and dentoalveolar complex include persistent oro-pharyngitis (Table 22.3), change in taste sensation with aversion to food, dental caries, trismus, ankyloglossia (thickening of tongue) with smoothening and thinning of the tongue mucosa, osteoradionecrosis and chronic pigmentation or even tissue defects leading to fistula formation (Fig. 22.3). Loss of taste and food aversion especially for protein-rich foods occur towards the end of radiotherapy schedule and may take up to year to resolve.

Trismus is defined as any restriction in the mouth opening and usually occurs when the field involves the temporomandibular joint, pterygoids or masseter muscle as in cases of tumours involving the nasopharynx, base of the tongue, salivary gland and maxilla/mandible and patients treated with concurrent chemotherapy [26]. Radiation doses in excess of 60 Gy increase the chances of trismus. Trismus usually sets in 8–12 weeks after the completion of treatment and leads to poor oral hygiene

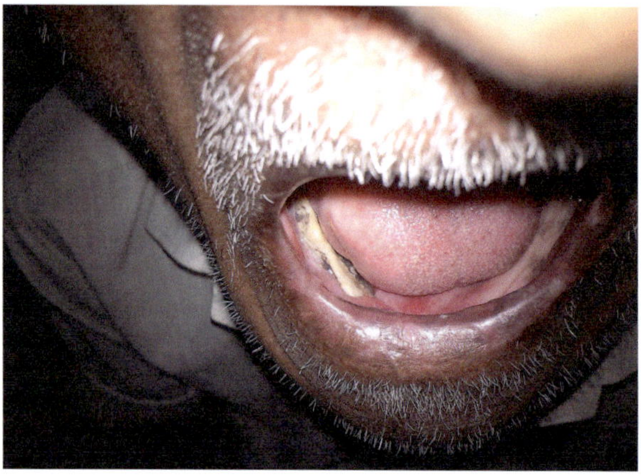

Fig. 22.4 Osteoradionecrosis of mandible

and reduced access for oral examination and dental procedures, dysphagia, malnutrition and speech deficits. Management comprises of diet modification, manual pressure, massage, exercises [27] and devices such as Dynasplint and TheraBite, clothespins and screws.

22.5 Osteoradionecrosis (ORN)

The phenomenon of osteoradionecrosis or ORN is defined as *exposed bone through an opening in the overlying skin or mucosa, persisting as a non-healing wound for 3 months or more* [28] (Fig. 22.4). The occurrence of gross pathological changes in the bone matrix after exposure to significant doses of ionizing radiation can happen late over a period of a few months develop but the initial injury in the bone is to the remodelling system comprising of osteocytes, osteoblasts and osteoclasts. Osteoblasts have been found to be more radiosensitive than osteoclasts, and their inactivation or destruction shifts the balance towards osteoclast activity, resulting in increased bone lysis. This initial injury to the bone cells (osteoblasts) could occur either by direct irradiation injury to the cells themselves or indirectly by vascular injury or by a combination of both mechanisms. The resultant weakened bone is then rendered susceptible to trauma and infection which can further compromise blood supply resulting in necrosis. The most common bone-developing ORN is the mandible because of its single artery blood supply, and the incidence varies from 2.6 to 22% [29, 30]. A typical presentation of **ORN** could be defined as *an initial small area of mucosal breakdown causing exposure of the underlying bone, which progresses with occurrence of trismus, neuropathic pain and chronic drainage* [28]. In these patients, along with ORN, we also note very commonly other features of late irradiation-induced tissue damage such as xerostomia, chronic trismus, dysgeusia, dysphagia and decreased tongue mobility.

Staging: Marx's staging system, proposed in the 1980s, is the most widely used and stages ORN based on response to treatment [28]. According to this staging system, the causal event in the occurrence of ORN is endarteritis. This could lead to subsequent tissue hypoxia which then causes hypocellularity and hypovascularity, resulting in tissue breakdown and chronic non-healing wounds [28]. In recent times, another staging system has been proposed by Kagan and Schwartz based on clinical and radiological findings, based on which present treatment guidelines have been formulated [31]. According to this system, in **stage I**, there is minimal soft tissue ulceration with minimal exposure of the cortical bone. In this stage, most patients respond to conservative management. **Stage II** is divided into groups IIa and IIb and broadly includes patients with localized mandibular cortical involvement as well as that of underlying medullary bone. In **stage IIa** there is minimal soft tissue ulceration, while in **stage IIb** there is extensive soft tissue involvement with even development of oro-cutaneous fistula as well as mild soft tissue necrosis. In **stage III** there is full thickness involvement and devitalization of the bone. The inferior border of the mandible can be resorbed, or there may be fistula formation or even pathological fracture.

Influencing factors/conditions: A number of factors can influence the development of osteoradionecrosis or ORN. These include total dose of radiation to the bone (whether it is limited below or more than 60 Gy), volume of the bone (commonly mandible) receiving dose more than 60 Gy, the part of the mandible that is irradiated and dose fractionation (fraction sizes >2 Gy) [32–34]. ORN does not occur commonly when mean doses to the mandible are restricted below 60 Gy. However use of brachytherapy can increase the risk of occurrence of ORN especially if the target volume abuts or lies in contact with the bone, as the high doses used with steep gradients could result in severe tissue damage [28, 35]. Additionally the presence of conditions affecting the teeth such as dental conditions or periodontal disease, dental extractions/surgery or injury soon after radiation therapy can also lead to the development of ORN [36]. ORN is seen to more commonly occur in the first 2–4 years after completion of treatment in as many as 70–94% of cases [37]. *Early-onset* ORN (occurring within 2 years after completion of radiation therapy) is commonly associated with either radiation doses higher than 70 Gy or surgical trauma, whereas *late-onset* ORN could result from trauma experienced by an irradiated bone which is already suffering from a compromised vasculature postirradiation due to fibrosis or damage to microvasculature [37]. Another type is *spontaneous ORN* which is associated with doses above 60 Gy and can occur in 5–15% of cases treated with older techniques where tissue sparing may not be possible, while with newer techniques like 3D conformal therapy and IMRT in which the mandible can be contoured as an organ at risk and a dose constraint given, this condition may be seen in less than 6% of cases treated [38, 39].

22.6 Management of Oral and Oropharyngeal Mucosal Reactions

The prevention and treatment of oral and oropharyngeal mucositis are important issues for radiation oncologists as its occurrence is one of the major reasons for both treatment break and noncompliance as well as an important reason for resultant poor response/survival, poor nutrition and cachexia, loss of weight and poor quality of life post-therapy. Pre-radiotherapy care minimizes the sequelae and should include thorough clinical history, physical examination and radiographic examination. This is done to assess before starting radiation therapy if there are any inflammatory periapical abnormalities as well as any other dental disease or tumour invasion of the bone. An assessment of the periodontal status is also made. A panoramic X-ray of the teeth along with selected periapical or bitewing films (or both) should be done for pre-radiotherapy dental assessments. Also patients should be advised to give up tobacco chewing and alcohol intake during treatment and after. Another commonly used prophylactic strategy to avoid radiation treatment breaks and bypass any mucositic reaction is to plan the use of feeding tubes, which would allow for continuous enteral nutrition even when patients on radiation therapy develop mucositis and cannot chew properly or swallow their food. This can help to prevent malnutrition and dehydration and some of their secondary effects.

Dental extraction before radiotherapy: Dental extraction is carried out for the teeth which show [40] nonrestorable caries, active periapical disease in symptomatic teeth, moderate to severe periodontal disease, lack of opposing teeth, compromised hygiene, partial impaction or incomplete eruption and extensive periapical lesions (if not chronic or well localized). Time period between dental extraction and the start of radiotherapy is important. In cases of uncomplicated tooth extraction, patient can be started on radiotherapy in 7–14 days of extraction. In cases where the tooth extraction was extensive or the tooth had an acute infection associated with it, a gap of 4–6 weeks is recommended between extraction and radiotherapy.

Care for oral mucositis: The principles of all treatment protocol for oral mucositis are based on mitigating an adverse oxygen environment, avoiding tissue injury, promoting oxygenation and repair and symptomatic relief as well as control of inflammation/infection. The various steps involved include avoidance of chronic mucosal-irritating factors, maintaining local hygiene and tissue moisture/oxygenation, relief of pain and inflammation and prevention/treatment of infection [41, 42]. Mucosal damage by irritating factors such as sharp or rough dental fillings must be smoothened or polished before radiotherapy to avoid damage to the inflamed mucosa, and continuation during radiotherapy of prosthetic appliances should be decided upon [27]. Plaque control and maintaining good oral hygiene are actions which must be encouraged [41]. A few practitioners also discourage either wearing of dentures during radiotherapy or removing them at night with regular assessments to ensure hygiene and prevent these denture surfaces from being colonized with *Candida* species [43, 44]. Also the use of foods with astringent properties such as tobacco and alcohol as well as spicy or acidic foods is discouraged to prevent irritating the inflamed mucosa [45].

Symptomatic relief of pain or local inflammation can be realized by the use of topical anaesthetics, analgesics and mucosal-coating agents. Agents such as benzydamine (by indirect action) or sucralfate (by direct action) which act as cytoprotectants by forming a protective coating over the inflamed mucosa are commonly used and recommended [45]. Local pain relief can be affected by periodic use of mouth rinses containing topical anaesthetics such as viscous xylocaine or benzydamine [46]. A simple mouthwash comprising of equal amounts of salt and of baking soda mixed in water can be effective for managing early stage oral mucositis [40]. Sucralfate suspensions form a protective viscous coating over the oral mucosa and provide relief from pain and allow the underlying inflamed mucosa to heal by preventing its coming in contact with food irritants or salivary secretions, and this line of treatment has shown encouraging results in some studies. However there is no demonstrable benefit of either prophylactic antibiotic lozenges or sucralfate according to recent clinical practice guidelines for prevention and treatment of oral mucositis [47, 48]. Studies using polymyxin E/tobramycin/amphotericin B (PTA) have shown encouraging results with benefit from narrow-spectrum antibiotics in a curative setting but not prophylactic role [45, 48, 49]. There also have been some studies made to assess the effect of using colony-stimulating factors to reduce mucositis and promote healing, but there are no definite recommendations [49, 50]. Radioprotectors (amifostine) [51] have also shown encouraging results in decreasing the intensity of mucositis, but doubts remain on its efficacy and risk of promotion of tumour growth.

According to existing guidelines, oral mucositis has best responded to interventions like maintaining a proper oro-dental hygiene including the use of topical fluoride pastes as well as benzydamine mouth rinses. Other recommendations for treatment of oral mucositis include using cryotherapy (use of ice cubes orally) 30 min especially before 5FU or high-dose melphalan infusions to cause local vasoconstriction and prevent local drug concentration and a newly available molecule which is a keratinocyte growth factor-1 (palifermin) with recommended doses of 60 μg/kg/day given as conditioning and prophylactic therapy for 3 days prior and 3 days post-transplant in patients with haematological malignancies who require autologous stem cell transplant and are treated with high-dose chemotherapy with or without total body irradiation. This drug is thought to prevent onset of oral mucositis in these patients. Palifermin has also in clinical trials shown effect in reducing incidence of ulcerative mucositis in patients with haematologic cancers [52]. However its efficacy and safety in other cancers causing oral mucositis, principally in head and neck cancers, have not been proven, though phase III trials are currently underway in the USA and Europe.

Care of dental caries: Before radiotherapy is started, unhealthy or carious teeth must be removed, and ill-fitting dentures should be corrected. Any sharp or jagged teeth edges should also be smoothened. A patient's ability and willingness to cooperate in this initial dental assessment and preventive regimen should be assessed, and instructions regarding proper diet to be taken as well as dental and oral care during radiotherapy must be explained to the patient. During radiotherapy, recommended measures include scrupulously maintaining a good oral hygiene, applying fluoride toothpastes or oral creams daily, daily flossing teeth and interdental regions to prevent residual foods from decaying and causing caries, using rinses to dissolve oral and dental plaques, limiting foods which would predispose to increased dental caries such as foods rich in acidic content and sugar or high-residue foods as well as using mucosal protecting and mineral-rich mouth rinses or artificial saliva preparations [53–55]. In fact it is possible, despite low salivary output, in irradiated patients, to achieve almost complete freedom from dental caries by daily using fluoride along with strict oral hygiene [56].

Care of loss of taste: Efforts are made during irradiation to maintain or improve food intake by improving the taste, colour and smell of food, as well as helping patients adapt to their changed taste sensation with dietary counselling. The patient's caloric requirements during the radiotherapy course should be planned before starting irradiation, and the meal plan should include supplementary feedings as well as mineral and protein supplements which can be started at the beginning of therapy and followed during the course of therapy. This part is explained subsequently in detail in Chap. 28. Zinc supplements can be beneficial in improving taste in some patients [57], especially in the post-radiotherapy period.

Treatment of ORN: It is based on the staging of the condition, and goals of therapy include removing the dead necrotic bone and improving both concentration and penetration of the vascularity of the remaining irradiation-affected tissues [29, 30]. The primary modality of treatment for ORN is surgery, while the use of hyperbaric oxygen (HBO) therapy may have an adjunctive role. As described before in this chapter, Marx protocol stage I condition is highly localized and can be initially treated by local debridement and HBO. Surgery may not be required in these cases. Stage I cases that do not respond as well as stage II cases can be treated primarily by local excision (marginal mandibulectomy in case of oral ORN) of the involved region, after which HBO treatment may be instituted. In case of stage III where the defect may involve the inferior border of the mandible or there is presence of an oro-cutaneous fistula or pathologic fractures, the line of management would entail extensive surgery with resection of the involved portion of the mandible along with a margin of the healthy bone and stabilizing the resultant defect by extra-oral fixation.

Care of Dental implants: During the radiotherapy of a patient with head and neck tumours, the inflamed oral mucosa is more prone to injuries, and patients with dental implants are to be managed carefully to avoid further injury to the mucosa. If possible implants should be avoided completely, while those with permanent implants, careful planning of fields and radiation dose and maintaining oral hygiene are important [58].

References

1. Elting LS, Bodey GP, Keefe BH. Septicemia and shock syndrome due to viridans streptococci: a case-control study of predisposing factors. Clin Infect Dis. 1992;14:1201–7.
2. Carl W. Oral complications in cancer patients. Am Fam Physician. 1983;27(2):161–70.
3. Jansma J, Vissink A, Spijkervet FK, et al. Protocol for the prevention and treatment of oral sequelae resulting from head and neck radiation therapy. Cancer. 1992;70:2171–80.
4. Sonis ST, Sonis AL, Lieberman A. Oral complications in patients receiving treatment for malignancies other than of the head and neck. J Am Dent Assoc. 1978;97:468–72.
5. Woo SB, Sonis ST, Monopoli MM, Sonis AL. A longitudinal study of oral ulcerative mucositis in bone marrow transplant recipients. Cancer. 1993;72:1612–7.
6. Guggenheimer J, Verbin RS, Apple BN, et al. Clinico-pathologic effects of cancer chemotherapeutic agents on human buccal mucosa. Oral Surg Oral Med Oral Pathol. 1997;44:58–63.
7. Lockhart PB, Sonis ST. Alterations in the oral mucosa caused by chemotherapeutic agents. A histologic study. J Dermatol Surg Oncol. 1981;7:1019–25.

8. Squier CA. Mucosal alterations. NCI Monogr. 1990;9:169–72.
9. Sonis ST. Mucositis as a biological process: a new hypothesis for the development of chemotherapy-induced stomatotoxicity. Oral Oncol. 1998;34:39–43.
10. Sonis ST, Lindquist L, Van Vugt A, et al. Prevention of chemotherapy-induced ulcerative mucositis by transforming growth factor beta 3. Cancer Res. 1994;54:1135–8.
11. Sonis A, Sonis S. Oral complications of cancer chemotherapy in pediatric patients. J Pedod. 1979;3:122–8.
12. Waterfield MD. Epidermal growth factor and related molecules. Lancet. 1989;1:1243–6.
13. Sonis S, Clark J. Prevention and management of oral mucositis induced by antineoplastic therapy. Oncology (Huntingt). 1991;5:11–8; discussion 18–22
14. Plevova P. Re: mucositis as a biological process: a new hypothesis for the development of chemotherapy-induced stomatotoxicity. Oral Oncol. 1999;35:225–6.
15. Schubert MM. Measurement of oral tissue damage and mucositis pain. In: Chapman CR, Foley KH, editors. Current and emerging issues on cancer pain: research and practice. New York: Raven; 1993. p. 247–65.
16. Cox JD, Stetz J, Pajak TF. Toxicity criteria of the Radiation Therapy Oncology Group (RTOG) and the European Organization for Research and Treatment of Cancer (EORTC). Int J Radiat Oncol Biol Phys. 1995;31(5):1341–6.
17. WHO handbook for reporting the results of cancer treatment. Geneva: WHO Offset Publications; 1979, Series number 48. (Albany, NY: sold by WHO Publications Centre USA).
18. DCTD, NCI, NIH, DHHS. Cancer Therapy Evaluation Program: common toxicity criteria version 2.0. 1998. http://ctep.info.nih.gov/CTC3/ctc.htm.
19. Eilers J, Berger A, Petersen M. Development, testing, and application of the oral assessment guide. Oncol Nurs Forum. 1988;15:325–30.
20. Trotti A, Bellm LA, Epstein JB, et al. Mucositis incidence, severity and associated outcomes in patients with head and neck cancer receiving radiotherapy with or without chemotherapy: a systematic literature review. Radiother Oncol. 2003;66:253–62.
21. Leahy D, St Germain J, Varrichio C. The nurse and radiotherapy. St Louis: CV Mosby; 1979.
22. Kashima HK, Kirkham WR, Andrews JR. Postirradiation sialadenitis: a study of the clinical features, histopathological changes, and serum enzyme variations following irradiation of human salivary glands. Am J Roentgenol Radiat Ther Nucl Med. 1965;94:271–91.
23. Coppes RP, Zeilstra LJW, Kampinga HH, Konings AWT. Early to late sparing of radiation damage to the parotid gland by adrenergic and muscarinic receptor agonists. Br J Cancer. 2001;85:1055–63.
24. Mossman KL. Gustatory tissue injury in man: radiation dose response relationship and mechanism of taste loss. Br J Cancer. 1986;53:9–11.
25. Tomita Y, Osaki T. Gustatory impairment and salivary gland pathophysiology in relation to oral cancer treatment. Int J Oral Maxillofac Surg. 1990;19:299–304.
26. Goldstein M, Maxymiw WG, Cummings BJ, Wood RE. The effects of antitumour irradiation on mandibular opening and mobility. A prospective study of 58 patients. Oral Surg Oral Med Oral Pathol Endod. 1999;8:365–73.
27. Engelmeier RL, King GE. Complications of head and neck radiation therapy and their management. J Prosthet Dent. 1983;49:514–22.
28. Marx RE. A new concept in the treatment of osteoradionecrosis. J Oral Maxillofac Surg. 1983;41:351–7.
29. Constantino PD, Friedman CD, Steinberg MJ. Irradiated bone and its management. Otolaryngol Clin North Am. 1995;28:1021–38.
30. Epstein JB, van der Meij EH, McKenzie M, Wong F, Lepawsky M, Stevenson-Moore P. Postradiation osteonecrosis of the mandible. A long-term follow-up study. Oral Surg Oral Med Oral Pathol Oral Radiol Endod. 1997;83:657–62.
31. Schwartz HC, Kagan AR. Osteoradionecrosis of the mandible: scientific basis for clinical staging. Am J Clin Oncol. 2002;25:168–71.
32. Marx RE, Johnson RP. Studies in the radiobiology of osteoradionecrosis and their clinical significance. Oral Surg Oral Med Oral Pathol. 1987;64:379–90.

33. Glanzmann C, Gratz KW. Radionecrosis of the mandibula: a retrospective analysis of the incidence and risk factors. Radiother Oncol. 1995;36:94–100.
34. Ahmed M, Hansen VN, Harrington KJ, Nutting CM. Reducing the risk of xerostomia and mandibular osteoradionecrosis: the potential benefits of intensity modulated radiotherapy in advanced oral cavity carcinoma. Med Dosim. 2009;34:217–24.
35. Thorn JJ, Hansen HS, Specht L, Bastholt L. Osteoradionecrosis of the jaws: clinical characteristics and relation to the field of irradiation. J Oral Maxillofac Surg. 2000;58:1088–93; discussion 1093–5
36. Store G, Boysen M. Mandibular osteoradionecrosis: clinical behaviour and diagnostic aspects. Clin Otolaryngol Allied Sci. 2000;25:378–84.
37. Reuther T, Schuster T, Mende U, Kubler A. Osteoradionecrosis of the jaws as a side effect of radiotherapy of head and neck tumour patients – a report of a thirty year retrospective review. Int J Oral Maxillofac Surg. 2003;32:289–95.
38. Vissink A, Jansma J, Spijkervet FK, Burlage FR, Coppes RP. Oral sequelae of head and neck radiotherapy. Crit Rev Oral Biol Med. 2003;14:199–212.
39. Studer G, Gratz KW, Glanzmann C. Osteoradionecrosis of the mandibula in patients treated with different fractionations. Strahlenther Onkol. 2004;180:233–40.
40. Pamela J. Hancock, Joel B. Epstein, Georgia Robins Sadler. Oral and Dental Management Related to Radiation Therapy for Head and Neck Cancer. J Can Dent Assoc. 2003;69(9):585–90.
41. Scully C, Epstein JB. Oral health care for the cancer patient. Oral Oncol Eur J Cancer. 1996;32B:281–92.
42. Miaskowski C. Management of mucositis during therapy. NCI Monogr. 1990;9:95–8.
43. Lockhart PB. Oral complications of radiation therapy. In: Peterson DE, Elias EG, Sonis ST, editors. Head and neck management of the cancer patient. Boston: Martinus Nijhoff; 1986. p. 275–97.
44. Epstein JB. Infection prevention in bone marrow transplantation and radiation patients. NCI Monogr. 1990;9:73–85.
45. Sutherland SE, Browman GP. Prophylaxis of oral mucositis in irradiated head and neck cancer patients: a proposed classification scheme of interventions and meta-analysis of randomized controlled trials. Int J Radiat Oncol Biol Phys. 2001;49:917–30.
46. Dreizen SA, Daly TE, Drane JB, Brown LR. Oral complications of cancer radiotherapy. Postgrad Med. 1977;61:85–92.
47. Spijkervet FKL, van Saene HKF, van Saene JJM, Panders AK, Vermey A, Mehta DM. Mucositis prevention by selective elimination of oral flora in irradiated head and neck cancer patients. J Oral Pathol Med. 1990;19:486–9.
48. Symonds RP, McIlroy P, Khorrami J, Paul J, Pyper E, Alcock SR, et al. The reduction of radiation mucositis by selective decontamination antibiotic pastilles: a placebo-controlled double-blind trial. Br J Cancer. 1996;74:312–7.
49. Farrell CL, Rex KL, Kaufman SA, Dipalma CR, Chen JN, Scully S, et al. Effects of keratinocyte growth factor in the squamous epithelium of the upper aerodigestive tract of normal and irradiated mice. Int J Radiat Biol. 1999;75:606–20.
50. Mascarin M, Franchin G, Minatel E, Gobitti C, Talamini R, de Maria D, et al. The effect of granulocyte colony-stimulating factor on oral mucositis in head and neck cancer patients treated with hyperfractionated radiotherapy. Oral Oncol. 1999;35:203–8.
51. Antonadou D, Pepelassi M, Synodinou M, Puglisi M, Throuvalas N. Prophylactic use of amifostine to prevent radiochemotherapy-induced mucositis and xerostomia in head-and-neck cancer patients. Int J Radiat Oncol Biol Phys. 2002;52:739–47.
52. Spielberger R, Stiff P, BensingerWet a. Palifermin for oral mucositis after intensive therapy for hematologic cancers. N Engl J Med. 2004;351:2590–8.
53. Daly TE, Drane JB. Prevention and management of dental problems in irradiated patients. J Am Soc Prev Dent. 1976;6:21–5.
54. Regezi JA, Courtney RM, Kerr DA. Dental management of patients irradiated for oral cancer. Cancer. 1976;8:994–1000.
55. Toljanic JA, Saunders VW. Radiation therapy and management of the irradiated patient. J Prosthet Dent. 1984;52:852–8.

56. Jansma J, Vissink A, Gravenmade EJ, Visch LL, Fidler V, Retief DH. In vivo study on the prevention of post-radiation caries. Caries Res. 1989;23:172–8.
57. Matsuo R. Role of saliva in the maintenance of taste sensitivity. Crit Rev Oral Biol Med. 2000;11:216–29.
58. Weischer T, Mohr C. Ten-year experience in oral implant rehabilitation of cancer patients: treatment concept and proposed criteria for success. Int J Oral Maxillofac Implants. 1999;14(4):521–8.

23 Management of Skin Reactions

23.1 Pathophysiology

The skin is the largest organ in the body and one of the most visible targets for assessing radiotherapy-induced reactions. In the orthovoltage era, the dose at which skin reaction occurred was taken as a measure of dose fractionation and for calculation of NSD [1]. The advantage of megavoltage beams lies in their ability for skin sparing (Chap. 9, Part II). Factors affecting skin reactions are total radiotherapy dose delivered, fraction size, volume of field treated, use of radiosensitizers (like chemotherapy drugs, e.g. Adriamycin, cisplatin, gemcitabine) as well as volume of normal structures involved [2].

The skin has been classified by Casarett et al. as an acutely reacting tissue with the epidermis consisting of rapidly dividing basal layer cells [3]. These suffer lethal damage following irradiation and undergo apoptosis. The most sensitive cells are those lining the hair follicles because of the limited number of cells in the functional subunits (FSUs) and hence its limited reparative potential compared to the skin [4]. Thus after the start of radiotherapy, the first reaction seen is alopecia. The main site of radiation damage to the skin is at the basal layer cells of the epidermis. The effects are not immediately seen but start occurring once the superficial layers have been shed when the damage has exceeded the regenerative potential of the basal layer. Skin reactions vary from mild erythema to moist desquamation and even ulceration. The extent of the severity of the reactions also depends in addition to the factors described previously on the area of skin treated. Areas where the skin is thin, overlying bone or cartilage or near body folds (e.g. inguinal or perineal area, inframammary folds) can show more severe reactions than other areas. The pathophysiology of the initial skin changes is due to capillary dilatation caused by the loss of pericytes. Over a period of time, the changes lead to dry desquamation of the skin which is due to the destruction of the sebaceous and sweat glands. This happens 2–4 weeks after onset of erythema in presence of continuing radiation injury.

A. Mukherji, *Basics of Planning and Management of Patients during Radiation Therapy*, https://doi.org/10.1007/978-981-10-6659-7_23

23.2 Clinical Effects

The first major effect seen in most patients is the gradual thinning out and loss of hair. But unlike chemotherapy, this treatment-induced alopecia is localized to the treatment field and occurs due the sensitivity of the rapidly dividing hair follicles to irradiation. Depending on the dose delivered, this effect can be transient or permanent. There is initially an increase in hair loss beginning at a dose of 15–20 Gy (third or fourth week) which progresses to complete alopecia over treated area over the next 2–3 weeks. Recovery starts usually 2–3 months after completion of therapy.

Skin changes can occur as early as within 2–3 weeks into radiotherapy and either may resolve, remain stable or even progressively worsen over the next 2 weeks. Skin erythema is the first clinical sign of a skin reaction. In most cases the skin changes begin as localized erythema and usually proceed to a dry desquamation in most cases after which they gradually resolve over the next 3–4 weeks depending on the size of field, any concurrent chemotherapy used, use of tangential fields or bolus and depth of dose prescription.

As explained before, the phase of dry desquamation is caused by loss of sweat and sebaceous gland function with patients complaining of increased itchiness, flaking and cracking of the skin as well as loss of hair. These effects are affected both by time-dose effects and total dose received. This phase of dry desquamation is followed by wet desquamation where inflammation, oedema and denudation of the skin are apparent, leaving behind raw surfaces which can be covered by fibrinous exudates (Figs. 23.1 and 23.2) At this stage, the treatment needs to be stopped to allow the tissue to repair and regenerate. Beyond this stage there is severe skin denudation with loss of skin integrity and formation of deep-seated ulcers. At this stage the patient needs urgent treatment as they are at increased risk of life-threatening infections and severe pain. Treatment at this stage requires inpatient care, local treatment and systemic treatment for infections and any existing protein or fluid-electrolyte imbalance. In patients receiving concurrent chemo-radiation, the grade of skin reactions is even more severe for a particular dose of radiation received. According to the RTOG, a grading system for skin reactions is listed in Table 23.1.

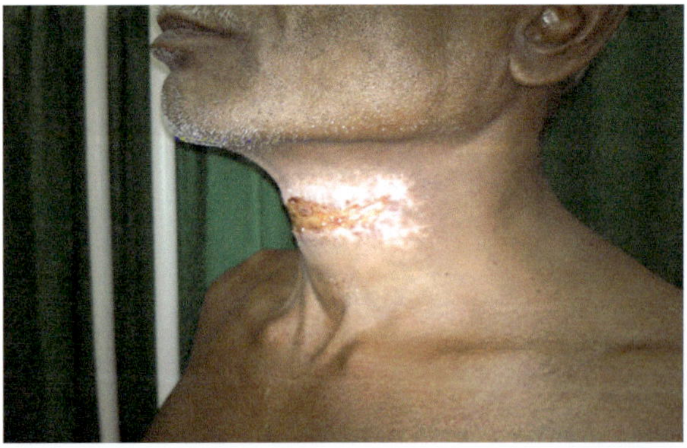

Fig. 23.1 Grade 2 Skin reaction with radiotherapy

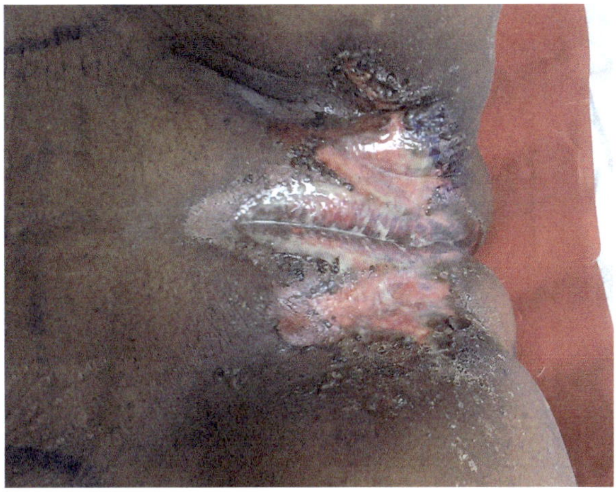

Fig. 23.2 Grade 3 Skin reaction with radiotherapy

Table 23.1 RTOG grading system [5] used for assessing skin reactions

Grade	RTOG criteria
Grade 0 (none)	None
Grade 1 (mild)	Follicular reactions/mild erythema/epilation/dry squamation/no sweating
Grade 2 (moderate)	Tender or bright erythema/patchy moist desquamation or moderate oedema
Grade 3 (severe)	Confluent moist desquamation other than skin folds, pitting oedema
Grade 4 (life-threatening)	Ulceration, haemorrhage or necrosis

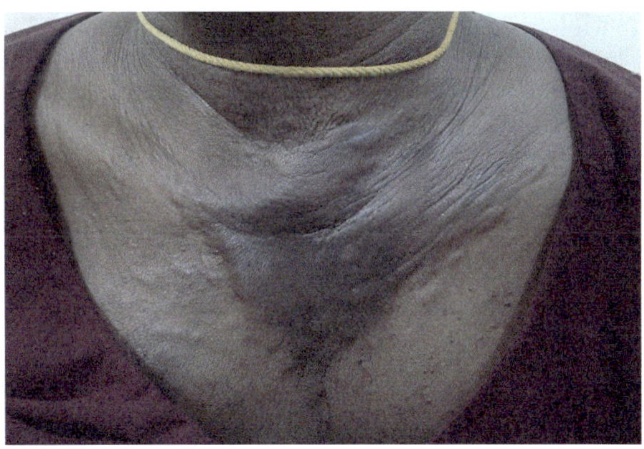

Fig. 23.3 Post radiotherapy cutaneous kelosis with subcutaneous fibrosis

Late effects of irradiation include permanent alopecia, cutaneous and subcutaneous fibrosis with or without kelosis especially with megavoltage radiation (Fig. 23.3), contractures, lymphangitis and lymphoedema (Fig. 23.4), telangiectasias due to capillary dilatation, formation of fibrous bands as well as loss of function of sweat and sebaceous glands or even deep-seated ulcers with necrosis of underlying tissues

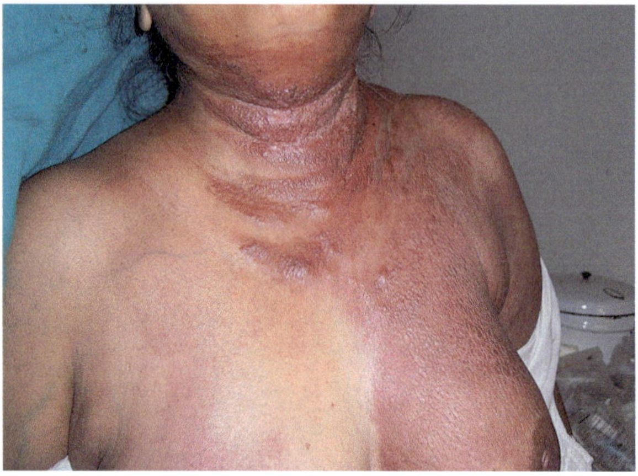

Fig. 23.4 Post-radiotherapy lymphangitis of skin

and even bones/cartilage. There is also increased risk over longer follow-up periods to develop second cancers like angiosarcomas.

23.3 Radiation Recall Phenomenon

Use of certain chemotherapeutic agents like doxorubicin, daunorubicin or actinomycin D post-radiotherapy leads to onset of skin reactions which resemble those seen earlier during treatment with external beam radiotherapy. Thus the chemotherapeutic agent "recalls" the reactions caused earlier by the external beam radiotherapy received by the patient. These reactions are not dose dependent and may occur idiosyncratically. Thus patients receiving these agents especially after radiotherapy should be carefully monitored for skin reactions. Treatment is usually symptomatic and as per standard recommendations for skin reactions caused by radiotherapy.

23.4 Care of Skin Reactions

Care of skin reactions is directed towards maintaining the integrity of the skin if still present and preventing further exacerbation of the reactions and symptomatic management towards resolution of present lesions. It is important to counsel patients before starting therapy towards expected reactions and measures to be taken to avoid them as far as possible. Moist skin can lead to more severe reactions, and it is important to keep the skin clean and dry. Scrubbing the skin and use of soap should be avoided during radiotherapy; the person should bathe regularly and use a soft cloth to dry himself/herself using gentle patting motions. If powder is used, then talcum powder or other commercial preparations should be avoided and baby powder used. Also perfumed skin creams/lotions should be avoided as they contain astringents which may further damage the labile skin [6].

During treatment it is important to avoid extremes of temperature and excess exposure. Cosmetics and lotions should not be used. Clothing should be loose and

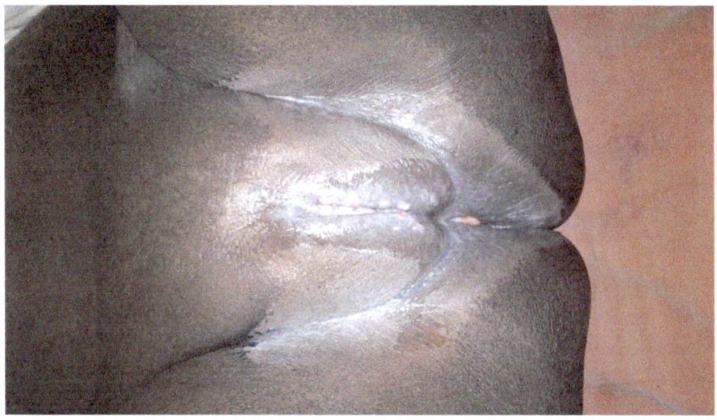

Fig. 23.5 Skin reactions after healing with thinning of skin

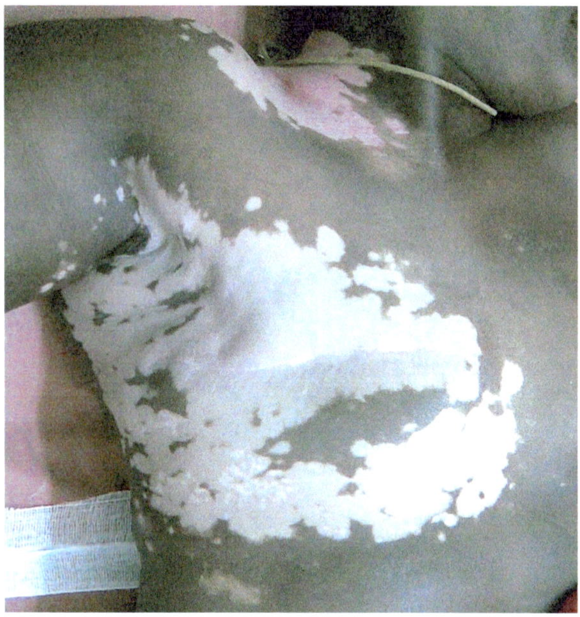

Fig. 23.6 Post-radiotherapy depigmentation of skin over treated field

non-constricting with no elastic bands present. Material should be cotton or linen. In case of mild skin erythema or itching, 1% hydrocortisone is used [7]. If moist desquamation takes place, active care is required to avoid infection. Hydrocortisone lotion, 1% gentian violet or peroxide lotion can be applied over affected area which should be kept clean and dry. Systemic or topical antibiotics can be prescribed if required based on swab culture sensitivity reports. Non-adherent dressings are applied for moist desquamation both during and after radiotherapy. Even after completion of therapy, patient should continue to wear loose and soft clothing to avoid abrasions. Use of scrubbing or non-pH neutral soaps should be avoided at least for the first 3 months.

Post-therapy, the skin over the treated area will remain thinner and dryer for many months (Fig. 23.5). There may also be either hypo- or hyperpigmentation over the treated area (Fig. 23.6). In case of severe reactions having occurred during radiotherapy, there may not be healing having taken place resulting in formation of

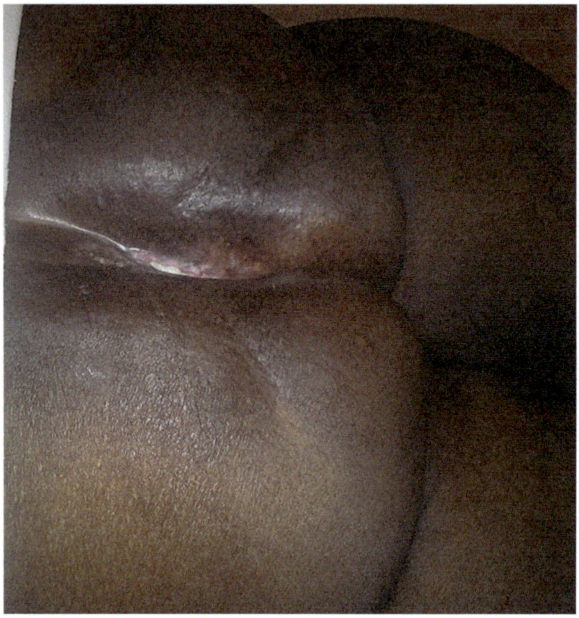

Fig. 23.7 Post-radiotherapy deep seated ulceration and necrosis over the posterior aspect of sacrum in this case of cervical cancer

deep-seated ulcers with necrosis of underlying tissues and even bones/cartilage (Fig. 23.7). There is increased risk even after treatment for the first 3–6 months of abrasions leading to erythema and further reactions, and hence use of razor or exposure to harsh climate and fabrics is to be avoided during this period.

References

1. Cohen L, Creditor M. Iso-effect tables for tolerance of irradiated normal human tissues. Int J Radiat Oncol Biol Phys. 1983;9:233–41.
2. Gorodetsky R, Mou X, Fisher DR, et al. Radiation effect in mouse skin: dose fractionation and wound healing. Int J Radiat Oncol Biol Phys. 1990;18:1077.
3. Rubin P, Casarett GW. Clinical radiation pathology, Vols. 1 and 2. Philadelphia: WB Saunders; 1968.
4. Withers HR, Taylor JMG, Maciejewski B. Treatment volume and tissue tolerance. Int J Radiat Oncol Biol Phys. 1988;14:751.
5. Cox JD, Stetz J, Pajak TF. Toxicity criteria of the Radiation Therapy Oncology Group (RTOG) and the European Organization for Research and Treatment of Cancer (EORTC). Int J Radiat Oncol Biol Phys. 1995;31(5):1341–6.
6. Campbell I, Illingworth M. Can patients wash during radiotherapy to the breast or chest wall? A randomized controlled trial. Clin Oncol. 1992;4:78–82.
7. Thomas S. Wound management and dressings. London: The Pharmaceutical Press; 1990.

24 Management of GI Complications

24.1 Pathophysiology

As described in Chap. 21, tissues are supposed to be composed of functional subunits (FSUs), which are the minimum clonogenic entity required for regeneration of a structure. This concept of functional subunits can explain why some tissues require tolerance doses as a mean value and why for some other tissues the tolerance dose is limited by a maximal cut-off point dose. Organs with acinar or alveolar architecture (like the kidney, salivary glands, pancreas, sweat glands, testis, mammary epithelium, lung and even liver) have structurally defined FSUs, while the target cells in the dermis, CNS, various mucosae, gut and epidermis are less restricted by physical barriers, and cellular migration may influence regeneration. Also the concept of volume effect is important in normal tissue sparing especially in tissues with serial FSUs like the spinal cord, the nerve tracts or the small bowel where the loss of one subunit may result in an overt expression of injury, regardless of the state of the other subunits in the series. The probability of a serious injury increases with the volume exposed (i.e. the number of FSUs exposed) and has been demonstrated for small bowel obstruction [1].

The mucosa of the oesophagus is contiguous with the oropharyngeal mucosa and suffers also from irradiation to the lower neck or thorax and upper abdomen. The radiation beams affect the rapidly dividing cells of the oesophageal mucosa and also the cells of the crypts in the small bowel. The damage is not immediately apparent as the well-differentiated superficial layers are relatively undamaged. The initial site of damage is the capillary network of these cells with loss of pericytes and increased capillary dilatation and leakage resulting in pericellular oedema. This along with the DNA damage to the basal cells themselves results not only in loss of reproductive ability of these cells but also in the loss of cellular membrane integrity.

In the small and large intestines and stomach, after the superficial layers are lost as a result of the continuous turnover that these tissues are subjected to, anatomical damage to the mucosa starts becoming apparent with loss-of-function postirradiation of the basal or cryptic cells which are then unable to replenish the losses the gut mucosa

A. Mukherji, *Basics of Planning and Management of Patients during Radiation Therapy*, https://doi.org/10.1007/978-981-10-6659-7_24

Table 24.1 RTOG grading system [2] used for assessing oesophageal reactions

Grade	RTOG criteria (oesophagus)
Grade 0 (none)	No changes
Grade 1 (mild)	Mild dysphagia/odynophagia, requires soft diet
Grade 2 (moderate)	Moderate dysphagia/odynophagia, requires liquid diet
Grade 3 (severe)	Severe dysphagia/odynophagia with dehydration or weight loss requiring NG feeding/IV fluids or hyperalimentation
Grade 4 (life-threatening)	Complete obstruction/ulceration/perforation/fistula

is subject to. These cells are very rapidly dividing with a turnover every 2 days, and radiation damage can lead to delayed or arrested mitosis or loss of cell membrane integrity. Initial changes present as punctate follicles and superficial ulcers along with submucosal oedema which may gradually deepen and coalesce with continuing radiation damage to give rise to deep-seated ulcers or patchy areas of raw mucosa followed by confluent areas of raw mucosa and surrounding erythema. Further injury can result in large-scale necrosis with perforation or even stricture formation, the results of which can be catastrophic. As the lesions become apparent anatomically and increase in severity, the patient starts complaining of local pain with progressive difficulty in food or fluid intake, with rapid decrease in general body nutrition and hydration.

Radiation-induced damage to the stomach is usually dose dependent. The damage to gastric and intestinal mucosa like oesophageal mucosa is also due to capillary damage followed by loss of the dividing cells resulting in the appearance of symptoms of radiation damage (Table 24.1).

24.2 Clinical Importance

In irradiation of the chest and abdomen, common early effects seen are oesophagitis and enteritis which if not controlled can progress to chronic inflammatory lesions and even stricture formation. Oesophagitis usually starts after completion of the second or third week of therapy, usually at a dose of 20–30 Gy, and can worsen towards the end of treatment. Clinical symptoms of oesophagitis range from mild substernal burning or discomfort to severe angina-like pain or severe dysphagia or even life-threatening mediastinitis, causing sudden collapse of patient [3]. Common symptoms are sore throat, feeling of "lump" in throat, pain or difficulty in swallowing and burning retro- or substernal pain. The incidence and severity of these symptoms are dependent on the dose, presence of oesophageal disease and whether concurrent chemotherapy is given [4, 5]. The symptoms can resolve over the next 6–7 weeks, about the end of the second month post-radiotherapy in many cases, but can also develop into a chronic problem requiring break in treatment as well as alimentation.

Another important intervention in the initial stages of both oesophagitis and enteritis is the control of radiation-induced nausea and vomiting. This occurs especially when large abdominal, chest or head fields are irradiated and have both central and local components. Various factors affecting this set of symptoms include fraction size (the larger the fraction, the more is the symptom), field size, age of patient, level of anxiety and site of irradiation. The mildest symptoms are described as indigestion, while more severe episodes can be accompanied by weakness, palpitations, sweating, increased respiratory rate and tachycardia. These symptoms usually start within the first 3 weeks of therapy, but in cases where concurrent chemotherapy is being given, they may start immediately after chemotherapy itself and therefore are described as chemo-induced vomiting.

In the stomach, after 2 weeks of radiotherapy, there is a reduction in all gastric secretions, followed by the development of gastritis with resultant hyperaemia, punctate haemorrhages and oedema. This is followed by the development of symptoms by the end of the third week of radiotherapy and may lead to pyloric spasm, anorexia and weight loss. Similarly enteritis starts towards the end of the third or fourth week of therapy beyond 25 Gy dose and can resolve over the next 4–5 weeks. If the area being irradiated is large and proper anti-emetic prophylaxis as well as fluid support not given, patients can develop moderate to severe diarrhoea with resultant break in treatment. Also in moderate to severe cases of enteric reactions to radiotherapy, there can be loss of villi and microvilli over a large part of the bowel mucosal surface especially in the large intestine which can lead later to the onset of malabsorption syndromes [6].

24.3 Care of Reactions

Aims for treatment of radiation-induced oesophagitis include prevention of further damage to mucosa, starting treatment for repair of already damaged mucosa, symptomatic treatment and maintenance of nutrition and hydration. General measures for care of a patient with dysphagia and regurgitation include:

- Elevation of head end of bed while in supine position to prevent aspiration. It is important to remember that in most of these patients, the gag reflex is decreased, and the risk of these patients developing aspiration pneumonitis is very high.
- Food should be avoided within 2–3 h of going to bed.
- Putting in a Ryle's tube for aspiration if required or maintaining nutrition by a feeding gastrostomy/jejunostomy.
- Providing high-calorie, high-protein liquid or semisolid diet composed either of medicinal preparations or bland food which is soft in consistency. Foods which are spicy or irritating (like carbonated drinks, alcohol, raw juices, hard biscuits) should be avoided. But high-protein foods should be avoided in the acute phase of reactions as proteins stimulate gastrin secretion which can worsen reactions.
- Single large meals should be avoided and replaced by small frequent meals to avoid stretching and further damage to the mucosa as well as damage from reflux due to the radiation-induced laxity of the lower oesophageal sphincter.
- Preventing stressful stimuli such as odours or sights which precipitate emesis and use of prophylactic measures for control of emesis, pain, dehydration or decreased oral intake.

- Nutritional counselling to be provided to all patients and hydration and weight to be monitored on a weekly basis. In case of severe deficiencies, to institute early parenteral nutrition so as to avoid long treatment breaks as these are directly correlated with response and survival.

Symptomatic therapy involves use of pro-motility drugs like metoclopramide to decrease reflux and antacids to decrease or counteract gastric acid secretion, and preparations of alginic acid help by forming a coat over the mucosa and preventing contact with acidic secretions allowing the mucosa time to heal. Similarly other liquid preparations are also used including aluminium hydroxide and local anaesthetic combinations (e.g. Mucaine™) to also coat and heal the damaged mucosa. Drugs like nifedipine are used for treating oesophageal spasm [7]. After managing the acute phase, it is important as previously discussed to maintain hydration and nutrition so as to avoid as far as possible treatment breaks. Late effects of radiation-induced damage include formation of strictures and stenosis leading to obstruction, ulceration and oesophageal perforation due to both radiation-induced damaged and local tumour necrosis. Other effects not commonly seen are heart decompensation especially if the dose to more than 60% of heart volume exceeds 40 Gy. Treatment includes use of aspirin and corticosteroids for treatment of myocarditis and pericarditis as well as monitoring for pericardial tamponade and myocardial dysfunction.

Treatment for nausea and vomiting includes symptomatic management, relief of precipitating factors, administering anti-emetics as a prophylactic measure, control of hypoglycaemia and dehydration, nutritional supplementation, monitoring of fluid and electrolyte balance and preventing exposure to pro-emetic stimuli like odours or sights. Various drugs used include metoclopramide, haloperidol, pyridoxine, phenothiazines, 5HT3 receptor blocking drugs like ondansetron, antihistaminic drugs like cyclizine as well as steroids. Other general measures followed include those described in this section previously. Antidiarrhoeal drugs such as loperamide or octeotride are used to bring down frequency and severity of loose motions. First loperamide should be started every 2–3 hourly for a maximum of 48 h. If the diarrhoea has not responded, then switch to octreotide at dose of 50 μg SC every 8 h, and increase dose to 100 μg if response not noted. Antibiotics are rarely required. Abdominal cramps are common and can be treated with dicyclomine.

Management of bowel toxicities depends on site irradiated and field volume as well as dose delivered. Most of these cases present with mild to moderate diarrhoea. The principal line of management is in maintaining fluid balance, monitoring fluid and electrolyte levels, taking care of spasmodic pain and emesis and later managing malabsorption syndromes if any as well as other late toxicities like strictures and adhesions causing obstructions, ulcerations and perforations. In case of the rectum, local care in the form of enemas (steroid-sucralfate) or commercially available creams can be used. Laser coagulation of telangiectasias and punctate haemorrhages is another method. An important point is to ensure high-roughage, low-residue diet so as to decrease the bowel transit time and allow reactions to heal. In case of severe reactions with deep-seated ulcerations, temporary diversion colostomy is done to allow passage of faecal matter and allow lesion to heal.

Patients should be encouraged to drink a minimum of 2.5–3 L of fluids per day. Foods rich in roughage and calcium as well as potassium should be advised. In case of parenteral nutrition for bowel rest or severe reactions, low-osmolality, low-residue formulae should be used. If IV fluids are used more than 72 h, then IV amino acids should be added. After patients are put back on oral nutrition, they are given frequent small meals of easily digestible food which is bland and non-irritating to the mucosa. Milk and milk products are usually avoided as lactase deficiency can lead to lactose intolerance with resultant surge in distension, flatulence and cramps. However yoghurt or curd can be given if neutropenia is absent as the lactobacilli help in fermentation of food material (milk products) in the gut decreasing flatulence.

Recent recommendations state that sulfasalazine taken orally twice a day can reduce the incidence and severity of radiation-induced bowel changes in patients on radiotherapy. However 5-amino salicylic acid (5-ASA) compounds cannot prevent GI mucositis. According to other recommendations, sucralfate enemas can control or heal chronic radiation-induced proctitis and rectal bleeding, while systemic glutamine shows no benefit in the prevention of GI mucositis. Octreotide at doses above 100 μg given subcutaneously twice daily after failure of loperamide can control chemotherapy-induced diarrhoea.

References

1. Letschert JG, Lebesque JV, Aleman BM, et al. The volume effect in radiation-related late small bowel complications: results of a clinical study of the EROTC Radiotherapy Cooperative Group in patients treated for rectal carcinoma. Radiother Oncol. 1994;32:116.
2. Cox JD, Stetz J, Pajak TF. Toxicity criteria of the Radiation Therapy Oncology Group (RTOG) and the European Organization for Research and Treatment of Cancer (EORTC). Int J Radiat Oncol Biol Phys. 1995;31(5):1341–6.
3. Finkelstein E. Nifedipine for radiation and esophagitis. Lancet. 1986;i:1205–6. (Letter to Editor).
4. Cooper JS, Guo MD, Herskovic A, et al. Chemoradiotherapy of locally advanced esophageal cancer: long-term follow-up of a prospective randomized trial (RTOG 85-01)—Radiation Therapy Oncology Group. JAMA. 1999;281:1623–7.
5. Stahl M, Stuschke M, Lehmann N, et al. Chemoradiation with and without surgery in patients with locally advanced squamous cell carcinoma of the esophagus. J Clin Oncol. 2005;23:2310–7.
6. Jervis HR, Donati M, Stromberg LR, Sprinz H. Histochemical investigation of the mucosa of the exteriorized small intestine of the rat exposed to x-irradiation. Strahlentherapie. 1977; 138:326–9.
7. Unsawadi T, Valdiviesco M, Barkley HT. Esophageal complications from combined chemradiotherapy (cyclophosphamide + Adriamycin + cisplatin + XRT) in the treatment of non-small cell lung cancer. Int J Radiat Oncol Biol Phys. 1985;11:511–9.

25 Managing Local Pain

25.1 Pathophysiology of Pain

Pain in cancer patients may be a result of tissue damage by the tumour, such as bone destruction by a metastasis or invasion of the nerve plexus by cancer, or from the treatment received (like radiotherapy or surgery). At the time of diagnosis, about one-third of cancer patients suffer from pain, while in advanced stages, at least two-thirds suffer. Cancer itself causes about 80–90% of pain syndromes, while in 20–40% of cases, pain is therapy induced. Only 2–4% of cancer patients suffer from chronic pain unrelated to cancer. Irradiation of normal tissues, especially those with a rapid growth turnover rate, causes cell death and triggers a cascade of pro-inflammatory cytokines, thrombotic factors and growth factors, causing local painful reactions [1]. Both early and late stages of cancer can result in patients presenting with severe pain, though it is more common in advanced stages. Current medical management of pain is one of the many modalities and is based on the World Health Organization (WHO)'s principle of an "analgesic ladder" that involves a stepwise intensification in the class of analgesic drugs used for cancer pain relief. This "ladder" is basically more of a set of guiding principles rather than a rigid protocol [2].

25.2 Types of Pain

Pain is generally defined as either nociceptive or non-nociceptive. Nociceptive pain is the response of the nervous system proportionate to the tissue damage initiating the response and is divided into somatic pain and visceral pain, depending on the location and symptoms of the painful stimulus. Typically, somatic pain presents as a well-localized, sharp, stabbing (knife-like) and achy pain as a response to skin, muscle and connective tissue damage. On the other hand, visceral pain is difficult to localize and often presents as a cramping or a dull ache [3].

Non-nociceptive pain includes both neuropathic and psychogenic (or idiopathic) components where the nervous system responses are not related to the damage

A. Mukherji, *Basics of Planning and Management of Patients during Radiation Therapy*, https://doi.org/10.1007/978-981-10-6659-7_25

causing the response and responses may occur without tissue damage. Neuropathic pain involves abnormal pain processing by the peripheral or central nervous system. Patients may complain of burning, shooting, tingling or numbness, which generally occurs along a nerve distribution [4]. Patients may also experience pain that is out of proportion to their physical injury. Psychogenic causes (i.e. depression and anxiety) may exacerbate the perception of painful stimuli.

25.3 Management of Pain

The *2005 APS Guideline for the Management of Cancer Pain in Adults and Children* discusses cancer pain management algorithms, psychological strategies, supportive therapy, integration of non-medical and medical treatments as well as other modalities like nerve blocks, surgical strategies, radiation therapy and chemotherapy as well as patient education and adherence to the pain management plan, as well as improving quality of care [1, 5]. Modalities include use of medicines (opioids, non-opioids or anti-inflammatory agents), radiotherapy, chemotherapy, adjuvant drugs and surgical methods like tumour debulking, nerve blocks, plexus blocks as well as use of bisphosphonates. Radiotherapy is also a valuable modality in the treatment of cancer pain. It is commonly used in the palliative setting when a radiosensitive cancer invades the bone, soft tissue or nerves [6].

25.4 Pain Palliation by Oral Medication

Management of pain especially that induced by cancer in modern practice by the use of medications is still traditionally based on the World Health Organization (WHO)'s "analgesic ladder", which allows the practitioner an important flexibility in the choice of drugs. A very important part of this WHO stepladder method is an increased encouragement on the correct use of oral opioids for both moderate and severe pain. Also the use of analgesics is combined with both disease-modifying therapies and nondrug measures so as to achieve greater analgesic effect for dosages prescribed. Oral administration of drugs has been proven to be safe, effective and easy, supporting the autonomy of patients and keeping them independent of specific medical or technical help. Drugs are administered according to the duration of their activity. This means that medication needs to be taken at fixed time intervals. *For dose titration as well as for breakthrough pain, normal-release (NR) or immediate-release (IR) preparations are preferred. After determination of the dose for pain control, sustained-release (SR) formulations can be useful.* Pain therapy is built up stepwise (the "WHO analgesic ladder"). Pain therapy is initiated with non-opioids. Weak opioids are added in step 2. If pain control remains insufficient, weak opioids are replaced by strong opioids. Non-opioids should be continued in steps 2 and 3. Depending on the pain modality, co-analgesic and adjuvant drugs may be added at each level. Frequent and serious unwanted side effects should be treated prophylactically.

25.5 WHO Ladder

The "WHO analgesic ladder" is basically a sequence of instructions involving a three-step drug class escalation depending upon a patient's response to each class of analgesic started. Every cancer patient, and especially those in advanced stages, should be evaluated for presence and severity of pain which should be accordingly treated using the three-step ladder, and the response of these patients' to such therapy should be reassessed and recorded periodically at short intervals with interventions made if such response is not deemed adequate.

First step (phase I non-opioids): The first analgesic intervention is by prescribing oral non-opioids (aspirin or paracetamol) for mild pain; an adjuvant drug for treatment of other associated symptoms can be added. Nonsteroidal anti-inflammatory drugs (NSAIDs) have excellent anti-inflammatory properties [7]. Therefore, they have some advantages in pain caused by bone or periosteal metastasis and in inflammatory processes. These include acetaminophen, non-specific cyclooxygenase inhibitors (including ibuprofen, diclofenac and aspirin) and cyclooxygenase-2 inhibitors (celecoxib and meloxicam). Their gastrointestinal toxicities increase with the concomitant administration of corticosteroids or aspirin.

Second step (phase II mild opioids): After the use of the initial non-opioid analgesics, if the pain is not relieved, then the practitioner can escalate to the next class of drugs which are weak opioids such as codeine. However the use of adjuvant drugs for associated symptoms should still be continued as required.

Third step (phase III strong opioids): If the pain has not responded to use of weak opioids, then strong opioids like oral morphine should be considered. The various steps in the introduction and titration of the optimum morphine dose and preparation are explained in the subsequent section. It is however important to remember that the dose of morphine should be increased stepwise till relief of pain is achieved or side effects cannot be tolerated by the patient. Usually opioids such as morphine are commonly used, while drugs such as pethidine (has a short duration of action and has accumulation of toxic metabolite) or pentazocine (has weak analgesic effect with a ceiling dose and may cause withdrawal effects) are better avoided. As in the previous steps, in this step also, adjuvant drugs are used to further enhance pain relief and take care of other symptoms. In case of a patient presenting with moderate to severe pain, the practitioner can straight away start with step 3, and if pain is continuous, immediate-release morphine should be started at 4-h intervals around the clock.

25.6 Barriers to Pain Relief

Good pain relief in cancer patients can translate into multiple benefits for the patient and the treating team. In cases where cure or control is possible, pain relief can result in improved compliance as well as a feeling of wellness which can translate into improved response and survival. In advanced cases where palliation is the aim, good pain relief will result in improved quality of life and dignity on part of the patient.

However, many times because of many factors, such desired pain relief is not achieved resulting in distress for the patient and frustration felt by the treating team. The reasons for such failure include lack of education and training, fear of addiction, as well as restricted availability of morphine because of strict regulation.

- A common factor is the lack of knowledge or awareness in both health professionals and patients about the importance of pain management can result in selection of inadequate drugs or dosages.
- Hence because of specific administering steps to be followed, it is recommended that the prescription and administration of morphine should be given by doctors and nurses who are properly trained in pain management as well as palliative care.
- Also fears and concerns about possible risk of addiction and non-intended diversion of morphine on part of unexposed medical practitioners can result in limitation in the proper use and availability of morphine. However this fact has not been supported by data which in fact reports that addiction is rare when morphine is used to treat cancer pain (WHO Technical Report Series, No. 804). But for many practitioners not properly trained, addiction is often confused with physical dependence, which is an expected result of morphine use, and results in limitations in the use of opioids to treat cancer pain [2].
- Similarly strict regulation of morphine use and distribution as well as complicated bureaucratic procedures can discourage the development of manufacturing capabilities. This limits availability of morphine for cancer patients and results in shortages which necessitate rationing of morphine to patients. As a result dose optimization is restricted leading to poor pain relief.

This WHO ladder approach if used correctly is a proven safe and effective method of achieving cancer pain control and is simple as well as inexpensive and can achieve pain relief in 80–90% of patients [2]. But for utilizing this system effectively, it is important that health professionals be properly trained in the use and distribution of morphine to avoid loss or unauthorized use.

25.7 Recommendations for Prescribing Morphine

While starting morphine for pain not relieved by phase I and II methods, we have to remember the following points [8]:

1. Morphine is basically a step 3 analgesic and should only be prescribed for pain after there has been minimal or no relief even after maximal dose usage of a step 2 drug or in cases where the patient presents initially with severe pain.

2. The prescribed dose of morphine needs to be titrated to achieve good pain control. Oral morphine is initially given as an oral solution or standard formulation tablets. Calculation of the starting dose of morphine is based on the analgesic already being used so as to provide greater pain relief than existing drug. Thus there is no fixed starting dose; a low dose of 5–10 mg can be sufficient to improve pain relief compared to a weaker drug like NSAID or paracetamol, though higher doses of 20–50 mg may be required if the patient is already on a stronger analgesic.
3. One-third of patients can experience nausea in the first few days of taking morphine. An anti-emetic (e.g. cyclizine) should always be prescribed with morphine.
4. Most patients can develop constipation on morphine. Hence a regular laxative (e.g. senna + docusate) should always be prescribed with morphine.
5. Some patients will experience mild sleepiness in the first few days of taking morphine. This almost always wears off. Drowsiness/fatigue in a patient with advanced disease is almost certainly disease related.
6. If signs of opioid toxicity occur (confusion, twitching, hallucinations), the opioid dose should be reduced by one-third.
7. The aim is to choose the lowest possible dose of morphine that achieves pain relief. If the initial dose of morphine provides no benefit over the previous analgesic, the dose should be increased by 30–50% every 2–3 days till pain relief is achieved for a dosage schedule. It is important to remember that the frequency of each dose for standard formulation tablets is 4 h (*by the clock*) [8]. To further augment the response, an adjuvant analgesic (antidepressants or anticonvulsant agents) may be added.
8. Since the dose scheduling of the standard morphine tablets is four hourly, it may be necessary to provide a double dose at bedtime to allow for 6–8 h of pain-free sleep to the patient. Whenever pain reoccurs in between regular doses of morphine (*breakthrough pain*), additional doses, which are equal in strength to the regular dose (*rescue dose*) as either oral solution or standard formulation tablets, are given and are then included in the total daily calculated dose [9].
9. Once pain is controlled and a final estimate by repeated titration of the patient's daily morphine requirement is calculated, this dose can then be given divided into 12-hourly doses in the form of modified-release (MR) or sustained-release (SR) capsules instead of the standard tablet formulations. The first dose of this MR or SR morphine should be given 4 h after the last dose of the standard formulation [8].

Normal-release preparations of morphine are preferred during dose titration as they have a rapid onset but a short duration of action. This allows for a quick establishment of a steady state, and peak plasma concentrations are seen within the first hour after oral administration (Hoskin et al.) [10], while onset of analgesia then lasts for about 4 h. This then allows calculation of the strength required per dose to obtain adequate analgesia, and once this amount has been calculated for a 24-h period, it is then converted to two 12-h doses as MR/SR capsules.

25.8 Indications for Subcutaneous or Intravenous Morphine

The above-mentioned guidelines for morphine prescription are for the oral route of administration. However there may be situations where the patient cannot take medications orally. In such a situation, usually, the preferred route of morphine administration is subcutaneous, rather than an intramuscular injection which may be more painful when repeated for multiple doses.

Another option is of intravenous infusion of morphine, for which there are very definite indications. Intravenous morphine infusion is specifically indicated in patients with an indwelling intravenous line requiring chronic sustained analgesia and poor general condition; patients with generalized edema or those who have developed erythema, soreness or sterile abscesses with subcutaneous administration; patients with coagulation disorders; as well as patients with poor peripheral circulation where absorption of the drug from the subcutaneous capillary system may not be assured.

The next point to remember while opting for parenteral administration of morphine is the dosage to be given. As a general rule, the relative potency ratio of oral morphine to both the subcutaneously administered morphine and intravenous morphine is between 1:2 and 1:3 (i.e. 20–30 mg of oral morphine is equianalgesic to 10 mg by SC/IV injection) [11].

25.9 Alternates to Oral Morphine

In addition to the previously mentioned alternatives to oral morphine (viz. subcutaneous and IV morphine), various other alternatives to oral morphine also exist. These are spinal or intrathecal morphine; other opioids like hydromorphone, oxycodone or methadone given orally; and intrathecal or transdermal fentanyl. The oral alternatives of hydromorphone/methadone or oxycodone are not very popular because of pronounced differences in their plasma half-life, relative analgesic potency and duration of action from patient to patient, and therefore the optimum doses cannot be easily titrated, and hence their use by non-specialist practitioners is not recommended. Methadone is a long-acting opiate receptor antagonist and also acts as an NMDA (*N*-methyl-D-aspartate) receptor antagonist, preventing morphine tolerance [12]. Also whenever a patient has to be shifted from oral morphine to any of these drugs or to study the relative efficacy of these drugs to morphine, conversion factors are used (e.g. *2 mg of PO methadone is roughly equivalent to 30 mg of PO morphine, while 2 mg of PO methadone is about equivalent to 1 mg of IV methadone*). Finally it is important to remember that when changing from one opiate to another, a reduction factor is sometimes initially applied (which may be 25–75% of the original drug's dose) because of reduced tolerance to the new medication.

Spinal (epidural or intrathecal) use of opioid analgesics along with local anaesthetics or clonidine is usually contemplated in patients with inadequate analgesia from regular optimum treatment or in those suffering intolerable adverse effects. **Intrathecal morphine (ITM)** can provide significant and safe analgesia for between 12 and 24 h and is especially indicated after procedures such as total hip replacement, total knee replacement and laparotomies for frail, elderly patients. The recommended dose is 100–200 μg, which may be increased up to 0.3 mg (300 μg) in selected cases. The onset of action is within 30–60 min, and thus ITM is given by the anaesthetist immediately before surgery.

However intrathecal morphine (ITM) has its limitations. It is relatively contraindicated in patients with a known history of postoperative nausea and vomiting and absolutely contraindicated in patients with known sensitivities to morphine, advanced respiratory disease or obstructive sleep apnoea or those already receiving high-dose opioids or CNS depressants. Though the risk of serious respiratory depression requiring intervention is low, such risk increases with patient age and ASA (anaesthetic risk classification) status.

Transdermal fentanyl usually administered as an adhesive patch is an effective alternative to oral morphine especially for patients with stable opioid requirements. Fentanyl has a low molecular weight with high lipid solubility and is easily absorbed through the skin. Post-application, the drug first enters the circulation which may take up to 1–2 h, after which the serum levels rise gradually. The analgesic effects start within 8–16 h after application, and a steady state is achieved at 72 h [13]. Each patch may be applied for 3 days during which, with continued use, an intradermal depot is formed which allows maintenance of the analgesic effect for up to 16 h even after removal of the patch.

Intrathecal fentanyl is another alternative to morphine with very few significant side effects. A dose of about 25 μg may provide analgesia for 80–130 min. Addition of a small amount (1–2 mL) of 0.5% bupivacaine to intrathecal fentanyl can help by significantly speeding up the onset of analgesia to within 10 min, and this analgesic action also lasts for same duration (2–4 h). An important side effect is the risk of early respiratory depression, occurring within 2 h of administration, though no late respiratory depression has been reported. Other effects commonly include pruritus, nausea and vomiting, which may be managed conservatively. Adding an epidural local anaesthetic to intrathecal fentanyl could be more effective in managing movement-related pain [14], while adding clonidine could help in neuropathic pain [15].

25.10 Side Effects of Opioid Therapy

Nausea and vomiting: Within the first 2 weeks of opioid therapy, 40–60% of patients suffer from nausea and vomiting. This can be caused by different mechanisms: irritation of the dopaminergic D2 receptor-binding site in the area postrema, delayed gastric emptying and constipation. Therefore, it seems advisable to offer some anti-emetics, prophylactically, preferably with D2 receptor antagonistic activity during this period.

Sedation/delirium: Sedation is expected when opioid therapy is started. It is more pronounced in elderly and cachectic patients and is intensified by co-medication with other centrally acting drugs (e.g. benzodiazepines, antidepressants, neuroleptics and antihypertensive drugs). In the majority of patients, sedation is reduced or even disappears in the course of treatment. If it persists or is complicated by delirium or confusion, lowering the dose or changing the opioid needs to be considered.

Constipation: Constipation is the most common and persistent side effect of opioids. It causes nausea, vomiting and loss of appetite and weight; it impairs general well-being and activity; and it can be dangerous when it leads to bowel obstruction. Constipation is mediated by the central nervous system (brain and spinal cord) as well as by the intestinal nervous system. Constipation increases rather than decreases in the course of treatment, and its prophylactic treatment is obligatory.

Respiratory depression: The respiratory depressant potency of opioids is correlated with their intrinsic activity at the μ receptor and is characterized by rapid tachyphylaxis. Respiratory depression hardly ever occurs if the dose has been titrated correctly with oral therapy.

Antitussive effect: Suppression of the protective cough reflex is maximal at dosages below those required for analgesia. It is not correlated with μ-receptor binding.

Urinary retention: Urinary retention occurs predominantly in patients with pre-existing disorders, such as neurogenic dysuria or benign prostatic hypertrophy. This can be treated medically with carbachol (10–40 mg/day) or phenoxybenzamine (10–40 mg/day). Sometimes, a urinary catheter is necessary.

Pruritus: Opioids may cause pruritus, especially within the perioral zone, without any skin reaction. This side effect is more frequent in spinal opioid therapy and usually disappears gradually. Patients must be instructed that this phenomenon is different from allergy.

25.11 Role of Adjuvant Therapy

Using the WHO ladder, most pain related to cancer can be managed with oral medications in 70–85% of patients [16, 17]. At any point of the WHO analgesic ladder, adjuvant therapy can be initiated to supplement NSAIDs and opioid treatment. *Benefits of adjuvant therapy include use of medications tailored towards specific causes of nociceptive responses (i.e. neuropathic) and reduction of opiate side effects.* Neuropathic pain is generally not responsive to opiate medications, unless significantly high doses are used, so other classes of drugs are often prescribed [18]. Anticonvulsants, such as gabapentin, carbamazepine and pregabalin, are known to be effective in managing neuropathic symptoms [4]. Both gabapentin and pregabalin are excreted by the kidneys and have minimal drug-drug interactions and are effective for first-line treatment for neuropathic pain [4].

Antidepressants are another broad category of medications that stabilize neurons involved in neuropathic pain. Tricyclic antidepressants in low doses, such as amitriptyline, have been well studied for pain relief [19]. Serotonin reuptake inhibitors and newer classes of antidepressants, including selective serotonin and norepinephrine reuptake inhibitors (duloxetine and venlafaxine), are also commonly prescribed for neuropathic pain because many patients also have depressive or anxiety symptoms, and thus antidepressants have a dual role to play resulting in improved efficacy [19].

In a patient with neuropathic pain, the radiation oncologist may prescribe an anticonvulsant at low doses, titrating the dose to improve analgesia while monitoring side effects. Antidepressant treatment can be also started especially if patients exhibit signs of depression or anxiety, and then add the anticonvulsant as a secondary medication. In any case, both medications can be used synergistically to improve analgesia for neuropathic pain. Ketamine, a specific NMDA receptor antagonist, is also used to relieve cancer and neuropathic pain, especially refractory pain [20]. Other adjuvant analgesic drug classes used in cancer therapy include local anaesthetics, steroids, muscle relaxants, benzodiazepines, adrenergic agonists and bisphosphonates [20].

25.12 Surgical and Neuroablative Techniques

Although most pain symptoms can be managed with oral and intravenous medications, the regimen may become insufficient or side effects become intolerable. A variety of neurolytic procedures with the goal of reducing pain medication requirements can be used. Bulky tumours can press on nerve plexuses or visceral organs and cause pain which can be relieved simply by tumour debulking by surgical excision or by chemotherapy in case of chemosensitive tumours. The release of pressure by the tumour can result in almost immediate relief from pain. Also in advanced tumours where surgery is not possible, radiotherapy is an important modality for pain palliation. Radiotherapy can result both in tumour shrinkage relieving pain or in strengthening of the skeletal frame in lytic bone metastases after tumour disappearance [6, 21]. But radiotherapy can also give rise to treatment-induced pain by causing mucositis, stricture, lymphoedema or fibrosis, which can be present in up to half the patients treated and has to be managed symptomatically [21].

Peripheral nerves after leaving the spinal cord can be exposed to various types of neurolytic procedures. Common nerves that are neurolysed include intercostal nerves (for thoracotomy pain), maxillary and mandibular nerves (for postherpetic neuralgia) and median branch nerves (for back pain) [22]. Cryoanalgesia techniques involve the application of subzero temperatures to induce Wallerian degeneration of neurons but allowing normal regrowth of axons. Radiofrequency techniques apply heat to nerves to cause damage. Chemical neurolysis can be achieved with phenol or alcohol preparations. Pain originating from the perineal, pelvic and abdominal regions is supplied by pain fibres following sympathetic fibres innervating the region. Along with the pain fibres, these sympathetic nerves coalesce at specific ganglia (impar, hypogastric and celiac, respectively). At these sites, image-guided neurolytic procedures can be performed with alcohol or phenol [23]. As the pain fibres are destroyed, the associated region is also sympathetically denervated.

Sympathetically mediated pain may present at an extremity with initial symptoms of swelling, redness and temperature change. Chronic skin changes, hair loss and muscle atrophy and disuse may follow [2]. Along with pharmacologic treatment, neuroablative techniques targeting sympathetic fibres to the upper extremity (stellate ganglion) and lower extremity (lumbar sympathetics) can be used to treat these syndromes [24]. Another technique of disrupting the flow of pain signals in the spinal cord involves electrostimulation techniques. Transcutaneous electrical nerve stimulation, spinal cord stimulators at thoracic and lumbar regions and deep-brain stimulators at the thalamus or motor cortex can interfere with the conduction of pain signals. The stimulation of large motor fibres inhibits the conduction of pain signals by small nerve fibres and has shown efficacy for various pain syndromes [25].

Neurosurgical techniques are used to treat refractory pain and in specific situations. Plexus root avulsions may be responsive to dorsal root entry zone lesions, but indications and success rates are limited [26]. More specific procedures at the spinal cord and central nervous system (e.g. thalamotomy and deep-brain stimulation) have also been used with variable success and significant side effects [27].

References

1. Gordon DB, Dahl JL, Miaskowski C, et al. American Pain Society recommendations for improving the quality of acute and cancer pain management: American Pain Society Quality of Care Task Force. Arch Intern Med. 2005;165:1574–80.
2. World Health Organization, Cancer Pain Relief: With a Guide to Opioid Availability, Second edition. 1996.
3. Besson JM, Chaouch A. Peripheral and spinal mechanisms of nociception. Physiol Rev. 1987;67:67–186.
4. Irving GA. Contemporary assessment and management of neuropathic pain. Neurology. 2005;64(12 Suppl 3):S21–7.
5. Miaskowski C, Cleary J. Guideline for the management of cancer pain in adults and children. Glenview: American Pain Society; 2005.
6. Friedland J. Local and systemic radiation for palliation of metastatic disease. Urol Clin North Am. 1999;26:391–402.
7. Bruera E. Mechanism of action of nonsteroidal anti-inflammatory drugs. Cancer Invest. 1998;16:538–9.
8. Hanks GW, et al. Morphine and alternative opioids in cancer pain: the EAPC recommendations. Br J Cancer. 2001;84(5):587–93.
9. Twycross RG. Control of pain. J R Coll Physicians Lond. 1984;18:32–9.
10. Hoskin PJ, Hanks GW, Aherne GW, Chapman D, Littleton P, Filshie J. The bioavailability and pharmacokinetics of morphine after intravenous, oral and buccal administration in healthy volunteers. Br J Clin Pharmacol. 1989;27:499–505.
11. Twycross RG. The therapeutic equivalence of oral and subcutaneous/intramuscular morphine sulphate in cancer patients. J Palliat Care. 1988;4:67–8.
12. Inturrisi CE. Pharmacology of methadone and its isomers. Minerva Anestesiol. 2005;71:435–7.
13. Lehmann KA, Zech D. Transdermal fentanyl: clinical pharmacology. J Pain Symptom Manage. 1992;7:S8–S16.
14. Mercadante S. Problems of long term spinal opioid treatment in advanced cancer patients. Pain. 1999;79:1–13.
15. Eisenach JC, DuPen S, Dubois M, Miguel R, Allin D. Epidural clonidine analgesia for intractable cancer pain. Pain. 1995;61:391–9.
16. Ventafridda V, Tamburini M, Caraceni A, et al. A validation study of the WHO method for cancer pain relief. Cancer. 1987;59:850–6.
17. Zech DF, Grond S, Lynch J, et al. Validation of World Health Organization Guidelines for cancer pain relief: a 10-year prospective study. Pain. 1995;63:65–76.
18. Milch RA. Neuropathic pain: implications for the surgeon. Surg Clin North Am. 2005;85: 225–36.

19. Hainline B. Chronic pain: physiological, diagnostic, and management considerations. Psychiatr Clin North Am. 2005;28:713–35.
20. Lussier D, Huskey AG, Portenoy RK. Adjuvant analgesics in cancer pain management. Oncologist. 2004;9:571–91.
21. Pignon T, Fernandez L, Ayasso S, et al. Impact of radiation oncology practice on pain: a cross-sectional survey. Int J Radiat Oncol Biol Phys. 2004;60:1204–10.
22. Trescot AM. Cryoanalgesia in interventional pain management. Pain Physician. 2003;6:345–60.
23. NIH Consensus Conference. Acupuncture. JAMA. 1998;280:1518–24.
24. Mekhail N, Kapural L. Complex regional pain syndrome type I in cancer patients. Curr Rev Pain. 2000;4:227–33.
25. Rushton DN. Electrical stimulation in the treatment of pain. Disabil Rehabil. 2002;24:407–15.
26. Sindou M, Mertens P. Neurosurgical management of neuropathic pain. Stereotact Funct Neurosurg. 2000;75:76–80.
27. Slavik E, Ivanovic S. Cancer pain (neurosurgical management). Acta Chir Iugosl. 2004;51:15–23.

Managing Bone Marrow Toxicities

26

26.1 Pathophysiology

Bone marrow is the principal haematopoietic tissue in the body, and in young patients, it is distributed in almost all bones, while in older people, it is mainly present in flat bones like the sternum, iliac crest and ribs. Bone marrow suppression following radiotherapy is generally not as severe as following chemotherapy as the effects post-radiotherapy are seen mostly locally in the exposed marrow and are usually compensated by the hyperactivity of remaining marrow. Severe reactions develop when chemotherapy and radiotherapy are given concurrently which affect marrow both locally and globally.

Unlike chemotherapy, radiotherapy affects both haematopoietic and stromal cells resulting in the disruption of bone marrow architecture, fibrosis and scarring of tissue, resulting in long-term effects like hypoplasia or aplasia. Studies have shown that regeneration of bone marrow is severely affected at doses above 30 Gy to marrow and goes into aplasia at doses above 45–50 Gy to marrow involving more than 25% of that particular bone marrow volume (Table 26.1).

26.2 Effect of Radiotherapy on Circulating Blood Cells

Anaemia: It is commonly seen in cancer patients and is generally mild but can be exacerbated by chemotherapy and radiotherapy as well as compounded by nutritional deficiencies as a result of reduced oral intake and absorption which may be a result of therapy-induced side effects. The life span of red blood cells (RBCs) is long at about 120 days, and hence the effects of therapy may not be immediately evident, taking some time to develop in the presence of continuing injury to red cell producing marrow and decrease in compensatory activities. Patients first present with signs and symptoms suggestive of tissue hypoxia as anaemia reduces oxygen transport to the tissues. Symptoms include easy fatigability, decrease in appetite, irritability, shortness of breath, headache, dizziness or constipation. Skin and

A. Mukherji, *Basics of Planning and Management of Patients during Radiation Therapy*, https://doi.org/10.1007/978-981-10-6659-7_26

Table 26.1 Percent bone marrow irradiation with standard radiotherapy portals

Site of irradiation	Percent bone marrow irradiated (%)
Chest wall	15–20
Abdomen	20–25
Lung fields/mediastinum	20–25
Pelvis	15–25
Mantle	20–50
Cranial	25–45
Craniospinal	60–75
Total lymphatic	60–70
Total body	100

mucous membranes become pale and listless. In severe cases, renal and circulatory functions are affected leading to life-threatening situations like sudden anasarca, angina due to myocardial hypoxia, renal tubular necrosis and even heart failure. Older people suffer more severe symptoms than younger age groups.

Leucopenia: This condition seriously decreases the body's ability to mount an immune response to stimuli and leads to an increase in the risk of susceptibility to infection. Leucopenia risk is increased by infection, chemotherapy, age, use of steroids and other immune-suppressants as well as recent surgery. Febrile neutropenia (FN) is defined as the condition when a cancer patient receiving either chemotherapy or radiotherapy presents with fever with body temperature at or above 38.3 °C as well as neutrophil counts less than 1000 cells/mm^3. This condition is considered serious occurring either during the initial cycles of chemotherapy or with concurrent chemo-radiation [1–6], with effects ranging from life-threatening infections, organ damage, decrease in quality of life [7–9] to interruption in cancer treatment leading to limitation or loss of benefits of therapy [10–16]. Various factors like tumour stage and type, chemotherapy regimen being followed, whether more than one treatment modality is being simultaneously given, patient's age, general condition, any medical co-morbidities as well as availability of supportive facilities can affect both susceptibility and response of the patient [8, 17, 18]. The common approach in the management of these patients who develop febrile neutropenia consists of admission, evaluation and administration of broad-spectrum parenteral antibiotics [9].

Thrombocytopenia: Platelets have a rapid turnover time (8–9 days) and are very sensitive to damage by radiotherapy. *Thrombocytopenia may be the first sign of bone marrow suppression* and is due to damage by irradiation or replacement by tumour cells. Purpuric spots and petechiae are the first signs suggestive of thrombocytopenia and usually appear over the gums, mucosal membranes and skin of extremities. This can be followed by overt bleeding either from the aerodigestive tract or genitourinary tract. The risk of spontaneous bleeding increases with platelet counts of below 20,000 cu mL^{-1}, while occult bleeding can occur at counts below 50,000 cu mL^{-1}. Spontaneous bleeding however occurs in presence of other precipitating factors like fever or infection (Table 26.2).

Table 26.2 RTOG criteria [19] for grading of acute haematological reactions

Blood parameter	Grade 0	Grade 1	Grade 2	Grade 3	Grade 4
Haematologic WBC (×1000)	≥4.0	3.0 to <4.0	2.0 to <3.0	1.0 to <2.0	<1.0
Platelets (×1000)	≥100	75 to <100	50 to <75	25 to <50	<25 or spontaneous bleeding
Neutrophils	≥1.9	1.5 to <1.9	1.0 to <1.5	0.5 to <1.0	<0.5 or sepsis
Haemoglobin (g%)	>11	11–9.5	<9.5 to 7.5	<7.5–5.0	–
Haematocrit (%)	≥32	28 to <32	<28	Packed cell transfusion required	–

26.3 Management of Haematological Toxicities

The most effective way of management lies in prevention of haematological toxicities and in prophylactic compensation for expected toxicity during therapy. Anaemia can be treated effectively maintaining adequate nutrition and treatment of underlying disease. Adequate rest is advised for these patients as they tire easily. If anaemia has already developed, then it should be corrected with blood transfusions, for which packed cell transfusion is more beneficial. Psychological support is also essential to allow these patients to maintain a positive outlook and thus maintain good appetite.

In patients with leucopenia, the main aim of treatment is to protect from infections till the body has recovered with blood counts back to normal. Granulocyte-stimulating factors can be given prophylactically to prevent development of leucopenia or fasten recovery once neutropenia has developed as well as prevent associated complications [8, 20]. The use of prophylactic antibiotic has been thought to cause a decrease in neutropenia incidence, severity as well as mortality, a fact which has been borne out from studies, systemic reviews and meta-analyses [21–24]. These colony-stimulating factors are now also being used to build up counts in prophylactic use to support dose-dense and dose-intense chemotherapy regimens which have shown survival benefits [25–29] but could not be previously undertaken because of the high risk of severe neutropenia and its life-threatening complications. While previous guidelines from the American Society of Clinical Oncology (ASCO) recommended starting G-CSF support if there was more than 40% risk of developing neutropenia following chemotherapy [8], present recommendations suggest starting of such prophylaxis if the risk of fever and neutropenia is more than 20% [30]. However use of G-CSF in established febrile neutropenia is still not recommended [30].

The Infectious Diseases Society of America (IDSA) has released guidelines [30] for patients of neutropenia which basically divides all cases into a high-risk and a low-risk category. Patients at high risk include those in whom there is an anticipation of prolonged neutropenia for more than 7 days with greater severity of fall of counts [absolute neutrophil count (ANC) below 100 cells/mm^3] with cases may or may not having significant medical co-morbid conditions, such as hypotension, pneumonia, new-onset abdominal pain or neurologic changes. These patients require immediate admission, inpatient care and support with parenteral antibiotics which can be either monotherapy or combination therapy. Commonly recommended drugs include antipseudomonal β-lactam agents such as cefepime, carbapenem (meropenem or imipenem-cilastatin) or piperacillin-tazobactam, while drugs like aminoglycosides, fluoroquinolones and/or vancomycin may be added later if there is suspicion of drug resistance or in case complications develop.

Patients who are at a lower risk of developing severe neutropenia or its complications include cases where chemotherapy would cause short and mild episodes of neutropenia, while the patients themselves would have little co-morbidity. These patients are the candidates for oral empirical antibiotic therapy in which a combination of ciprofloxacin in combination with amoxicillin-clavulanate is recommended. Other oral regimens may include levofloxacin or ciprofloxacin monotherapy or a combination of ciprofloxacin and clindamycin, but these regimens are not as well studied but still used. However the same drug should not be used both for prophylaxis and therapeutic coverage even if empirically. In these cases, for diagnosing the causative pathogen, the treating team should collect at least two sets of blood cultures of which one set each should be collected simultaneously from each existing central venous catheter (CVC) and/or from a peripheral vein site whichever is present. Also a chest X-ray should be done wherever patients have respiratory signs or symptoms.

26.3.1 Initial Antibiotic Therapy

The following are the accepted recommendations for selecting an antibiotic to treat febrile neutropenia according to the Infectious Disease Society of America [30].

- The initial regimen should include a broad-spectrum antibiotic as well as one targeting gram-negative bacilli or cocci.
- Drugs which are active against aerobic gram-positive cocci such as vancomycin should not be given as a standard initial antibiotic regimen for patients on chemotherapy presenting with fever and neutropenia.
- Vancomycin or drugs against gram-positive cocci should be considered only in special clinical situations such as in suspected catheter-related infection, skin or soft tissue infection, pneumonia or in presence of haemodynamic instability.
- The initial empirical antibiotic therapy can be modified especially in patients with unstable condition, in cases where the blood culture results show organisms like methicillin-resistant *Staphylococcus aureus* (MRSA), vancomycin-resistant enterococcus (VRE), extended-spectrum β-lactamase (ESBL)—producing gram-negative bacteria—and carbapenemase-producing organisms, such as *Klebsiella pneumoniae* carbapenemase (KPC). These are commonly seen either in hospital-acquired situations or in cases of repeat infection. Drugs of choice for these organisms include the following:
  - MRSA: Vancomycin, linezolid or daptomycin may be added to existing regimen after full culture reports.
  - VRE: Linezolid or daptomycin.

– ESBLs: Carbapenems are used for these organisms.
– KPCs: Polymyxin-colistin or tigecycline.

26.3.1.1 Indications for Change/Addition in Antibiotic Prophylaxis [30]

- In cases where the initial antibiotic coverage included vancomycin or drugs active against gram-positive organisms, after 48–72 h, if there is no evidence of such organisms on culture reports, then these drugs may be stopped.
- In cases where even after initiating the empirical antibiotic therapy the condition remains haemodynamically unstable, the antibiotic coverage should be expanded then to include drugs active against resistant gram negative and gram positive such as those mentioned in previous section as well as cover for anaerobic bacteria and fungi.
- A change in the antibiotic regimen from an intravenous drug to an oral drug may be considered where the patients are clinically stable with adequate GI absorption. Patients, whose condition is classified as low-risk on either IV or oral antibiotics in the hospital, if they are clinically stable, can be considered for outpatient-based care.
- However in these cases if the fever persists or recurs within 48 h after they have been shifted to outpatient care, readmission to the hospital is advised, and these patients should then be reclassified as in high-risk group and hence treated accordingly.
- Also cases where the fever has not responded to after 4–7 days of the initial empirical antibiotic therapy, with the duration of neutropenia having lasted more than 7 days, should be suspected of having fungal infections also, and hence such coverage should be initiated.

26.3.1.2 End Point for Antibiotic Prophylaxis [30]

- Required antibiotics should be continued in patients with clinically or microbiologically documented infections, for at least the duration of neutropenia or longer if clinically necessary.
- The end point for stopping antibiotics is the recognition of signs of marrow recovery. Traditionally this means an absolute neutrophil count of more than 500 cells/mm^3 and showing an increasing trend. Otherwise antibiotics with or without regimen addition/modification should be continued till there is fever.
- In case the recommended course duration of the given antibiotic regimen has been completed with patient showing signs and symptoms of resolution of the documented infection, oral fluoroquinolones may be started in patients who remain neutropenic until there is marrow recovery.

Protective measures for patients with neutropenia include following barrier nursing methods, use of positive pressure isolation chambers to prevent airborne infections from entering the environment, monitoring blood counts, screening of blood and body fluids for infections, rigid monitoring of personal hygiene, increased fluid intake preferably orally and nutritional supplementation.

Management of thrombocytopenia involves monitoring for any occult bleeding and avoiding situations which increases risk of bleeding. Symptoms of internal bleeding include pallor, weakness, rapid deep respiration, rapid weak pulse and hypotension. Use of intramuscular injections, constipation, use of NSAIDS as well as minor injuries increase risk in thrombocytopenic patients and should be avoided [31]. Platelet transfusions are indicated when counts fall below 20,000 cu mm^{-1}, though risk continues until bone marrow has recovered.

References

1. Lyman GH, Dale DC, Crawford J. Incidence and predictors of low dose-intensity in adjuvant breast cancer chemotherapy: a nationwide study of community practices. J Clin Oncol. 2003;21:4524–31.
2. Lyman GH, Morrison VA, Dale DC, et al. Risk of febrile neutropenia among patients with intermediate-grade non-Hodgkin's lymphoma receiving CHOP chemotherapy. Leuk Lymphoma. 2003;44:2069–76.
3. Wolff DA, Crawford J, Dale DC, Poniewierski MS, Lyman GH. Risk of neutropenic complications based on a prospective nationwide registry of cancer patients initiating systematic chemotherapy. Proc Am Soc Clin Oncol. 2004;23:547 (abstract 6125).
4. Lyman GH, Delgado DJ. Risk and timing of hospitalization for febrile neutropenia in patients receiving CHOP, CHOP-R, or CNOP chemotherapy for intermediate-grade non-Hodgkin lymphoma. Cancer. 2003;98:2402–9.
5. Vogel CL, Wojtukiewicz MZ, Carroll RR, et al. First and subsequent cycle use of pegfilgrastim prevents febrile neutropenia in patients with breast cancer: a multicenter, double-blind, placebo-controlled phase III study. J Clin Oncol. 2005;23:1178–83.
6. Timmer-Bonte JN, de Boo TM, Smit HJ, et al. Prevention of chemotherapy-induced febrile neutropenia by prophylactic antibiotics plus or minus granulocyte colony-stimulating factor in small-cell lung cancer: a Dutch randomised phase III study. J Clin Oncol. 2005;23:7974–84.
7. Padilla G, Ropka ME. Quality of life and chemotherapy induced neutropenia. Cancer Nurs. 2005;28:167–71.
8. Ozer H, Armitage JO, Bennett CL, et al. Update of recommendations for the use of haematopoietic colony stimulating factors: evidence-based, clinical practice guidelines. J Clin Oncol. 2000;18:3558–85.
9. Hughes WT, Armstrong D, Bodey GP, et al. 2002 Guidelines for the use of antimicrobial agents in neutropenic patients with cancer. Clin Infect Dis. 2002;34:730–51.
10. Budman DR, Berry DA, Cirrincione CT, et al. Dose and dose intensity as determinants of outcome in the adjuvant treatment of breast cancer. The Cancer and Leukemia Group B. J Natl Cancer Inst. 1998;90:1205–11.
11. Kwak LW, Halpern J, Olshen RA, Horning SJ. Prognostic significance of actual dose intensity in diffuse large-cell lymphoma: results of a tree-structured survival analysis. J Clin Oncol. 1990;8:963–77.
12. Bonadonna G, Valagussa P, Moliterni A, Zambetti M, Brambilla C. Adjuvant cyclophosphamide, methotrexate and fluorouracil in node-positive breast cancer: the results of 20 years of follow-up. N Engl J Med. 1995;332:901–6.
13. Lepage E, Gisselbrecht C, Haioun C, et al. Prognostic significance of received relative dose intensity in non-Hodgkin's lymphoma patients: application to LNH-87 protocol. The GELA. (Groupe d'Etude des Lymphomes de l'Adulte). Ann Oncol. 1993;4:651–6.
14. Chang J. Chemotherapy dose reduction and delay in clinical practice: evaluating the risk to patient outcome in adjuvant chemotherapy for breast cancer. Eur J Cancer. 2000;36(Suppl. 1):S11–4.

15. Mayers C, Panzarella T, Tannock IF. Analysis of the prognostic effects of inclusion in a clinical trial and of myelosuppression on survival after adjuvant chemotherapy for breast carcinoma. Cancer. 2001;91:2246–57.
16. Wood WC, Budman DR, Korzun AH, et al. Dose and dose intensity of adjuvant chemotherapy for stage II, node-positive breast carcinoma. N Engl J Med. 1994;330:1253–9.
17. Crawford J, Dale DC, Lyman GH. Chemotherapy-induced neutropenia: risks, consequences, and new directions for its management. Cancer. 2004;100:228–37.
18. Lyman GH, Lyman CH, Agboola O. Risk models for predicting chemotherapy-induced neutropenia. Oncologist. 2005;10:427–37.
19. Cox JD, Stetz J, Pajak TF. Toxicity criteria of the Radiation Therapy Oncology Group (RTOG) and the European Organization for Research and Treatment of Cancer (EORTC). Int J Radiat Oncol Biol Phys. 1995;31(5):1341–6.
20. Komrokji RS, Lyman GH. The colony-stimulating factors: use to prevent and treat neutropenia and its complications. Expert Opin Biol Ther. 2004;4:1897–910.
21. Cullen M, Steven N, Billingham L, et al. Simple investigation in neutropenic individuals of the frequency of infection after chemotherapy +/antibiotic in a number of tumours (SIGNIFICANT) trial group. Antibacterial prophylaxis after chemotherapy for solid tumors and lymphomas. N Engl J Med. 2005;353:988–98.
22. Bucaneve G, Micozzi A, Menichetti F, et al. Gruppo Italiano Malattie Ematologiche dell'Adulto (GIMEMA) Infection Program. Levofloxacin to prevent bacterial infection in patients with cancer and neutropenia. N Engl J Med. 2005;353:977–87.
23. Gafter-Gvili A, Fraser A, Paul M, Leibovici L. Meta-analysis: antibiotic prophylaxis reduces mortality in neutropenic patients. Ann Intern Med. 2005;142:979–95.
24. van de Wetering MD, de Witte MA, Kremer LC, Offringa M, Scholten RJ, Caron HN. Efficacy of oral prophylactic antibiotics in neutropenic afebrile oncology patients: a systematic review of randomised controlled trials. Eur J Cancer. 2005;41:1372–82.
25. Gregory SA, Trumper L. Chemotherapy dose intensity in non-Hodgkin's lymphoma: is dose intensity an emerging paradigm for better outcomes? Ann Oncol. 2005;16:1413–24.
26. Pfreundschuh M, Trumper L, Kloess M, et al. Two-weekly or 3-weekly CHOP chemotherapy with or without etoposide for the treatment of elderly patients with aggressive lymphomas: results of the NHL-B2 trial of the DSHNHL. Blood. 2004;104:634–41.
27. Pfreundschuh M, Trumper L, Kloess M, et al. Two-weekly or 3-weekly CHOP chemotherapy with or without etoposide for the treatment of young patients with good-prognosis (normal LDH) aggressive lymphomas: results of the NHL-B1 trial of the DSHNHL. Blood. 2004;104:626–33.
28. Thatcher N, Girling DJ, Hopwood P, Sambrook RJ, Qian W, Stephens RJ. Improving survival without reducing quality of life in small-cell lung cancer patients by increasing the dose intensity of chemotherapy with granulocyte colony stimulating factor support: results of a British Medical Research Council Multicenter Randomised Trial. Medical Research Council Lung Cancer Working Party. J Clin Oncol. 2000;18:395–404.
29. Steward WP, von Pawel J, Gatzemeier U, et al. Effects of granulocyte-macrophage colony-stimulating factor and dose intensification of V-ICE chemotherapy in small-cell lung cancer: a prospective randomised study of 300 patients. J Clin Oncol. 1998;16:642–50.
30. Friefeld AG, et al. Clinical practice guidelines for the use of antimicrobial agents in neutropenic patients with cancer. Clin Infect Dis. 2011;52:e56–93.
31. Haeuber D, Spross JA. Alterations in protective mechanisms: haematopoiesis and bone marrow depression. In: Baird SB, McCorkle R, Grant M, editors. Treatment modalities part III from cancer nursing: a comprehensive textbook. London: WB Saunders; 1991.

Managing Complications: Lymphoedema and Fibrosis

27

27.1 Radiation-Induced Late Fibrosis

Radiation fibrosis (RF) is used to describe the slow fibrotic tissue sclerosis that often occurs in response to radiation exposure, while radiation fibrosis syndrome (RFS) describes the clinical presentations of progressive fibrotic tissue sclerosis resulting from radiation treatment [1]. In this condition, the earliest presenting feature is usually the loss of tissue elasticity which is followed by mild induration [2]. Occurrence of higher grades of skin or mucosal reactions during radiotherapy can result in increased extent and severity of irradiated tissue induration, as a result of which the surface layers will become rigid and may even retract due to underlying loss of elasticity caused by the fibrosis of the dermis and subcutaneous tissues (Fig. 27.1).

In addition to this rigidity and fibrosis, other changes like hyperpigmentation, epilation and hyper- or hypoplasia (thickening or thinning out) of the epidermis with loss of vascularity and dryness are also seen which may be caused by damage to the overlying epithelium by radiation-derived free radicals as well as post reaction healing disuse atrophy. In cases where patients' reactions during irradiation have been very severe, late effects may include ulceration and necrosis which could be because of the extravasation of fibrinous exudate from damaged tissue or from vascular compromise further worsened by local trauma or infection. This radiation-induced fibrosis can be found co-existing with local or regional lymphoedema (described in the next section), because of which the tissue induration can worsen further and result in loss or limitation of functionality.

It has been noted clinically that the most commonly affected anatomic regions after irradiation include the breast, the head and neck and the connective tissues [3–12]. Risk of occurrence of radiation-induced fibrosis is further exacerbated in situations like addition of surgery and/or chemotherapy to radiotherapy, treatment plans for radiotherapy which involve larger irradiated volumes or with higher total dose or hypofractionated regimens employing higher dose per fraction and concurrently

A. Mukherji, *Basics of Planning and Management of Patients during Radiation Therapy*, https://doi.org/10.1007/978-981-10-6659-7_27

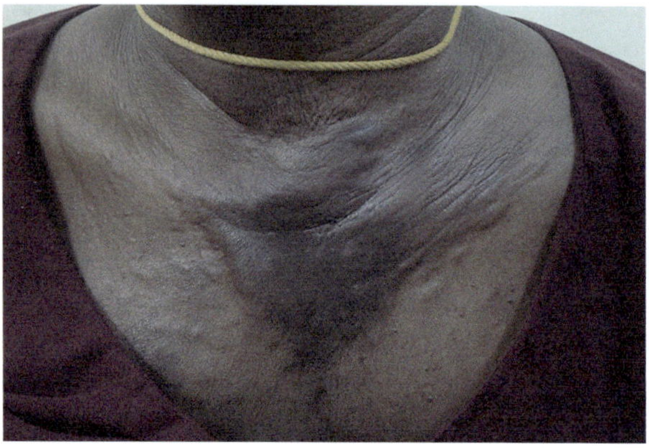

Fig. 27.1 Post radiotherapy cutaneous kelosis with subcutaneous fibrosis

occurring infection during irradiation or operative complications (e.g. seroma, wound drainage and extensive haematoma). Also presence of dose inhomogeneity because of poorly defined match zones or field abutments thus causing localized overdosing can increase the risk of late-occurring radiation-induced fibrosis.

Pathophysiology of radiation-induced fibrosis: The theories accounting for late radiation reactions include injury to vascular/endothelial damage causing vascular insufficiency leading to permanent hypoxia and nutritional damage and also effect on normal tissue response due to radiosensitivity of target cells and predicted by the linear quadratic equation [2].

Three histopathological phases of radiation-induced fibrosis are:

1. A prefibrotic phase characterized by chronic inflammation where major changes may occur in the endothelial cells.
2. After the prefibrotic phase, there is a phase of organization of the fibrosis in which there is formation of patchwork areas showing active as well as dense fibrosis in which areas with a high concentration of myofibroblasts lying in unorganized matrix intermingle with areas having low cellularity with senescent fibrocytes embedded in a densely sclerotic stroma.
3. Finally, phase of late fibro-atrophy, where there is loss of stromal tissue cells and tissue retraction due to dense stromal fibrosis is seen [13].

Exposure to irradiation and its' resultant formation of free radicals leads to the institution of an organized response from the body tissues, which may involve various interactions between growth factors, inter- or intracellular signaling pathways and molecules with their receptors as well as the extracellular matrix in which the principal target includes collagen. TGF-β1 from the progenitor fibroblasts has been thought to be one of the principal targets responsible for the fibrotic reaction seen which is caused by the proliferation of collagen-producing postmitotic fibrocytes [14–16]. The various pathways postulated to cause connective tissue fibrosis include (Fig. 27.2):

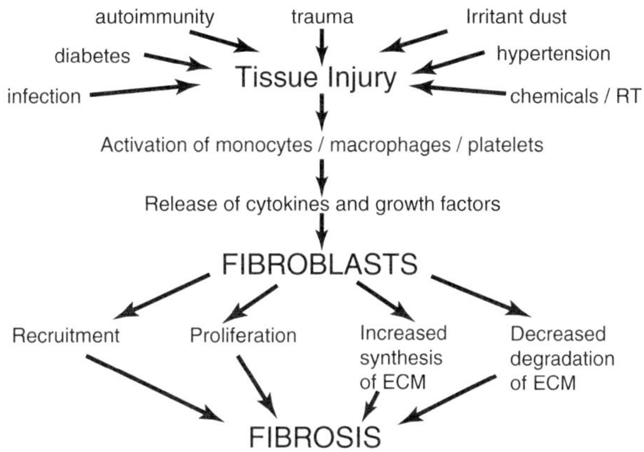

Fig. 27.2 Processes leading to radiation induced fibrosis

- Exudation occurring repeatedly from the irradiated tissues can result in deficiency of tissue plasminogen activator as a result of which there would be an increased deposition of fibrin which may not respond to body immune mechanisms or conventional therapies.
- Endothelial cell injury and their detachment lead to exudation of plasma causing fibroblast growth factor (FGF) activation which then causes stimulation of collagen synthesis, loss of mitogenic control of smooth muscle cells (SMCs) and overproduction of collagen.
- Radiation-induced action on the endothelial cells can lead to an increased expression of factors such as TNF-alpha and platelet-derived growth factors (PDGF) which are known to exacerbate smooth muscle cell proliferation and collagen synthesis.
- Downregulation of endothelial cell nitric oxide synthase and thrombomodulin activity resulting in unopposed smooth muscle cell proliferation, TGF-β caused epithelial breakdown, chronic subepithelial inflammation with fibroblast proliferation.
- Late effects of irradiation-induced tissue damage may result in permanent phenotypic changes in the stromal fibroblasts which may then result not only in an increased production and accumulation of postmitotic fibrocytes but also in increased production of matrix elements and their resultant fibrosis and organization.

Management options: Limited management options are available clinically to resolve this fibrotic tissue response to radiotherapy. Most of these options are in the experimental stage or have little clinical evidence. Options include use of drugs like pentoxifylline with or without vitamin E; use of hyperbaric oxygen; use of steroids, interferon-α and colchicine; as well as use of non-pharmacologic methods such as physiotherapy and microcurrent therapy.

Medical management: Since free radical injury to the endothelium and fibrocytes has been postulated as the main event initiating radiation-induced fibrosis, treatment options revolve around use of antioxidants, improving vascularity, increasing tissue repair mechanisms and reducing the effect of released cytokines.

Copper or zinc superoxide dismutase (SOD) in a liposomal carrier molecule is a potent antioxidant and was the first identified agent found to be effective in managing and rolling back chronic fibrosis seen as a late effect of radiotherapy [17]. SOD captures oxygen free radicals and then by enzymatic processes converts these radicals to hydrogen peroxide which is then metabolized further. SOD has been shown to decrease TGF-β1 expression in myofibroblasts, both during transcription and translation affecting messenger RNA and formed protein, and thus plays an important role in downregulation of production of collagen chains.

Pentoxifylline (PTX) is a methylxanthine derivative which is a phosphodiesterase inhibitor and acts mainly on the vascular system. It is responsible for many dose-related haemorrhagic effects, lowering of blood viscosity, improving erythrocyte deformability and malleability and increasing oxygenation of affected tissues as well as promoting platelet deaggregation. This lowering of blood viscosity and improved ability to fit into narrowed or fibrosed arterioles and capillaries allows for better oxygen delivery to the irradiated tissue and thus helps combat the onset of hypoxia and resultant late effects like necrosis or fibrosis. PTX also helps decrease radiation-induced tissue injury by preventing cytokine-induced neutrophil activation, decreasing oxygen radical formation and quenching free radicals already formed. It also increases release of prostacyclins from normal endothelial cells and thus helps inhibit the cytokine cascade caused by tissue injury, while, at the same time, PTX indirectly inhibits the production of thromboxane which is a potent vasoconstrictor and platelet aggregation stimulator. Some studies have shown more benefit with use of PTX in prevention of radiation-induced soft tissue necrosis than in developed fibrosis [18]. Concurrent use with tocopherol (vitamin E), a very strong antioxidant, in treatment of radiation-induced fibrosis has shown benefit [19] though the results have not been reproducible worldwide, and therefore widespread use of this combination has not occurred.

Corticosteroids have been thought to have an ameliorative effect on irradiation-induced injuries, mainly because of their anti-inflammatory agents, and therefore have been in clinical use in the past, but it is uncertain in the presence of developed radiation-induced fibrosis whether the use of steroids would have any benefit. A study by Hirota et al. [9] has reported on the effect of use of steroids in which patients given corticosteroids along with their chemotherapy had significantly lower incidences of severe tissue fibrosis compared with those not receiving. Another class of agent that has been used is the angiotensin-converting enzyme (ACE) inhibitors [20] which act by blocking conversion of angiotensin I to angiotensin II and thereby help in combating tissue fibrosis by not both increasing the production and cutting down the breakdown of extracellular matrix (ECM) components.

Hyperbaric oxygen therapy: Apart from use in osteoradionecrosis of the bone following radiotherapy, hyperbaric oxygen is also used for laryngeal necrosis post-RT, proctitis, cystitis and colitis. Hyperbaric oxygen (HBO) therapy helps in arresting or countering radiation-induced fibrosis by various mechanisms which may include increasing oxygen diffusion into the tissues, effect on collagen synthesis as well as neo-vascularization. Thus HBO increases vascular density thereby decreasing the capillary filtration pressure which results in reduction in tissue oedema [21]. Use of HBO has also shown benefit in radiation-induced neuropathies and plexopathy though randomized trials have not shown objective improvements [22].

Physiotherapy: Regular guided physical exercises help in preventing the formation of contractures and in counteracting the advent of tissue fibrosis.

Impedance-controlled microcurrent therapy: This therapy is thought to act by influencing movement of extracellular calcium ions across the cell membrane. This allows an increase in cellular synthesis of ATP which plays an important role in various cellular processes such as protein synthesis, cell repair and replication.

27.2 Radiation-Induced Lymphoedema

Lymphoedema is the condition in which there is increased collection of lymph (high-protein fluid) in the third space (interstitial spaces) which is caused by damage to normal lymphatic transport. This accumulation of proteinaceous fluid as explained in the previous section on fibrosis will lead to increased fibrin deposition as well as set off various body immune processes resulting in release of cytokines and other factors which would cause dermal fibrosis and chronic inflammation with resultant poor healing. This phenomenon of lymphatic obstruction with resultant oedema is called lymphoedema and is usually noted to occur in tissues where the drainage is more linear with lack of space such as in the extremities, breast, face, neck or trunk. A study by Petrek et al. reported that 6–30% of breast cancer survivors develop lymphoedema [23], while another study by Armer reported occurrence of lymphoedema in 22–43% of cancer patients after completion of their treatment, with the risk of developing lymphoedema in these patients related to the number of lymph nodes removed operatively [24]. But all studies have not validated such finding with another study [25] disputing any correlation of occurrence of lymphoedema with factors such as age, smoking status, co-morbidities like diabetes or hypertension, chemotherapy given, disease stage as well as number of metastatic lymph nodes.

27.2.1 Clinical Manifestations

The onset of lymphoedema is usually slow though a sudden or acute exacerbated condition may be noted if there is coincident injury or tissue inflammation or even infection. The classical definition of a lymphoedema is the occurrence of a non-pitting swelling, usually of an extremity, and which may involve the digits. However in its early stages, until fibrosis occurs, lymphoedema can present with pitting oedema. This swelling may be seen both in the proximal and distal portion of the limb but is usually restricted in extent. Because of the stasis in lymph flow and subsequent tissue injury, these patients are at an increased risk of developing recurrent skin infections [26]. Lymphoedema can also occur on the body or chest wherever use of radiotherapy has resulted in the blocking of dermal lymphatics.

Various other clinical presentations seen in patients with lymphoedema include a feeling of heaviness or fullness as if the affected limb has gradually become heavier, the skin starting feel increasingly tight as well as reduced range of movement (ROM) and flexibility of the affected joint. The skin look and texture become hyper-keratotic, with superficial skin lesions ranging from verrucous to nodular to vesicular types of lesions. Other presenting complaints may include in case of upper limb lymphoedema symptoms such as difficulty in wearing previously fitting clothes or rings, watches or bracelets, while in lower limbs, symptoms may include sensation of tightness over the skin of the lower limb or difficulty in wearing shoes, loss of hair over the skin, itching or burning sensation in the legs or toes or sleep disturbance. Regular movements including fine and coarse movements as well as the ability to perform acts of daily living might be affected because of the increased size and weight of the affected limb.

27.2.2 Evaluation and Staging of Lymphoedema

Observation: One should note appearance of the skin for the following features: thickness, tautness, shine, whether the skin appears fibrosed or puckered or hard, whether there is any discolouration of the skin and also whether the oedema is present and if present then whether it is pitting or non-pitting. Location and appearance of scars and wounds should be noted.

Skin and scar assessment: The clinician during his/her assessment should note the presence, location of scars and tissue adhesions. The clinician should then first describe the texture of the examined tissue (describing it as brawny/fibrous/soft or pliable). Then the type and extent of scars (whether they are hypertrophic or keloid and localized or widespread), texture of scars, presence of contractures or adhesions and mobility of scars should be described. The clinician should be especially alert to the presence of the skin texture resembling an orange peel, which would be suggestive of the malignant process involving the dermal lymphatics as in patients with inflammatory breast cancer.

After this an assessment is made of the limb girth in case of lymphoedemas affecting extremities so as to grade the severity of the condition. The measured girth of the affected side should be compared to non-affected side using a tape measure at set marks on the skin. These points of matched markings on both limbs can be located at fixed points. A difference of 2 cm or more at any measured point compared with the other limb is considered clinically significant. This could be done by several ways. One method would include marking the skin at the proximal tip of the ulnar styloid process and at every 5 and 10 cm proximally for the full length of the arm and leg, respectively. Another method could involve taking measurements at four fixed points on both arms: the metacarpal-phalangeal joints, the wrist, 10 cm distal to the lateral epicondyles and 15 cm proximal to the lateral epicondyles. Another method is to measure the water displaced on immersing the measured and the contralateral limb in water wherein a difference of 200 mL or more is used to define presence of lymphoedema [27].

27.2.3 Classifying Severity of Lymphoedema

A common method for grading the severity of lymphoedema especially in the upper limbs in breast cancer patients has been described by Mondry et al. [27]. According to this system, in *stage I*, the lymphoedema is reversible, and the presenting features include pitting oedema, increase in limb girth and a feeling of heaviness in the limb. In *stage II*, the texture of the affected tissue becomes spongy, but there is no pitting oedema. Later on as a part of this stage, there is a gradual fibrotic change occurring in the tissue which causes it to harden and increase in size [27]. The next stage is also called lymphostatic elephantiasis and is the most advanced stage (*stage III*) in which the involved limb increases in size significantly along with dermal fibrosis and hardening as well as presence of skin papillomas, acanthosis, fat deposits and even warty overgrowths in some cases.

Another commonly used approach is the Common Terminology Criteria for Adverse Events (CTCAE) v3.0 [28]. This approach benefits from including both objective measures (interlimb discrepancy) and subjective, clinical assessments in diagnosing lymphoedema (Table 27.1). The grading by this method is described as follows:

27.2.4 Management of Lymphoedema

Management of lymphoedema primarily aims at decongesting the blocked lymphatics of the affected area and hence is called complete decongestive therapy (CDT), or decongestive lymphatic therapy (DCT). This includes a gamut of interventions such as dedicated care of the affected skin, manual draining of lymphatics, exercise therapy, compression bandaging as well as use of compression garments. Studies have reported on the benefit of these interventions such as by Ko and colleagues who reported 59% and 67% reductions, respectively, in lymphoedema of the upper and lower limbs subsequent to complete decongestive therapy. This study also reported a continuation of

Table 27.1 Modified from CTCAE grading system [28] used for assessing lymphoedema

Grade	Common Terminology Criteria for Adverse Events (CTCAE) v3.0 (lymphoedema) findings
Grade 0	No changes
Grade 1	There is a 5–10% difference in volume or circumference at the point of greatest visible difference between two measured limbs; the swelling causing obscuration of anatomic architecture on close inspection and pitting oedema
Grade 2	The interlimb difference in volume/circumference is between 10 and 30%; there is easily visible obscuration of local anatomy, obliteration of skin folds and readily apparent deviation from normal anatomic contour
Grade 3	The interlimb difference in volume/circumference is more than 30% with lymphorrhea present with the normal tissue anatomy grossly deformed causing interference with daily acts of living
Grade 4	Progression to malignancy (e.g. lymphangiosarcoma) with amputation indicated or presence of disabling lymphoedema

benefit following this therapy over a period of 9 months in 90% of subjects who were compliant with home programs that included wearing a daytime compression garment, night-time bandaging and continuing home exercises [29]. Studies have also reported on the benefits of use of compression bandaging and especially short-stretch bandages in reducing limb size whether they are used alone [30–32], in combination with compression garments [30] or along with manual lymphatic drainage [31, 32]. The highest amount of benefit using this decongestive therapy is seen to occur in the first 2 weeks of treatment with an average reduction in the limb volume ranging between 26 and 38% [31], while adding manual lymphatic drainage to compression bandaging caused a further limb volume reduction by 7–7.5% [31, 32].

Positional changes as single modality treatment interventions such as keeping the affected part elevated has not shown to significantly reduce lymphoedema, though when used along with measures such as compression bandaging or garments can be used as measures to sustain benefit from the active decongestant therapy and prevent any subsequent increase in lymphoedema. Such benefit was noted in a study by Swedborg et al., wherein a 1–3% tissue volume reduction occurred after performing 1–5 h of elevation [33]. This reduction in the tissue volume caused by maintaining the limb or affected part elevated is however mainly seen in cases with mild grades [32, 34], and therefore it is imperative to recognize early signs of lymphoedema and institute prompt therapeutic measures.

27.2.5 Indications for Treatment

While generally mild lymphoedema may be transient and may subside with restoration of normal lymph flow and increased ambulation, higher grades may require specialized treatment. Treatment for lymphoedema should be instituted in the following situations:

1. When the functioning of a limb is affected because of change in size or weight of the affected limb as well as loss of motion.
2. During assessment measurement of limb girth between affected and unaffected sides being more than 2 cm at at least three measured points along the limb length.
3. Presence of scar tissue resulting in limitation of the normal range of motion (ROM) and function for that limb. Also when a patient cannot assume the proper treatment position for receiving radiotherapy.
4. Treatment may be started to afford limb care and pain relief and prevent further loss of limb function.

27.2.6 Contraindications/Precautions for Treatment by Manual Lymphatic Drainage

General precautions: Caution should be exercised in the use of techniques for enabling manual lymphatic drainage in some situations such as when the lymphoedema increases very rapidly or there is an onset of fresh erythema. These signs may be indicative of either a deep vein thrombosis or disease progression in the cancer or even infection in a background of unmanaged lymphoedema.

Contraindications: Treatment techniques of manual lymphatic drainage should not be used when there is active infection like cellulitis (patient may present with erythema, warmth, local osedema, tenderness to touch as well as fever, chills and myalgias), when there is compromised arterial perfusion and in areas where there is potential or known untreated cancer or early-stage cancer. Such patients should receive 2–3 cycles of chemotherapy before initiating treatment.

References

1. O'Sullivan B, Levin W. Late radiation-related fibrosis: pathogenesis, manifestations, and current management. Semin Radiat Oncol. 2003;13(3):274–89.
2. Hill RP, Rodemann HP, Hendry JH, et al. Normal tissue radiobiology: from the laboratory to the clinic. Int J Radiat Oncol Biol Phys. 2001;49:353–65.
3. Johansson S, Svensson H, Denekamp J. Dose response and latency for radiation-induced fibrosis, edema, and neuropathy in breast cancer patients. Int J Radiat Oncol Biol Phys. 2002;52:1207–19.
4. Borger JH, Kemperman H, Smitt HS, et al. Dose and volume effects on fibrosis after breast conservation therapy. Int J Radiat Oncol Biol Phys. 1994;30:1073–81.
5. Krishnamurthy R, Whitman GJ, Stelling CB, et al. Mammographic findings after breast conservation therapy. Radiographics. 1999;19:S53–62.
6. Olivotto IA, Weir LM, Kim-Sing C, et al. Late cosmetic results of short fractionation for breast conservation. Radiother Oncol. 1996;41:7–13.
7. Bentzen SM, Dische S. Morbidity related to axillary irradiation in the treatment of breast cancer. Acta Oncol. 2000;39:337–47.
8. Trotti A. Toxicity in head and neck cancer: a review of trends and issues. Int J Radiat Oncol Biol Phys. 2000;47:1–12.
9. Hirota S, Tsujino K, Oshitani T, et al. Subcutaneous fibrosis after whole neck irradiation. Int J Radiat Oncol Biol Phys. 2002;52:937–43.
10. Wratten CR, Poulsen MG, Williamson S, et al. Effect of surgery on normal tissue toxicity in patients treated with accelerated radiotherapy. Acta Oncol. 2002;41:56–62.
11. Peters LJ, Ang KK, Thames HD Jr. Accelerated fractionation in the radiation treatment of head and neck cancer. A critical comparison of different strategies. Acta Oncol. 1988;27:185–94.
12. van Kampen M, Eble MJ, Lehnert T, et al. Correlation of intraoperatively irradiated volume and fibrosis in patients with soft-tissue sarcoma of the extremities. Int J Radiat Oncol Biol Phys. 2001;51:94–9.
13. Delanian S, Lefaix JL. Current management for late normal tissue injury: radiation-induced fibrosis and necrosis. Semin Radiat Oncol. 2007;17:99–107.
14. Border WA, Noble NA. Transforming growth factor beta in tissue fibrosis. N Engl J Med. 1994;331:1286–92.
15. Franklin TJ. Therapeutic approaches to organ fibrosis. Int J Biochem Cell Biol. 1997;29:79–89.
16. Leask A, Abraham DJ, Finlay DR, et al. Dysregulation of transforming growth factor beta signaling in scleroderma: overexpression of endoglin in cutaneous scleroderma fibroblasts. Arthritis Rheum. 2002;46:1857–65.
17. Delanian S, Baillet F, Huart J, et al. Successful treatment of radiation-induced fibrosis using liposomal Cu/Zn superoxide dismutase: clinical trial. Radiother Oncol. 1994;32:12–20.
18. Dion MW, Hussey DH, Doornbos JF, et al. Preliminary results of a pilot study of pentoxifylline in the treatment of late radiation soft tissue necrosis. Int J Radiat Oncol Biol Phys. 1990;19:401–7.

19. Delanian S, Balla-Mekias S, Lefaix JL. Striking regression of chronic radiotherapy damage in a clinical trial of combined pentoxifylline and tocopherol. J Clin Oncol. 1999;17:3283–90.
20. Molteni A, Moulder JE, Cohen EP, et al. Prevention of radiation-induced nephropathy and fibrosis in a model of bone marrow transplant by an angiotensin II receptor blocker. Exp Biol Med (Maywood). 2001;226:1016–23.
21. Plafki C, Carl UM, Glag M, et al. The treatment of late radiation effects with hyperbaric oxygenation (HBO). Strahlenther Onkol. 1998;174(Suppl 3):66–8.
22. Pritchard J, Anand P, Broome J, et al. Double-blind randomized phase II study of hyperbaric oxygen in patients with radiation-induced brachial plexopathy. Radiother Oncol. 2001;58:279–86.
23. Petrek JA, Heelan MC. Incidence of breast carcinoma related lymphedema. Cancer. 1998;83:2776–81.
24. Armer J, et al. Lymphedema following breast cancer treatment, including sentinel lymph node biopsy. Lymphology. 2004;37(2):73–91.
25. Ozaslan C, Kuru B. Lymphedema after treatment of breast cancer. Am J Surg. 2004;187(1): 69–72.
26. Bicego D, Brown K, Ruddick M, et al. Exercise for women with or at risk for breast cancer-related lymphedema. Phys Ther. 2006;86(10):1398–405.
27. Mondry TE, Riffenburgh RH, Johnstone PA. Prospective trial of complete decongestive therapy for upper extremity lymphedema after breast cancer therapy. Cancer J. 2004;10(1):42–8; discussion 17–9.
28. Cheville AL, McGarvey CL, Petrek JA, et al. The grading of lymphedema in oncology clinical trials. Semin Radiat Oncol. 2003;13(3):214–25.
29. Ko DSC, et al. Effective treatment of lymphedema of the extremities. Arch Surg. 1998;133:452–8.
30. Badger CMA, et al. A randomized, controlled, parallel-group clinical trial comparing multilayer bandaging followed by hosiery versus hosiery alone in the treatment of patients with lymphedema of the limb. Cancer. 2000;88:2832–7.
31. Johansson K, et al. Low intensity resistance exercise for breast cancer patients with arm lymphedema with or without compression sleeve. Lymphology. 2005;38(4):167–80.
32. McNeeley ML, et al. The addition of manual lymph drainage to compression therapy for breast cancer related lymphedema: a randomized controlled trial. Breast Cancer Res Treat. 2004;86:95–106.
33. Swedborg I, et al. Lymphedema post-mastectomy: is elevation alone an effective treatment? Scand J Rehabil Med. 1993;25:79–82.
34. Ramos SM, et al. Edema volume, not timing, is the key to success in lymphedema treatment. Am J Surg. 1999;178:311–5.

Dietary Care and Support During Radiotherapy

28

28.1 Effect of Cancer on Nutrition

Almost half of cancer patients worldwide with an even higher figure in the developing world present with weight loss, insufficient nutritional intake, a poor psychosocial outlook and dehydration. Weight loss is one of the most disabling aspects of cancer as it not only affects the patient's ability to withstand intensive cancer therapy, it may play a decisive role in deciding their modality of treatment; it may also worsen patient's reactions to treatment given and may result in increased late reactions and decreased quality of life. Weight loss leads to a marked decrease in body fat and muscle mass which leads to muscle wasting, physical weakness and susceptibility to infections. This condition is called "cachexia" [1].

Accompaniments of cachexia include anorexia; muscle wasting; early satiety; marked weight loss; anaemia; generalized oedema with progressive development of malabsorption; vitamin and protein deficiencies; disturbances in glucose, protein and fat metabolism; and gradual progressive organ dysfunction. All these can adversely affect quality of life and life expectancy as well as compliance and response to therapy [2].

28.2 Pathophysiology

Causes of malnutrition in a cancer patient include anorexia, taste alterations, dysphagia, food aversion, malabsorption, early satiety, metabolic disorders and emotional and psychological factors, and the extent and severity is influenced by location of cancer [2]. Protein energy malnutrition is the most common presentation and results in loss of subcutaneous fat and muscle mass along with loss of serum albumin and transferrin. In cancers, there is a net catabolic environment with increased loss of body stores, lack of proper replenishment and increased energy expenditure. This translates into decreased protein synthesis, increased mobilization of body glucose and glycogen stores, increase in fat catabolism and decreased bone mineralization.

A. Mukherji, *Basics of Planning and Management of Patients during Radiation Therapy*, https://doi.org/10.1007/978-981-10-6659-7_28

Many of these actions are mediated by a variety of cofactors and cytokines. These include interleukins (IL-1 and IL-6), interferons and tumour necrosis factor (cachectin) and tumour byproducts (e.g. proteolysis-inducing factor, lipolytic hormone) causing abnormalities in carbohydrate, protein and lipid metabolism [3].

These mediators cause nutrients to be shifted from the periphery to the liver with increased gluconeogenesis. A negative energy balance is demonstrated in many patients [3]. There is increased protein synthesis in the liver of acute-phase proteins rather than skeletal muscle protein. Fat stores are progressively depleted, and a tumour-derived lipolytic factor can cause fat breakdown, with the release of free fatty acids. Anaerobic glycolysis in tumour tissue produces lactic acid. This requires further energy to be processed further, through gluconeogenesis in the liver, and there is a reduced insulin response to the increased glucose turnover. Lactate together with substances such as tumour necrosis factor and interleukin-1 (IL-1) may directly suppress appetite [3]. Although the patient becomes progressively more malnourished, the normal physiological response to a state of starvation is lost and cannot be reversed by nutritional supplements. Other contributing factors in cancer malnutrition include reduced intake as a result of dysphagia, gastrointestinal obstruction or nausea and vomiting from any cause; treatment-related mucositis or enteritis further affects intake and absorption, and malabsorption of food may be due to surgery, biliary obstruction or direct involvement of the small bowel (e.g. in lymphoma). This may also be compounded by increased protein losses from the gut or frequent paracentesis.

Effect of radiotherapy: The site, total dose and duration of radiation therapy influence the severity of nutritional compromise and can be associated with both acute and long-term effects of radiation therapy [4, 5]. After radiotherapy of the oral cavity and pharynx, patients can experience either increased or suppressed taste sensation. Loss of taste is severe and rapid after oropharyngeal irradiation, but patients often regain preradiation taste sensitivity 2–4 months after therapy is completed. Radiation to the head and neck may inhibit adequate salivation, leading to changes in eating habits and even increased sensitivity of the teeth. Radiation to the abdomen is associated with various complications that may influence nutritional status. Low doses of gastric irradiation reduce gastric acidity, whereas higher doses may induce ulcer formation. Nausea, vomiting and diarrhoea are common in individuals undergoing radiation to the small and large bowel. In addition, chronic diarrhoea or bowel obstruction may develop due to radiation-induced enteritis following high-dose GI irradiation. Upper abdominal radiation may produce radiation-induced hepatitis, characterized by anorexia, nausea, vomiting and abdominal distention. This disorder is usually temporary. Radiation to the pancreas may similarly result in acute anorexia, nausea and vomiting.

Effect of chemotherapy: Many drugs produce nausea, vomiting and diarrhoea which can lead to anorexia, electrolyte imbalance and malnutrition. Mucosal toxicities (oral ulcerations, cheilosis, glossitis and pharyngitis) are seen with the use of some chemotherapeutic agents. This often leads to odynophagia and anorexia. Drugs such as actinomycin D, cytarabine, 5-fluorouracil, hydroxyurea and methotrexate can produce ulcerations of the entire GI epithelium [6]. Chemotherapy because of its side effects can aggravate the effect of tumour-related malabsorption syndromes [6]. Nutrition support is usually unnecessary in the initially well-nourished patient if the ill effects of chemotherapy are significantly limited in time and intensity. Multiple major organ systems are affected by chemotherapeutic agents which results in decreased efficiency of metabolism. The liver is especially vulnerable, and hepatic injury is commonly associated with anorexia. Diffuse hepatocellular damage often results in hypoalbuminemia.

Effect of cancer surgery: Cancer surgery once involved extensive resections with loss of large amounts of body tissues depending on the stage of the disease. In the present day, the focus has now shifted to organ and function preservation as far as possible, with resultant benefits both on patient cosmesis and functionality and on the general nutritional and psychological health. Nutritional status of a patient during and after surgery can affect surgical results as patients with good status develop fewer postoperative complications. Poor nutritional status can affect wound healing immune function, and several studies have shown that when patients with severe malnutrition receive nutritional support, the complication rate improves [7–9]. Complications also increase when many patients after surgery require adjuvant therapy either with chemo- or radiotherapy or both.

In addition, certain surgical procedures may require nutritional intervention such as surgery of the upper GI tract can compromise a patient's ability to take oral feedings. Conditions associated with oesophagectomy and oesophageal reconstruction may include delayed gastric emptying secondary to vagotomy, malabsorption and the development of a fistula or stenosis. Gastric surgery may result in dumping syndrome, malabsorption and/or hypoglycaemia. The site and extent of intestinal resection can result in a variety of nutritional complications. Jejunal resection can decrease the efficiency of absorption of carbohydrates, protein, fat, water and electrolytes. Ileum resection commonly results in vitamin B12 deficiency and bile salt losses. With extensive small bowel resection, malabsorption can result. Abnormalities in sodium and water balance are commonly associated with ileostomy and colostomy formation. In addition, gastric and intestinal bypass surgery can result in a blind loop syndrome with specific nutritional deficiencies.

Patients with pancreatic cancer should be nutritionally assessed because they frequently lose weight before their surgical intervention, and after pancreatectomy, malabsorption and endocrine and exocrine insufficiencies are common problems that may require insulin and pancreatic enzyme replacement. Patients with cancer undergoing uretero-sigmoidostomy may experience hyperchloremic acidosis and hypokalaemia in addition to other more common postoperative problems. If it is anticipated that nutritional intervention will be required postoperatively, a nasoenteric feeding tube can be placed intraoperatively. With patients in whom a longer recuperative course is anticipated, surgical placement of a gastrostomy tube or jejunostomy tube may be more appropriate.

Carbohydrate metabolism: *Abnormal glucose metabolism, a major source of caloric wasting, is a hallmark of cancer cachexia* [10] with increased glucose production and utilization as well as insulin resistance. Glucose intolerance may due to reduced tissue sensitivity to insulin [10]. There may be decreased pancreatic Î[2] cell receptor sensitivity in patients with cancer as well, leading to inadequate insulin release in response to a glucose load. *An increase in gluconeogenesis in the liver of the patient with cancer is a common finding* and can be the result of an increased release of glucogenic fuel substrates, such as lactate and alanine, as well as an increased induction of hepatic gluconeogenetic enzymes [10–12]. The energy drain created by increased hepatic gluconeogenesis leads to host depletion of protein and calories. Elevation level of hepatic glucose production in a tumour-bearing host requires energy with a drain on host energy. Patients with cancer who lose weight may exhibit increases in glucose flux and glucose oxidation rates [13, 14].

Protein metabolism: Cancer anorexia is accompanied by wasting of host protein mass, leading to fatigue, weakness and altered host cell-mediated immune response. Several studies have shown that in cancer-associated cachexia, there is an increased turnover of proteins and that the normal adaptation of reduced protein metabolism seen in starvation does not occur [15]. With nutritional depletion, patients with cancer anorexia continue to manifest elevated rates of skeletal protein mobilization rather than the normal response of decreased protein turnover and protein sparing. Protein turnover rates in cachectic patients with cancer are significantly higher compared with similarly malnourished control patients without cancer.

Lipid metabolism: The most common impairments in lipid metabolism seen in patients with cancer are hyperlipidaemia and depletion of fat stores [16–18]. Abnormal lipoprotein lipase activity alters the ability of fatty acids to be utilized as protein-sparing energy fuels and is a major cause of protein malnutrition. The hyperlipidaemia seen in patients with cancer is significant and may play a role in disease outcome as the elevated lipid levels have an inhibitory effect on monocytes and macrophages leading to immunosuppression. Cancer-associated reductions in plasma lipoprotein lipase are accompanied by normal or even increased insulin levels which represent a maladaptive host response. Impaired glucose and fat oxidation provide a sink for loss of gluconeogenic amino acids, therefore producing an energy deficit and malnutrition [19].

28.3 Management

The aim of nutritional care in a cancer patient is always supportive irrespective of the intent of primary therapy. Nutritional therapy intends to improve the patient's metabolic condition, body composition as well as functional status and, as a result, tries to improve the patient's quality of life. Nutrition support can prevent further deterioration in all of these parameters. Patients receiving either total parenteral nutrition (TPN) or enteral feeding show improved nitrogen balance as well as wound healing and outcomes of therapy. But TPN is generally not indicated for patients with advanced metastatic cancer who are not receiving antineoplastic treatment. Also the routine use of TPN in patients with cancer who can otherwise tolerate enteral nutrition is unjustified.

Nutritional support for patients receiving radiotherapy/chemotherapy: Enteral feedings can improve quality of life, reduce hospitalizations and reduce interruptions in treatment in these patients [4], although decision on the best mode of delivery is debatable [20, 21]. Routine use of nutritional support is usually not needed for all patients who undergo chemotherapy or radiation therapy; however, nutritional therapy should be considered for those patients who have severe malnourishment or a prolonged treatment-related anorexia or for patients whose malnutrition is a major obstacle to a continued reasonable quality of life [22]. Two older meta-analyses [23, 24] concluded that TPN provided no added benefits in terms of survival, tumour response or chemotherapy toxicity.

Nutrition support for patients with bone marrow transplantation: Bone marrow (BMT) or stem cell transplantation is performed usually after exposing a patient to high-dose myeloablative chemotherapy or even whole-body irradiation. This can lead to mucositis, oesophagitis, nausea, diarrhoea and graft versus host disease which may affect a patient's ability to maintain adequate oral intake. Many patients undergoing BMT are routinely started on parenteral nutrition. In a study, Weisdorf [25] reported increased survival in patients undergoing BMT who received TPN when compared with patients who only received maintenance intravenous fluids. But there have also been other studies that have associated TPN with higher rates of infections [26]. TPN was found to be associated with a significant preservation of weight compared with controls on oral diets and showed better quality of life and infections; therefore it has been suggested that in autologous BMT, TPN is better suited for patients with malnutrition or unable to take an oral diet [27].

Nutritional assessment of cancer patients: This is the first essential step towards nutritional management of cancer patients. This assessment draws up the nutritional status of the patient and an estimate of intervention required. The main steps are the following: (1) identify existing problems, (2) identify cause of problems, (3) generate baseline data for subsequent follow-up and (4) evaluate response to intervention. The main modalities are clinical examination, anthropometric data, biochemical analyses and dietary evaluation.

Clinical examination should include a complete general and systemic examination and evaluation of nutritional status and hydration. Special attention should be taken for examining the hair, skin, teeth, oral mucosa, general skin and muscle tone, body weight and height as well as a full mental and psychological evaluation.

Anthropometric evaluation will include body weight (provides base for all other data and a general indicator for body changes), height (represents chronic nutritional status), BMI, usual body weight (*is calculated from body weight using formulae and is an indicator of nutritional change*), mid-arm circumference (*reflects body protein and fat stores*), triceps skinfold thickness (*estimates subcutaneous fat and energy reserves*), mid-arm muscle circumference (*body energy and protein reserves*) and arm muscle area (*body energy and protein reserves*). Most of these tools measure subcutaneous fat which could account for, respectively, 30% and 33% of total body fat in men and women.

The weight should be taken early in the morning before any meals and with an empty bladder with same scale every time and wearing clothes. The height should be taken with patient barefoot or wearing socks, both heels together and touching the ground or board, patient standing erect and looking straight ahead and the handle bar of the chart lowered to rest on top of the head. The BMI is calculated from standard formulae, and a BMI of less than 22 may be indicative of possible protein calorie malnutrition, especially among patients with cancer, and a value less than 18 is consistent with significant malnutrition. Weight loss should be considered severe if there is a 5% loss of body weight in 1 month or a 10% loss within 6 months.

Biochemical analysis includes measurement of blood counts, electrolytes, urea/creatinine and serum ions as well as markers like albumin and transferrin. Serum albumin concentration is a commonly used index of nutritional status. Albumin has a half-life of about 20 days, and as a nutritional marker, serum albumin concentrations can be used for detecting malnutrition. In hospitalized patients, hypoalbuminemia is associated not only with anergic immune status but with increased morbidity and mortality and is a poor prognostic indicator [28]. But there are limitations to its use as a nutritional index especially for stressed and critically ill patients. During an acute illness or stress, such as injury, infection or surgery, serum albumin synthesis decreases. Albumin concentrations can also be affected by fluid status, volume repletion, heart disease, renal disease and liver disease. Also due to its long half-life, serum albumin does not respond on a daily or weekly basis to nutrition support. This has led to use of measuring prealbumin for short-term assessment of nutrition. The half-life of prealbumin is 1–2 days, and hence it can be used to monitor daily changes. Transferrin is a globulin which binds to elemental iron and is useful in its transport. Measurement of transferrin levels is a more sensitive method than measuring albumin to assess any change in nutritional status. But transferrin levels are unreliable for nutritional status in iron-deficient or iron-overloaded patients who tend to show high and low transferrin levels and in patients who have had multiple transfusions.

Evaluation of nutrition support requires assessment of several parameters and must differentiate an increase in weight caused by fluid retention from lean body mass. Malnourished patients who are suddenly overfed can develop an increase in intravascular volume, congestive heart failure and electrolyte abnormalities, which can be fatal [29]. The nitrogen balance determination is a dependable measure that can reflect the influence of nutrition support on lean body mass. *Nitrogen balance reflects the difference between nitrogen intake and output over a 24-h period.* If 1 g of nitrogen represents 6.25 g of protein, the nitrogen balance can be calculated by the following formula:

$$\text{Nitrogen balance} = [\text{Nitrogen intake} - \text{Nitrogen loss}$$
$$= \text{protein intake} / 6.25] - \left(\text{urine urea nitrogen} + 4\right)$$

The principal form of urine nitrogen is called urine urea nitrogen, which can be easily measured. Urea excreted in the urine reflects protein degradation. In addition to urea, other forms of nitrogen are excreted, including non-urea urine nitrogen, faecal nitrogen and integumental nitrogen. These are lost at a fairly constant rate except when diarrhoea is present. In calculating nitrogen loss, 4 g is added to the nitrogen output as an estimate of faecal and integumental losses.

Along with the nutritional balance, a nutritional assessment of the patient also has to be done to see if existing diet is sufficient and determine likes and dislikes, current and previous eating patterns, social-environmental-financial issues, factors inhibiting food consumption (aversion, oral mucositis, taste aberration, dysphagia, nausea, anorexia), any concurrent illness and any dietary change as a result of the cancer. Recommendations for nutritional supplementation include providing a high-energy, high-protein diet to counteract weight loss and increase repair of damaged tissues.

Nutritional adjuncts and immune boosters: In view of the needs of cancer patients, special enteral diets include concentrates of arginine as well as omega-3 fatty acids, nucleic acids and even glutamine. These nutrients are known to both preserve and improve host immune responses, and they may also reduce harmful and exaggerated inflammatory responses.

- Arginine is known to cause accentuation of macrophage-induced tumour cytotoxic effects and bactericidal activity. It also causes vasodilation by the action of nitric oxide. Arginine stimulates T cell proliferation as well as natural killer cell cytotoxic effects. It generates lymphokine-activated killer cells and modulates nitrogen balance and protein synthesis [30].
- Omega-3 polysaturated fatty acids are derived from fish oil. These compounds have very strong anti-inflammatory action mediated through the coagulation and can cause upregulation of the immune response.
- Glutamine helps transport of nitrogen between organs and can reduce the skeletal and intestinal protein waste during stress. It can also enhance macrophage and neutrophil phagocytosis as well as preserve the intestinal permeability. It is a major fuel for different cell types [31, 32].

Lipid requirements: The usual required body intake of lipid is 0.5–1.0 g/kg/day, with a maximum of 2.5 g/kg/day [33]. Lipid emulsions are usually formulated to provide approximately 30% of total nonprotein calories. A minimum intake of 0.5 mg/kg/day is enough to prevent essential fatty acid deficiency.

Protein requirements: The protein requirements for a mild to moderately stressed patient may be estimated at 1.5–2.0 g protein/kg based on ideal body weight. Protein requirements of cancer patients range from 0.2 to 0.3 g nitrogen/kg/day to maintain a positive nitrogen balance [34].

Fluid requirements: Fluid requirements depend on baseline requirements, losses and fluid deficits. The average person's fluid requirement varies from 1250 to 3000 mL/day, depending on body habitus, while an average cancer patient requires approximately 35 mL/kg/day. A range of fluid abnormalities can be seen in patients with cancer due to the disease process and therapies such as surgery, radiation therapy and chemotherapy.

Electrolytes: Electrolyte requirements for patients with cancer are essentially the same as for patients with nonmalignant forms of disease and depend on hormonal milieu, GI and pulmonary losses, disease state and renal and hepatic function [35]. In addition, treatment modalities (i.e. amphotericin B administration) can alter electrolyte requirements. A minimum of 20 meq of potassium phosphate per 1000 kcal will usually prevent hypophosphatemia [36].

Enteral nutrition: If patient's GI tract is intact and functioning, liquid formula diets are preferred. Oral supplements provide an excellent source of calories and protein to bolster oral intake or as complement to hyperalimentation. But many cancer patients suffer from anorexia, nausea, oropharyngeal obstruction or central nervous system pathology, cannot meet their caloric needs despite a functioning intestinal tract and can benefit from tube feeding. Small pliable nasogastric tubes are available and well tolerated by most patients. Delivery methods can be by either bolus feeding, gravity or mechanical pump systems. In the critically ill patient, the use of continuous rather than intermittent tube feeding is recommended as they have been associated with positive nitrogen balance and weight gain compared to intermittent tube feedings [37].

Parenteral nutrition: The aims for starting parenteral nutrition should be to:

- Minimize nutrition-related side effects
- Prevent or reverse nutrient deficiencies
- Allow a better modulation of fluid, electrolytes and other elements
- Preserve lean body mass
- Help patients better tolerate treatments
- Aid in recovery and healing
- Improve quality of life

The recommended daily nonprotein calorie intake is between 25 and 35 kcal/kg, and recommended daily nitrogen intake is between 200 and 250 mg/kg [38]. Usually, 60–70% of total nonprotein calories should be provided as dextrose and 30–40% in the form of an intravenous fat emulsion. Patients receiving PN should be monitored regularly by measuring weight, fluid balance, serum glucose, urea, electrolytes, plasma proteins and liver function tests. Serious complications from PN in these patients include catheter-related infections and metabolic complications (hyperglycaemia, electrolyte abnormalities and abnormalities in liver enzymes).

References

1. Kern KA, Norton JA. Cancer cachexia. JPEN J Parenter Enteral Nutr. 1988;12:286–98.
2. Bruera E. ABC of palliative care, anorexia, cachexia and nutrition. BMJ. 1997;315:1219–22.
3. MacDonald N, Easson AM, Mazurak VC. Understanding and managing cancer cachexia. J Am Coll Surg. 2003;197:143–61.
4. Lee JH, Machtay M, Unger LD, et al. Prophylactic gastrostomy tubes in patients undergoing intensive irradiation for cancer of the head and neck. Arch Otolaryngol Head Neck Surg. 1998;124:871.
5. Donaldson SS. Nutritional problems associated with radiotherapy. In: Newell GR, Ellison NM, editors. Nutrition and cancer: etiology and treatment. New York: Raven Press; 1981.
6. Mitchell EP, Schein PS. Gastrointestinal toxicity of chemotherapeutic agents. Semin Oncol. 1982;9:52–64.

7. Bozzetti F, Gavazzi C, Miceli R, et al. Perioperative total parenteral nutrition in malnourished, gastrointestinal cancer patients: a randomized, clinical trial. JPEN J Parenter Enteral Nutr. 2000;24:7.
8. Bozzetti F, Braga M, Gianotti L. Postoperative enteral versus parenteral nutrition in malnourished patients with gastrointestinal cancer: a randomised multicentre trial. Lancet. 2001;358:1487.
9. Heyland DK, Montalvo M, MacDonald S, et al. Total parenteral nutrition in the surgical patient: a meta-analysis. Can J Surg. 2001;44:102.
10. Heber D, Byerly LO, Chlebowski RT. Medical abnormalities in the cancer patient. Cancer. 1985;55:225–9.
11. Lundholm K, Edstrom S, Karlberg I, et al. Glucose turnover, gluconeogenesis from glycerol in estimation of net glucose cycling in cancer patients. Cancer. 1982;50:1142.
12. Waterhouse C. Lactate metabolism in patients with cancer. Cancer. 1974;33:66–71.
13. Norton JA, Burt ME, Brennan MF. In vivo utilization of substrate by human sarcoma-bearing limbs. Cancer. 1980;45:2934–9.
14. Warnold I, Lundholm K, Schersten T. Energy balance and body composition in cancer patients. Cancer Res. 1978;38:1801–7.
15. Shaw JHF, Humberstone DM, Douglas RG, et al. Leucine kinetics in patients with benign disease, non-weight losing cancer, and cancer cachexia: studies at the whole body and tissue level and the response to nutritional support. Surgery. 1991;109:37–50.
16. Kralovic RC, Zepp A, Canedella RJ. Studies of the mechanism of carcass fat depletion in experimental cancer. Eur J Cancer. 1977;13:1071–9.
17. Legaspi A, Jevanandam M, Staves HF, et al. Whole body lipid and energy metabolism in the cancer patient. Metabolism. 1987;36:958–63.
18. Beck SA, Tisdale MJ. Production of lipolytic and proteolytic factors by a Murine tumor producing cachexia in the host. Cancer Res. 1987;47:S919–23.
19. Vlassara H, Spiegel RJ, Doval DS, et al. Reduced plasma lipoprotein lipase activity in patients with malignancy-associated weight loss. Horm Metab Res. 1986;18:698–703.
20. Magne N, Marcy PY, Foa C, et al. Comparison between nasogastric tube feeding and percutaneous fluoroscopic gastrostomy in advanced head and neck cancer patients. Eur Arch Otorhinolaryngol. 2001;258:89.
21. Mekhail TM, Adelstein DJ, Rybicki LA, et al. Enteral nutrition during the treatment of head and neck carcinoma: is a percutaneous endoscopic gastrostomy tube preferable to a nasogastric tube? Cancer. 2001;91:1785.
22. Souba WW. Nutritional support. N Engl J Med. 1997;336(1):41–8.
23. Klein S, Simes J, Blackburn G. Total parenteral nutrition and cancer clinical trials. Cancer. 1986;58:1378–86.
24. McGeer AJ, Detsky AS, O'Rourke KO. Parenteral nutrition in cancer patients undergoing chemotherapy: a meta-analysis. Nutrition. 1990;6:233–40.
25. Weisdorf SA, Lysne J, Wind D, et al. Positive effect of prophylactic total parenteral nutrition on long-term outcome of bone marrow transplantation. Transplantation. 1987;43:833–8.
26. Szeluga DJ, Stuart RK, Brookmeyer R, et al. Nutritional support of bone marrow transplant recipients: a prospective randomized clinical trial comparing total parenteral nutrition to an enteral feeding program. Cancer Res. 1987;47:3309–16.
27. Roberts S, Miller J, Pineiro L, et al. Total parenteral nutrition vs oral diet in autologous hematopoietic cell transplant recipients. Bone Marrow Transplant. 2003;32:715–21.
28. Herrmann FR, Safran C, Levkoff SE, et al. Serum albumin level on admission as a predictor of death, length of stay, and readmission. Arch Intern Med. 1992;152:125–30.
29. Apovian CM, McMahon MM, Bistrian BR. Guidelines for refeeding the marasmic patient. Crit Care Med. 1990;18:1030–3.
30. Moncada S, Higgs A. The L-arginine-nitric oxide pathway. N Engl J Med. 1993;329:2002–12.
31. Hall JC, Heel K, McCauley R. Glutamine. Br J Surg. 1996;83:305–12.
32. Calder PC. More good news about glutamine. Nutrition. 2000;16:71–2.

33. Aspen Board of Directors. Guidelines for the use of total parenteral nutrition in the hospitalized patient. JPEN J Parenter Enteral Nutr. 1986;10:441–4.
34. Lowry SF, Brennan MS. Intravenous feeding in the cancer patient. In: Rombeau JL, Caldwell MD, editors. Parenteral nutrition. Philadelphia, PA: WB Saunders; 1986. p. 445–70.
35. Harrison LE, Brennan MF. The role of total parenteral nutrition in the patient with cancer. Curr Probl Surg. 1995;32(10):833–924.
36. Rombeau JL, Rolandelli RH, Wilmore DW. Nutritional support. In: Wilmore DW, Brennan MF, Harken AH, et al., editors. American College of Surgeons. Care of the surgical patient. New York: Scientific American; 1994. p. 1–40.
37. Parker P, Stroop S, Greene H. A controlled comparison of continuous versus intermittent feeding in the treating of infants with intestinal disease. J Pediatr. 1981;99:360–4.
38. Raynard B, Nitenberg G, Gory-Delabaere G, Bourhis JH, Bachmann P, Bensadoun RJ, Desport JC, Kere D, Schneider S, Senesse P, Bordigoni P, Dieu L. Summary of the standards, options and recommendations for nutritional support in patients undergoing bone marrow transplantation. Br J Cancer. 2003;89:S101–6.

29 Post-treatment Evaluation and Advice and Follow-Up Schedules

The responsibilities of a radiation oncologist do not end once the patient has completed his/her course of radiotherapy. Post-radiotherapy, significant sequelae can be expected in many patients depending upon the site and field size irradiated as well as radiation technique used and total dose delivered. In general, post-radiotherapy, the patient's reactions are expected to either progress further or remain the same for the first 6 weeks after which they slowly start resolving. Reactions which appear after 6 weeks but subside within 6 months are the subacute reactions, while those that appear after 6 months of completion of radiotherapy are called late reactions. The oncologist has to recognize the continuation of acute effects or appearance of subacute or late reactions and even to differentiate between late-onset sequelae and the early presenting features of a recurrence. Recurrences frequently develop within 1–2 years of completion of therapy and mostly within the first 5 years. Late recurrences are rarely seen and need to be addressed early so as to institute adequate salvage measures. Thus follow-up care in cancer involves regular medical assessments including a review of a patient's medical history, general physical examination, local examination, repeat biopsy/FNAC or other histopathological reviews, imaging, endoscopy and blood and other lab tests.

Follow-up care is important because it helps to identify changes in health. *The purpose of follow-up care is to check for recurrence or the cancer's response to the therapy given as well as identifying and managing sequelae of radiotherapy.* It is very important for healthcare providers dealing with cancer patients to ensure that all patients who are able to complete their therapy come for regular follow-up. The doctor or the medical team should also record details of those patients who have died or cannot come for follow-up. This is important so that the response of the patient to therapy may be assessed, sequelae may be studied and managed and lifestyle advice and supportive care may be offered to those who need it. These visits can be by the patient to their treating centre, or if required even home visits may be arranged. It is also necessary to have a proper follow-up data of patients treated to

A. Mukherji, *Basics of Planning and Management of Patients during Radiation Therapy*, https://doi.org/10.1007/978-981-10-6659-7_29

generate information on the natural history of the disease and its response to the therapy offered so that future research could be directed at improving irradiation protocols.

During each visit, the healthcare provider or the doctor should take a proper interview of the patient as well as examine the patient. The patients should be questioned and examined specifically with respect to the following points:

- Any symptom that has developed recently or any change in characteristic of existing symptom (pattern, severity, site).
- Any new pain and its location, intensity, character, frequency, association with time of day/body habit/activity or medication.
- New symptoms or exacerbation of pre-existing complaints which may have changed in intensity and character and are causing interference in activities of daily living such as lassitude or fatigue; difficulty with bladder, bowel or sexual function; difficulty in focussing or concentrating or even changes in memory/behaviour patterns/sleep or learning; and weight gain or loss.
- History of medicines, vitamins or alternative therapy they are taking.
- Emotional problems patients are experiencing, such as anxiety or depression.
- Family history should always be taken even at time of initial presentation as well as any changes occurring therein.

It is important also for the doctor or healthcare provider to keep the patient involved in these follow-up visits especially during the first 2–3 years after radiotherapy when the majority of the recurrences occur. It is important for the patient also to be vigilant at home so as to recognize early signs of disease relapse. Patients should report to their doctors any new finding even if it may seem unrelated and let the doctor decide whether or not the finding is of significance. The nature of the treatment given—its intent, dose of radiation, area treated, field and volume of tissue irradiated as well as technique used—will result in different sequelae and response, and based on this, the follow-up schedule of a patient can be individualized, and required attention may be paid to expected effects. *In general, schedule of follow-up visits is once every 1–2 months for the first 6 months, every 3 months for the next 2 years, then every 6 months for the next 2 years and thence yearly lifelong or till disease recurrence.*

Usually follow-up visits are to the same doctor who provided the cancer treatment, and therefore the patient should select a doctor for treatment with whom they are comfortable and to whom they can easily report to regularly for routine follow-up visits. These visits as explained before include not only history taking but also a careful examination, and based on these, the doctor can recommend various other investigations such as repeat FNAC/biopsy or regular imaging (ultrasound/CT/MRI or PET) or even tumour markers. The doctor may also recommend screening for haematological, biochemical and physiological functions to check for body health. Other coexisting or any health issues can be discussed with the treating doctor, but the patient may also have to follow up with their family physician or other specialists as required. Also in follow-up care, a nutritional specialist, physiotherapist, psychological counsellor along with the treating team of surgeon/radiation and medical oncologist should be in the loop.

Every cancer survivor should receive a comprehensive treatment summary and follow-up plan from their doctor once they complete their treatment. The treatment summary should include information on:

- Presentation of the cancer, staging, histopathological examination done including immunocytochemistry and report and imaging findings; all information with dates.
- Plan of treatment; modalities of treatment patient received including details of surgery done, name of surgeon, technique followed, intraoperative findings, intra- or postoperative complications and recovery period. Chemo details should include intent, timing (neoadjuvant/adjuvant/induction/maintenance/concurrent), dose, schedule, adjuvant drugs, patient tolerance, any acute events, pre- and post-grading, number of cycles and any breaks. Radiotherapy details should include intent, timing (neoadjuvant/adjuvant/concurrent), dose, schedule, technique used, machine used, beam energy, description of portals, total dose, duration of therapy, patient tolerance, any acute events, pre- and post-grading as well as any breaks.
- Response to therapy and expected remission to be explained to patient.
- Schedule of follow-up routine visits.
- Identify the doctors for follow-up cancer care.
- Chances of cancer recurrence or second malignancy.
- Follow-up tests that may be required, schedule of the tests and what results to expect.
- Symptoms to look out for in case of recurrences and plan of action in case symptoms appear.
- Common long-term and late effects of the treatment received should be explained.
- Steps to maintain health and well-being that have to be followed should be explained to the patient.
- Effects of cancer treatment taken on the social, professional and financial well-being need to be discussed with the patient. If required the patient can also be referred to local self-help groups and support forums.

Advice for patients: Cancer treatment can result in significant sequelae as well as mental, emotional, social and economic pressures. It is best that at this time, the patients should have someone to care for them and also the patients should join support groups for activities such as group discussions, physical exercises where possible, physiotherapy, counselling groups or even volunteer groups. Participating in volunteer activities can help people feel stronger and more in control of their lives. All patients may have daily changes in their routine lives, and if they feel that some changes are bothersome, they should make a note of these events and ask their doctor at the time of their follow-up visit. In fact all patients should be advised to record in writing or on tape any change in their daily activity pattern which they feel may be associated with their cancer treatment. People who have persistent emotional or physical distress after therapy should be however referred by their doctors to support groups or home healthcare providers after due assessment.

As explained in previously, the patient at the time of discharge from treatment should be given a full and proper record which would include details of treatment given, expected results and sequelae, care to be taken, follow-up protocol and contact details of support providers and doctor who will follow-up. Patients may not always see the same doctor for their follow-up care, so having this information available to share with another doctor can provide useful insight to the next doctor and save time in responding to the patient's presenting complaint during follow-up. In addition to the information described, it is important to keep the following information:

- Supportive care received (e.g. pain or nausea medication, emotional support and nutritional supplements)
- Identifying number and title of clinical trial (research study), if the patient participated in a clinical trial

Services that may be helpful as part of treatment as well as during follow-up care include counselling for genetic testing (if required), family relations and fertility/sexual queries. Support services would also include home care services, nutrition counselling, physical therapy, pain management and occupational or vocational therapy. Some patients may also need financial aid or assistance with transportation to and from appointments.

30 Psychological and Social Issues in Patients Undergoing Radiotherapy

30.1 An Introduction

Psycho-oncology is that subspecialty of oncology which recognizes the impact of cancer and cancer treatment on the patient as well as the patient's family's psychology. It also studies the impact of a declaration of cancer on the social standing as well as interrelationships of patients and their families. This discipline of cancer care also explores the need for holistic care of cancer patients which basically means considering all aspects of health, i.e. the physical, social as well as mental health and patients' being able to play their established role in society. This assessment is necessary as cancer and related changes in the physiology could significantly damage the patients' quality of life. Therefore cancer care must not only include the disease management and treatment of side effects/sequelae but also take care of psychosocial distress and institute rehabilitation as well as palliation where required. A diagnosis of cancer is a traumatic experience not only for the patients but also their families. An individual affected by cancer has to come face to face with issues such as loss of independence and ability to control one's life; increased health, social, emotional and sometimes even financial dependence on family and friends or even social organizations; and potential loss of financial security and self-esteem and professional as well as social standing. Patients thus are frequently psychologically imbalanced and depressed and sometimes even aggressively anti-social. This imbalance in the psychological health of the patient will decrease compliance to treatment and translate into a poor quality of life [1, 2].

Psycho-oncology hence assumes importance as it *addresses the psychosocial needs of patients and their family members across the continuum of care, from prevention and early detection through treatment and survivorship to palliative and end-of-life care* [3]. Therefore psychological support to cancer patients and their families can help by improving their coping abilities, decreasing distress, helping them become more responsive towards accepting medical and counselling benefits and also decreasing the stress on the doctors and nursing staff by making the patients or their families less aggressive. Hence psycho-oncology should be a necessary part

A. Mukherji, *Basics of Planning and Management of Patients during Radiation Therapy*, https://doi.org/10.1007/978-981-10-6659-7_30

of all oncological management whether curative or palliative and includes coordinating with not only oncological health staff but also psychiatrists, social workers, internists and even religious counsellors.

Psycho-oncology as a field is still in its early stages and has been fully integrated into regular oncological management in only a few and predictably developed countries [4]. Elsewhere its acceptance is dependent on local beliefs, cultural practices, economics and healthcare priorities for each country. While low-resource countries may focus more attention on cancer prevention and education to improve early detection of easily screened cancers such as cervical or oral cancers as well as on palliative care to optimally use their resources [3], in high-resource countries, cancer care is confronted with therapeutic alternatives presenting equivalent survival efficacy but different effects on quality of life. Physician-patient-shared decision making needs a high priority to prevent exacerbation of patients' psychological distress.

30.2 Effect of Social Impact and Psychological Factors

Quality of life: In the present era, an important goal of cancer therapy apart from achieving cure or prolongation of life remains preservation or improvement of quality of life. This term called *quality of life* is being now commonly used in the cancer literature and refers to the patient and their families' physical, mental, social and psychological health status including psychosocial adjustment, well-being and satisfaction with life. Psychologically for a patient, a diagnosis of cancer, even early-stage cancers, will raise fears of death, dependence, suffering, pain and disabilities and cause significant psychological distress. Mood disturbance (depression, anxiety) or cognitive abnormalities (poor concentration, memory impairment) are seen. Cancer treatment whether irradiation/chemotherapy or surgery is frequently associated with distressing sequelae and may develop during, immediately after or weeks/ months after treatment has ended [5]. As a result of the disease and its treatment, patients have decreased performance status and stamina, develop physical impairments and dysfunctionalities and develop decreased abilities in carrying out daily works of life. They also develop difficulties in responding to social and emotional situations and slowly disengage from society and family. Cancer patients frequently experience loneliness or lack of support and feel marginalized or even stigmatized by cancer and may encounter problems in returning to work.

Psychological distress and disorders: Psychopathological or psychosocial consequences of cancer and its treatment have to be addressed very specifically as usual diagnostic criteria for mental disorders may not adequately reflect the psychological disorders caused by cancer and its treatment [6]. As mentioned before, a diagnosis of cancer is in most cases a traumatic event for the patient and his/her family, and the resultant psychological stress could be considered by many as a "normal" reaction. Holland and colleagues [7] have explained this condition as a *distress* and not merely a *normal response to stress* to describe the psychological experience of oncology patients and to avoid further psychopathological stigmatization and have said that this situation requires specialized intervention. They have defined this term as a *multifactorial unpleasant emotional experience of a psychological (cognitive, behavioural, emotional), social, and/or spiritual nature that may interfere with the ability to cope effectively with cancer, its physical symptoms and its treatment. Distress moves along a continuum, ranging from common normal feelings of vulnerability, sadness and fears, to problems such as depression, anxiety, panic, social isolation and existential and spiritual crisis* [7].

Thus when people are first diagnosed as having cancer, they may react initially with shock and disbelief, along with anxiety, and then anger or depression. However in most cases, this initial reaction abates within a few weeks as patients adjust with their diagnosis and employ themselves with the modalities of disease management. But it has also been seen that a sizeable number of cancer patients develop pathological psychological disorders compared to the general population which may be persistent and would need professional attention [8]. Studies have noted that up to a third of all cancer patients have high levels of distress which could last for prolonged periods and which could result in difficulties in adjusting to their present situation as well as interfere with treatment compliance [9]. Cancer is one of the most common reasons of post-traumatic stress disorders with nearly one-fifth (19%) of breast cancer patients reporting this condition at the time of surgery [10]. Patients with advanced cancer stages fare even worse with more than half suffering psychological distress along with their physical symptoms [11]. Many of these advanced cancer patients progress into acute confusional state, and this causes added distress to their families [12]. This state may be due to the use of opioid analgesics and chemotherapy agents, cerebral tumours or encephalopathy.

Thus based on psychoanalytical and quality of life studies, predictors for these psychological problems have been identified, and these include disease stage, physical symptoms, pre-existing mental disease, emotional lability or personality, age and gender of patient, social and interpersonal record and education [1, 13–15]. It has been proposed, and there is now a growing consensus that cancer patients should be screened for these predisposing factors and should be put on support services at the earliest possible time [7, 16].

Sexual relations and parenting: A diagnosis of cancer affects a family as a whole and is not the patient's problem alone [17]. As consequent to a diagnosis of cancer, the interrelationships between various family members will have a significant impact on the patient's adjustment to his/her disease. The well-being of close relatives is of concern especially as this is usually the only source of support to patients. In cancer patients, marital relationships may also be affected. A marriage already plagued by pre-existing problems would likely give away causing the patient to withdraw away from society as well as be inconsistent with treatment; while a good marital relationship can act as a shock-absorber to the psychological and physiological stress of cancer and its treatment. Sexual functionality and ability is also an important but frequently insufficiently recognized complication of cancer and its treatment [18]. A multitude of sexual problems or inadequacies have been noted in cancer patients, which can occur both because of psychological and physiological injuries. Psychologically cancer-related anxiety or depression may play a major role in sexual withdrawal or inadequacies faced by cancer patients, while effects of treatment such as surgical injuries or cosmetic defects, presence of poorly located stomas, nerve damage, radical pelvic irradiation, as well as side effects of chemotherapy or hormone treatment can lead to inability by the patient to execute the sexual act or develop inadequacies in sexual behaviour. Treatment for prostate cancer such as prostatectomy or hormone therapy can diminish a man's self-esteem as a sexual partner [19]. Similarly fear of cosmetic defects in a substantial proportion of women who need to undergo mastectomy for breast cancer or hair loss or weight gain or loss from chemotherapy, increased mental lability and vaginal dryness after pelvic irradiation have led to feelings of poor self-esteem as well as apprehensions of poor cosmetic appearance and partner's difficulty in understanding patients' feelings [20]. This may adversely affect patient acceptance of and compliance with planned treatment course. Also breast cancer can affect the mother-daughter relationship, and daughters' distress levels have been found to be significantly related to mothers' distress levels [17]. Interactions and social bonding levels within a family also affect the children/adolescents' psychosocial outcomes, and maternal depression can affect parenting [21].

Effect of genetic risk: Newer modalities of testing and treatment while providing benefit to the health of individuals have their own psychosocial impact on patients' lives. In recent times this can be best exemplified by the increase in queries and worries in even healthy people regarding breast cancer genetic testing and subsequent treatment decisions for those at risk of higher incidence such as those with BRCA1 or BRCA2 mutation which indicates lifetime risk of breast cancer of 50–85% [22]. Testing and counselling for cancers like breast, prostate or rectum helps in early detection of such cancers by regular monitoring and increases the possibility of reducing cancer risk through chemoprevention or risk-reducing surgery, but it also increases stress in the population studied [23]. A screening test result could be classified as (1) **positive** in individuals who are not affected but are at increased risk due to familial mutation or are the first mutation in the family, (2) **negative** in the presence of a disease-related mutation identified in the family or (3) **uninformative or of uncertain significance**. A positive test result is not a diagnosis of cancer but merely an acknowledgement that the individual is at increased risk, but even this may cause increased anxiety of possible risk of genetic transmission to children. These individuals hence not only face the difficult choice on deciding for prophylactic therapy which may have marginal benefit but also may face potential insurance, employment or social discrimination. In case of the genetic test result being uninformative or of uncertain significance, the patient experiences further anxiety, depression or confusion as his/her true position becomes uncertain. A negative test result may reduce anxiety in the patient about personal cancer risk due to heredity but may result in strained family and social relationships or potential inappropriate routine surveillance.

Current research has not shown any potential psychological harm with positive screening results [23–25], but long-term information is lacking and needs to be carefully studied for long-term psychological impact. For example, while the use of screening mammography in women in general population has not negatively affected the psychological domains for those screened but in those who are recalled for further investigations for any abnormality, significant adverse long-term psychological effects were observed [26]. Similarly a subset of women postmastectomy have been shown to have developed high levels of psychological distress, sexual dysfunction and concern with body image [27].

Emotional and psychological problems in caregivers: In cancer care, it is very important to communicate properly with the patients and their families about their diagnosis, prognosis and potential therapeutic options as any lapse in doing so would make these people confused, frightened and in psychological distress. This will subsequently reflect on patient compliance and attitude towards their treatment and result in unsatisfactory outcomes, which would be stressful both for the doctor and the patient. It is these lapses which have frequently resulted in litigations and subsequent defensive medical practice as well as high levels of physician burnout [28].

Cancer treatment exacts a heavy toll on health givers as well as patients. Doctors frequently have to witness high levels of morbidity, mortality, difficult treatment decisions, emotionally labile patients and relatives, inter-staff conflicts as well as heavy work load. All this makes cancer care a highly stressful environment, and many healthcare professionals report feelings of helplessness, anger or occasional identification with the patient. Physicians and healthcare providers are often confronted during their interactions with cancer patients with a number of difficult issues such as delivering bad news, counselling and advising for surgical procedures which may be mutilating or highly risky, enrolling in clinical trials where the results may not be very clear, discussing treatment options and disease prognosis as risk percentages or survival/risk ratios which patient may not fully comprehend or even switching from curative treatment to supportive care when there is unsatisfactory response which the patient may find it difficult to accept or even may ask for experimental or untried treatments [29]. In cancer care, doctors and healthcare staff should understand the fact that even if cure is not possible, good quality care can be provided and all patients can be helped if not cured.

30.3 Management of Psychosocial Issues

Interventions targeted at healthcare professionals: Most training of healthcare providers in cancer care consists of training to diagnose, combat the disease and if cure is not possible to provide good palliation and quality of life. This mode of training can frequently miss out or lose focus on the psychosocial aspect of cancer care, and this lack is thought to be a significant barrier to evidence-based psychosocial care in oncology [2]. Studies have suggested that clinicians many times may not be able to identify patients with increased anxiety or depression [30–32] and need for psychosocial counselling [32]. Thus many patients who may not be otherwise readily forthcoming about their psychosocial problems and look towards the caregiving team for help may find that though their physical symptoms have been addressed, this lack of psychosocial support can leave the patient feeling unsupported [33]. Oncologists are expected to play an important role in identifying and preventing psychological distress to the patients and their families. Adequate communication skills are required to deal with issues that regularly arise in the cancer setting. Various such modes of assessment of the patient's psychological health have been designed with a view to provide for systems to detect physical and psychological problems and enable timely interventions. These include use of quality of life questionnaires [34], assessment tools [9] and guidelines for psychosocial management [7], as well as training healthcare professionals in psychosocial issues [35] and in communication skills [36, 37].

Psychological distress screening tools and psychosocial guidelines: Oncologists' estimation of severity of a patient's distress is often complicated by patient's denial [31] and also by the somatic symptoms such as pain, fatigue, weakness and reduced energy as well as appetite/weight changes. These symptoms are frequently mixed with the psychological symptoms such as breathlessness, muscle pain, dizziness; palpitation for anxiety and panic attack and fatigue or appetite/weight changes for depression. This creates difficulty in diagnosing depression or anxiety in cancer patients. In many such cases, if the clinician feels that the symptoms and the signs elicited do not match, then the patient should be evaluated for psychological issues such as depression, guilt, suicidal thinking or hopelessness [31]. Many countries have now put in place practice guidelines for evidence-based psychosocial interventions and also tools to define and provide a comparison for evaluating the quality of psychosocial care provided by a cancer or palliative care centre.

Communication skills training: A frequently overlooked but vital aspect of cancer care is maintaining a healthy doctor-patient relationship for which good communication is essential. Good communication improves the ability of patients to cope with their condition; enhances satisfaction with care, informed consent and cooperation with care providers thus reducing risk of malpractice litigation; and helps decrease professionals' burnout. The main features of a good doctor-patient interaction are creating a good interpersonal relationship; clear and precise exchange of information covering the patient's needs to make an informed choice and the doctor's requirements for making an assessment and helping the patient take difficult treatment-related decisions. It is important to maintain a patient-centred approach to encourage the patient to communicate more with the healthcare providers and allow the patient to understand medical information and help them in decision making.

Cancer patients may prefer to make their own informed choices or sometimes assume a passive role preferring their doctor to make the choices [38]. Therefore the healthcare provider should approach the patient with an open mind and be ready for both possibilities. They should be ready to provide all relevant information required to make an informed choice as well as provide supportive services. This is a difficult task as these skills are not necessarily taught in all medical schools, though many medical schools have now started including communication skills as part of their curriculum.

30.4 Interventions Targeted at Patients or Relatives

Improving quality of life: Quality of life is now an important determinant of the quality of cancer care and interventions aimed at improving or providing good quality of life which may be divided into preventive (includes identifying people at risk of developing psychological problems and focusing priority for these patients), treatment related (ensuring good standard of cancer care which does not cause more difficulties for the patient; treatment decisions should take into account patient health and tolerance) and supportive including cognitive, emotional, psychological and social. These supportive care interventions may include individual care or as part of group therapy or even family counselling [1], and such interventions last throughout the treatment and follow-up period and if necessary even into the bereavement period.

Cancer patients' psychological adjustments are a result of their interactions with their health caregivers, their personality, disease stage and symptoms and available support services. Providing psychological therapy to cancer patients and their families helps them in coping up with the disease. This psychological therapy helps in overcoming the negative thought processes in these people and thereby helps patients improve their compliance, follow-up and therefore their outcomes [39]. Such services can be in the form of individualized counselling or group therapy with other similar people which has the advantage of building up mutual support in the group between the patients towards each other [40]. Reinforcing positive emotional expressions can help adjust to the stress of cancer treatment and provide an emotional support in the face of a catastrophic event such as treatment failure. These also help in combating post-traumatic stress disorders especially in advanced cancers. These observations have led to the development of new forms of psychological therapy for advanced cancer patients [41].

Research evidence has pointed out that with respect to the effects of psychological therapy in oncology, while it does not promote survival it may affect survival outcomes by addressing patients' depression and hopelessness/helplessness and ensuring improved compliance with anti-cancer treatments. The relevant outcomes are indicators of quality of life such as anxiety and depression or mental/emotional adjustment to or rationalizing with one's condition, as well as aspects of interpersonal and social functioning. Newell et al. [26] in a study of 329 cases concluded that approaches such as group therapy, patient and family education, structured as well as unstructured counselling and cognitive behavioural therapy could provide benefit in many psychosocial outcomes which had been explored in this study. Customized designing of psychosocial interventions based on patients' customs, background and education needs to be studied more as it is a usual thought that more educated and better affordable patients choose psychological counselling [41], while poorer and less educated patients are often seen to have more advanced cancers with poorer compliance and results. Also it might be better if it is assessed as to what would be the best time to offer psychosocial support to cancer patients as not all patients will be initially responsive, being more interested in the primary cancer treatment. These patients may view offering of psychosocial support as an admission by the health caregivers of incurability of disease and may not be open in their discussions with their doctors [42].

30.5 Conclusions and Recommendations

Cancer and its treatment affect patients' physical and psychosocial functioning and hence affect the overall quality of life. Psycho-oncological practice now plays an important role throughout cancer care including prevention and early detection, diagnosis and first treatments, survivorship, recurrence, terminal stages and bereavement. Psychosocial interventions for cancer patients and their families have in recent years created a body of evidence, and these evidence-based approaches are being used in many countries to address the problems of the patients, their families and healthcare providers, thus improving patient outcomes. It is now recommended that psychosocial interventions in oncological care should be included in every national cancer care plan and these services made available in every cancer care service.

Healthcare professionals are being provided with validated psychosocial assessment tools, training and continuous supervision to respond to the psychosocial needs of patients and relatives. In a further attempt to institutionalize the many training and support programmes in psycho-oncology in different countries, the International Psycho-Oncology Society (IPOS) was started in 1984 to further education and research in psycho-oncology [7].

References

1. Aaronson NK, Ahmedzai S, Bergman B, et al. The European Organization for Research and Treatment of Cancer QLQ-C30: a quality of life instrument for use in international clinical trials in oncology. J Natl Cancer Inst. 1993;85:365–75.
2. Akizuki N, Yamawaki S, Akechi T, Nakano T, Uchitomi Y. Development of an impact thermometer for use in combination with the distress thermometer as a brief screening tool for adjustment disorders and/or major depression in cancer patients. J Pain Symptom Manag. 2005;29(1):91–9.
3. Akechi T, Okuyama T, Akizuki N, et al. Course of psychological distress and its predictors in advanced non-small cell lung cancer patients. Psychooncology. 2006;15:463–73.
4. Diagnostic and statistical manual of mental disorders: DSM-IV-TR. Washington, DC: American Psychiatric Association. 2000.
5. Brédart A, Bottomley A, Blazeby JM, Conroy T, Coens C, D'Haese S, et al. An international prospective study of the EORTC cancer in-patient satisfaction with care measure (EORTC IN-PATSAT32). Eur J Cancer. 2005;41(14):2120–31.
6. Breitbart W, Bruera E, Chochinov H, Lynch M. Neuropsychiatric syndromes and psychological symptoms in patients with advanced cancer. J Pain Symptom Manag. 1995;10(2):131–41.
7. Holland JC. IPOS Sutherland memorial lecture: an international perspective on the development of psychosocial oncology: overcoming cultural and attitudinal barriers to improve psychosocial care. Psychooncology. 2004;13(7):445–59.

8. Burgess C, Cornelius V, Love S, Graham J, Richards M, Ramirez A. Depression and anxiety in women with early breast cancer: five year observational cohort study. BMJ. 2005;330:702.
9. Carlson LE, Bultz BD. Efficacy and medical cost offset of psychosocial interventions in cancer care: making the case for economic analyses. Psychooncology. 2004;13(12):837–49; discussion 850–6.
10. Fobair P, Stewart SL, Chang S, D'Onofrio C, Banks PJ, Bloom JR. Body image and sexual problems in young women with breast cancer. Psychooncology. 2006;15(7):579–94.
11. Hack TF, Degner LF, Parker PA, SCRN Communication Team. The communication goals and needs of cancer patients: a review. Psychooncology. 2005;14(10):831–45; discussion 846–7.
12. Helgeson VS. Recent advances in psychosocial oncology. J Consult Clin Psychol. 2005;73(2): 268–71.
13. Cella DF, Tulsky DS, Gray G, Sarafian B, Linn E, Bonomi A, Silberman M, Yellen SB, Winicour P, Brannon J, et al. The functional assessment of cancer therapy scale: development and validation of the general measure. J Clin Oncol. 1993;11(3):570–9.
14. Eide H, Graugaard P, Holgersen K, Finset A. Physician communication in different phases of a consultation at an oncology outpatient clinic related to patient satisfaction. Patient Educ Couns. 2003;51(3):259–66.
15. Hewitt M, Rowland JH. Mental health service use among adult cancer survivors: analyses of the National Health Interview Survey. J Clin Oncol. 2002;20(23):4581–90.
16. Holland JC, Jacobsen PB, Riba MB, NCCN Fever and Neutropenia Practice Guidelines Panel. NCCN: distress management. Cancer Control. 2001;8(6 Suppl 2):88–93.
17. Hopwood P. Psychosocial aspects of risk communication and mutation testing in familial breast-ovarian cancer. Curr Opin Oncol. 2005;17(4):340–4.
18. Kash KM, Holland JC, Breitbart W, Berenson S, Dougherty J, Ouellette-Kobasa S, Lesko L. Stress and burnout in oncology. Oncology (Williston Park). 2000;14(11):1621–33; discussion 1633–4, 1636–7.
19. Kissane DW, Bloch S, Miach P, Smith GC, Seddon A, Keks N. Cognitive-existential group therapy for patients with primary breast cancer—techniques and themes. Psychooncology. 1997;6(1):25–33.
20. Kissane DW. Psychosocial oncology: present status, future directions. Multinational association of supportive care in cancer. In: 16th international symposium proceedings, 2004.
21. Lispscomb J, Gotay CC, Snyder C. Outcome assessment in cancer: measures, methods, and applications. Cambridge: Cambridge University Press; 2005.
22. Mehnert A, Koch U. Psychosocial care of cancer patients—international differences in definition, healthcare structures, and therapeutic approaches. Support Care Cancer. 2005;13:579–88.
23. Meiser B. Psychological impact of genetic testing for cancer susceptibility: an update of the literature. Psychooncology. 2005;14(12):1060–74.
24. Meiser B, Gaff C, Julian-Reynier C, et al. International perspectives on genetic counseling and testing for breast cancer risk. Breast Dis. 2006;27:109–25.
25. Merckaert I, Libert Y, Razavi D. Communication skills training in cancer care: where are we and where are we going? Curr Opin Oncol. 2005;17:319–30.
26. Newell SA, Sanson-Fisher RW, Savolainen NJ. Systematic review of psychological therapies for cancer patients: overview and recommendations for future research. J Natl Cancer Inst. 2002;94(8):558–84.
27. Newell S, Sanson-Fisher RW, Girgis A, Bonaventura A. How well do medical oncologists' perceptions reflect their patients' reported physical and psychosocial problems? Data from a survey of five oncologists. Cancer. 1998;83:1640–51.
28. Ong LM, de Haes JC, Hoos AM, Lammes FB. Doctor patient communication: a review of the literature. Soc Sci Med. 1995;40(7):903–18.
29. Osborn T. The psychosocial impact of parental cancer on children and adolescents: a systematic review. Psychooncology. 2007;16(2):101–26.
30. Ozalp E, Soygur H, Cankurtaran E, Turhan L, Akbiyik D, Geyik P. Psychiatric morbidity and its screening in Turkish women with breast cancer: a comparison between the HADS and SCID tests. Psychooncology. 2008;17(7):668–75.

31. Pascoe S, Edelman S, Kidman A. Prevalence of psychological distress and use of support services by cancer patients at Sydney hospitals. Aust N Z J Psychiatry. 2000;34:785–91.
32. Passik SD, Dugan W, McDonald MV, Rosenfeld B, Theobald DE, Edgerton S. Oncologists' recognition of depression in their patients with cancer. J Clin Oncol. 1998;16(4):1594–600.
33. Razavi D, Delvaux N, Farvacques C, Robaye E. Screening for adjustment disorders and major depressive disorders in cancer in-patients. Br J Psychiatry. 1990;156:79–83.
34. Razavi D, Merckaert I, Marchal S, Libert Y, Conradt S, Boniver J, et al. How to optimize physicians' communication skills in cancer care: results of a randomized study assessing the usefulness of posttraining consolidation workshops. J Clin Oncol. 2003;21(16):3141–9.
35. Sanson-Fisher R, Girgis A, Boyes A, Bonevski B, Burton L, Cook P. The unmet supportive care needs of patients with cancer. Supportive care review group. Cancer. 2000;88:226–37.
36. Santos FR, Kozasa EH, Chauffaille Mde L, Colleoni GW, Leite JR. Psychosocial adaptation and quality of life among Brazilian patients with different hematological malignancies. J Psychosom Res. 2006;60:505–11.
37. Schofield P, Carey M, Bonevski B, Sanson-Fisher R. Barriers to the provision of evidence-based psychosocial care in oncology. Psychooncology. 2006;15(10):863–72.
38. Sellick SM, Edwardson AD. Screening new cancer patients for psychological distress using the hospital anxiety and depression scale. Psychooncology. 2007;16(6):534–42.
39. Stead ML, Brown JM, Fallowfield L, Selby P. Lack of communication between healthcare professionals and women with ovarian cancer about sexual issues. Br J Cancer. 2003;88(5):666–71.
40. Söllner W, DeVries A, Steixner E, Lukas P, Sprinzl G, Rumpold G, Maislinger S. How successful are oncologists in identifying patient distress, perceived social support, and need for psychosocial counselling? Br J Cancer. 2001;84(2):179–85.
41. Strong V, Waters R, Hibberd C, et al. Emotional distress in cancer patients: the Edinburgh Cancer Centre symptom study. Br J Cancer. 2007;96:868–74.
42. Uchitomi Y, Mikami I, Nagai K, Nishiwaki Y, Akechi T, Okamura H. Depression and psychological distress in patients during the year after curative resection of non-small cell lung cancer. J Clin Oncol. 2003;21:69–77.

Index

A. Mukherji, *Basics of Planning and Management of Patients during Radiation Therapy*, https://doi.org/10.1007/978-981-10-6659-7

MIX
Papier aus verantwortungsvollen Quellen
Paper from responsible sources
FSC® C105338
FSC
www.fsc.org

If you have any concerns about our products,
you can contact us on
ProductSafety@springernature.com

In case Publisher is established outside the EU,
the EU authorized representative is:
Springer Nature Customer Service Center GmbH
Europaplatz 3, 69115 Heidelberg, Germany

Printed by Libri Plureos GmbH
in Hamburg, Germany